A Consumer
Approach to
Community Psychology

A Consumer
Approach to
Community Psychology

Edited with commentary by
James K. Morrison

Nelson-Hall nh Chicago

Library of Congress Cataloging in Publication Data
Main entry under title:

A Consumer approach to community psychology.

  Bibliography: p.
  Includes index.
  1. Community psychology. 2. Psychotherapy—
Philosophy. 3. Mental health services. I. Morrison,
James K.
RA790.5.C65   362.2'04'25   79-1172
ISBN 0-88229-458-X

Manufactured in the United States of America

10   9   8   7   6   5   4   3   2   1

To my parents: Emma and Harry Morrison

Contents

Chapter 3
Changing the Attitudes of Client-Consumers
and Service Providers

Chapter 4
Client Advisory Boards for Consumer Protection

Chapter 5
Client-Consumer Involvement in the
Delivery of Psychological Services

Chapter 6
Accountability to the Client-Consumer

Chapter 7
Consumer Independence from Service Providers

Chapter 8
A Community of Consumers

Chapter 9
The Ethical Problems of Service Providers

Contributors

As of April 1, 1977, when this manuscript was completed, the contributors to this volume held the following positions:

Robert R. Becker, Ph. D., clinical psychologist with the inpatient unit of the Capital District Psychiatric Center in Albany, N.Y.

Roy E. Becker, M.Ed., sociologist at the Centro del Barrio, Worden School of Social Service, San Antonio, Texas.

Margery Brown, Ph.D., clinical psychologist at the counseling center of Siena College, Loudonville, N.Y.

Johnel D. Bushell, B.A., mental health therapy aide with the Schenectady Unit of the Capital District Psychiatric Center.

Michael S. Cometa, Ph.D., assistant professor in the Psychology Department of Radford College, Radford, Virginia.

Michael J. Connelly, M.A., vocational rehabilitation counselor with the Schenectady Unit of the Capital District Psychiatric Center.

Norman Dovberg, D.O., staff psychiatrist at the Veteran's Administration Hospital in Albany, N.Y.

Morris E. Eson, Ph.D., professor in the Department of Psychology at the State University of New York at Albany.

Beverly L. Fasano, research assistant in Chicago, Illinois.

Mary Federico, group therapist, working at St. Catherine's Center for Children, Albany, N.Y.

Janet R. Fentiman, M.S.W., psychiatric social worker with the Albany City Unit of the Capital District Psychiatric Center.

Bernardo Gaviria, M.D., psychiatrist and the Chief of the Program Evaluation Unit of the Capital District Psychiatric Center in Albany, New York.

Gregory D. Hanson, Ph.D., clinical psychology intern with the Capital District Psychiatric Center in Albany, N.Y.

Michael S. Harris, R.N., community mental health nurse with the North Albany County Unit of the Capital District Psychiatric Center.

Susan Holdridge-Crane, Ph.D., clinical psychology intern with the Capital District Psychiatric Center.

Judith A. Libow, Ph.D., clinical psychology intern with the Texas Research Institute for Mental Sciences in Houston, Texas.

James C. Mancuso, Ph.D., professor in the Department of Psychology at the State University of New York at Albany.

James K. Morrison, Ph.D., chief of services with the North Albany County Unit of the Capital District Psychiatric Center, and assistant professor in the Department of Psychiatry at Albany Medical College.

Kathleen Liston Morrison, J.D., an attorney and Special Assistant to the General Counsel at the New York State Department of Environmental Conservation.

Jeffrey S. Nevid, Ph.D., an NIMH post-doctoral fellow in Mental Health Evaluation at Northwestern University.

Barbara Pitchford, M.A., school psychologist with Warren-Washington County BOCES of the State of New York.

Harold J. Rosenthal, J.D., staff attorney with Legal Aid Inc. of Albany.

Michelle P. Schwartz, B.S., registered nurse at Beth Israel Hospital in Boston, Massachusetts.

Frederick J. Smith, Ph.D., chief of services with the inpatient unit of the Capital District Psychiatric Center and associate professor in the Department of Psychiatry at Albany Medical College.

Jane E. Smith, B.S., research assistant with the Program Evaluation Unit of the Capital District Psychiatric Center in Albany.

Harold Yablonovitz, M.A., clinical psychologist and team leader with the North Albany County Unit of the Capital District Psychiatric Center.

Acknowledgments

One of the more difficult tasks facing an author is to properly acknowledge the contributions made by so many people to his book. It is not enough to simply thank the many coauthors listed in the table of contents. There are also many persons who had much to do with the type of conceptual paradigm which ultimately has influenced the author's overall consumer approach to community psychology. James C. Mancuso's keen and challenging ideas have always been at the heart of my approach. Certainly his insistence on the importance of a sound theoretical position underpinning any clinical intervention has strongly influenced my thinking.

It should also be obvious from reading this book that my overall approach owes much to the contributions of Thomas Szasz, Benjamin Braginsky, and George Kelly. They dared to lead the way toward new and more valuable ways of viewing the psychiatric client.

I owe special thanks to Frederick J. Smith who so often encouraged the development of innovative and sometimes controversial approaches to clients. Few administrators, I am afraid, would have been as supportive, let alone as open-minded.

The members of the community mental health team with whom I worked during the writing of this book, also deserve special mention. Without them and their help, little could have been accomplished. To Elizabeth Turpin, Millie Leonard, Michael Con-

nelly, Dottie Merwin, Hal Yablonovitz, Mike Harris, Janet Fentiman, Walter Friedman, Ann Shannon, Nancy Lill, Vance Hackel,
Esther Lawrence, Beth Rosetti, Gerald Montrym, Leta Georgiopou-
los, Arlene Armstrong, Diana Teta, Mark Banks and Dennis
Boyagian, my sincere thanks. And I would like to single out for
special acknowledgement Mary Anne Lyons, my superb typist and
team member, who has done such an excellent job typing the final
manuscript.

I also feel indebted to the administrators of the Capital District Psychiatric Center, Alan M. Kraft, N. Michael Murphy, and
William Gonzalez, for their support and encouragement of innovative approaches. And few colleagues have been as encouraging of,
and as quick to give support to, my consumer approach as Bernardo
Gaviria.

I would also like to thank the editors of those professional
journals which allowed me to reprint articles* originally published
in their journals. Specific acknowledgements will be made at the
beginning of each of those articles.

Finally, I owe much to those many clients, who must remain
nameless, who served on the client advisory board, filled out a
cornucopia of questionnaires, and provided me with a wealth of
new ideas.

---

*Note that a number of different journal styles are used in the articles in-
cluded in this book. This is necessary in order to fulfill the requirements of
journals that previously published articles be reprinted in the same style
in which they were originally published.

Preface

DECADES HAVE PASSED since mental health professionals first actively involved themselves in the clinical sphere; yet even today many clinicians persist in the assumption that, because of their training and experience, they are the best interpreters of the problems of psychiatric clients. And even when it appears true that professional caregivers understand the complexity of clients' problems better than the clients, such clinicians often then assume that they are justified in making unilateral decisions as to what type of treatment is best for such clients. Thus, one client is diagnosed as being "schizophrenic" and psychotropic medication is prescribed. Another is diagnosed as having an "anxiety neurosis" and is recommended for individual psychotherapy.

As if such assumptions were not presumptuous enough, it is not uncommon for mental health professionals to then ignore the client's role in the resolution of problems. Furthermore, almost as if to add insult to injury, when clinicians do happen to evaluate the effectiveness of their clinical strategies, they seldom ascribe much value to the opinions of the client-consumers related to the effectiveness of those strategies.

All of the above assumptions are open to question. It is the purpose of this book to question such traditional assumptions and to signal directions which are more challenging, more clinically effective, and more scientifically useful.

In my opinion, we have too long been caught in the scientifically arid, conceptual trap of construing most mental patients as bizzarre, irresponsible, semiaware, and ineffectual creatures whose total behavior patterns are quite incomprehensible. We have also implicitly assumed that the mental patient is either unable to give a decent account of his own problems—witness our endless search for psychopathology via the route of projective tests—or is not to be trusted in his account of those problems.

This book argues for a change in the way we construe psychiatric clients. Viewing them as persons with a variety of problems who are also capable, to some extent, of understanding and coping with their problems, leads to a different way of relating to clients within the mental health sphere. The importance of construct theory to the understanding of psychiatric clients has too long been neglected. The beauty and relevance of such a theory lie in its ability to clarify the differences between clients and to understand how each client's construct system leads us to expect many variations in the way persons think and respond. As delineated and applied in our own clinical setting, construct theory has led to client approaches that differ from those that would have emerged from either psychoanalytic or medical paradigms. Although the purpose of this book is not to outline construct theory, I believe the relationship between our overall consumer approach and construct theory will become more apparent with the reading of each article.

In an age characterized by proliferating demands for increased consumer protection, civil liberties, and accountability, a book focusing on the benefits of a consumer approach to community psychology is much needed. The vast majority of mental health professionals are well intentioned and basically humanistic in their concerns for client welfare. But the next step, actively and aggressively arguing for client advisory boards, client evaluation of services, and client evaluation of staff effectiveness, is a giant step indeed. Professionals in the field of community psychology and related disciplines need logical arguments that such client involvement is constructive, not destructive. Hopefully, the articles in this book will persuasively challenge the reader to conceptualize the delivery of services to clients in new and productive ways.

This book has been written for students of all the mental health professions—although psychology students may find the approach more comfortable than others—and for clinical professionals in the major mental health disciplines. Those readers seriously interested in civil liberties and consumer protection should find this book of assistance in arguing that a consumer approach to community psychology is operationally possible. Finally, as an administrator myself, I would hope that executive-directors, chiefs of service, hospital and clinic directors, and team leaders will also find this book of great utility in planning new systems of mental health service delivery and evaluation.

I have included in this book a number of already published articles, each of which I have either authored or coauthored. There are also a number of original contributions written by myself and a few colleagues. The articles included in each chapter are introduced by way of an "overview" in order to tie together more logically its contents. To the busy reader who only has the time to hit the book's highlights, I recommend first reading the overviews, and then focusing on articles or chapters of particular interest.

I would caution the reader that throughout the book certain key arguments are repeated over and over, sometimes unnecessarily so. Such repetition was unavoidable since the majority of articles in this book were previously published in different professional journals, thus necessitating a repetition of common themes. However, a possible blessing may emerge from such repetition, namely that the basic consumer approach of this book will periodically be brought into ever-clearer focus.

In conclusion, I feel the need to clearly state at the beginning of this book that the consumer approach to the problems of psychiatric clients is not the final solution, but rather a partial solution; and certainly not the only partial solution. However, in my enthusiasm, I find it difficult not to share with you my conviction that a total consumer approach can revolutionize the delivery of mental health services.

1
An Argument for a Consumer Approach

Overview

WHAT IS A "consumer approach to community psychology?" The answer to this question is begun with the first chapter in this book, and is pursued in the remaining chapters. In my opinion, the answer can never be completed because a valid consumer approach is always in the process of being defined and developed due to the different exigencies of each decade. Therefore, the consumer approach supported by this book is only one approach, and not necessarily the most valid and most useful one.

The consumer approach exemplified in the following chapters can be operationally defined by each of the chapters. Although such an approach will be argued in general terms in this first chapter, it is important to note here that the other chapters continue the argument in specific terms. Thus, the last eight chapters provide examples of specific ways in which the overall consumer approach described in Chapter 1 can be operationalized.

The first article in Chapter 1 argues that community mental health professionals should construe the psychiatric client differently in the light of the recent critique of the mental health establishment. It is furthermore argued that the client-consumer should have a role in the evaluation of the services he receives. The concept of a client advisory board is offered as one concrete way of giving the client an effective forum for making his opinions known. (The client board will be discussed in more detail later in the book.)

The second article in Chapter 1 addresses itself primarily to psychiatrists, but also, to a lesser extent, to other mental health professionals. No one would question that the psychiatric profession has always exerted a powerful influence on community mental health. If things are really to change in a consumer-oriented direction then psychiatrists must perceive value in the logic of a consumer approach. The article begins with a review of the charges by psychiatry's critics, and then attempts to provide some understanding of the reasons behind such charges. It is then suggested that a possible resolution to the conflict between the psychiatric establishment and its critics lies in the direction of a consumer approach. Many of the examples given of a consumer approach will be the focus of later articles in this book.

The purpose of this first chapter is quite simply to present the basic argument for a consumer approach. Actual evidence that such an approach can be useful and effective will be provided in subsequent chapters. The first article in Chapter 1 presents an argument for construing the psychiatric client as both consumer and evaluator of community mental health services.

The Client as Consumer and Evaluator of Community Mental Health Services*

James K. Morrison**

IN RECENT YEARS a new focus on the psychiatric client has clearly revealed a number of ethical issues for community psychologists (and professionals in related disciplines). A proliferating literature (APA, 1973; Beit-Hallahmi, 1974; Daniels, 1969; Ennis, 1972; Halleck, 1971; Hurvitz, 1973; Joseph, & Peele, 1975; Miron, 1970; Robinson, 1974; Schwitzgebel, 1973; Szasz, 1970a; Mancuso, & Eson, note 1) has raised questions about the ethics involved in involuntary commitment, uninformed consent to treatment, and the role of the psychologist as agent of the state (rather than of the client), to name but a few.

Many of these ethical issues appear to derive from a more careful look at the theoretical concepts (e.g., "mental illness") and clinical procedures (e.g., projective testing, diagnosis, psychotherapy) closely associated with traditional clinical and community psychology. Trenchant criticism of such concepts and procedures

*This article was published in *The American Journal of Community Psychology*, 1978, *6*, 147–155. Reprinted with the permission of Plenum Publishing Corporation.

**The author would like to thank Michael S. Cometa for his helpful comments during the preparation of this manuscript.

have issued from the disciplines of psychology (Braginsky, Braginsky, & Ring, 1969; Brown, 1973; Morrison, 1976a; Rosenhan, 1973; Sarbin, 1969; Sarbin & Mancuso, 1970), psychiatry (Breggin, 1975; Halleck, 1971; Laing, 1972; Szasz, 1961, 1970a, 1970b), and sociology (Becker, 1974; Goffman, 1961; Scheff, 1966). Often these critiques have centered on the questionable efficacy of various clinical procedures such as psychotherapy and hospitalization. Thus, if certain treatment does not work, how can one force these procedures on anyone? This type of criticism has led to periodic demands for the protection of what some (Ennis, 1972; Ennis & Siegel, 1973) in the legal profession currently view as patient rights (e.g., right to treatment after involuntary commitment, right to give informed consent to treatment).

Simultaneous with this demand for patient rights, a number of researchers have provided evidence which contradicts the assumption that clinical and community psychology are precise sciences incorporating a number of objective procedures. A series of studies (Braginsky & Braginsky, 1974; Dohrenwend & Dohrenwend, 1969; Haase, 1964; Levy & Kahn, 1970; Masling & Harris, 1969; Trachtman, 1973) indicate the extent to which client and clinician variables such as sex, social class, and political orientation are the key factors (rather than client behavior or psychodynamics) accounting for many of the different results of projective testing and diagnosis. Further, some (Breggin, 1975; Brown, 1973; Halleck, 1971) have objected that psychotherapy is too often used as a means of social control against various clients (e.g., poor, women, homosexuals). In summary, psychiatric clients appear to be in the precarious position of being the consumers of often ineffective and ethically questionable services.

The Changing View of the Client Consumer

Coincident with the raising of the above issues, recent studies (Morrison & Becker, 1975; Morrison & Nevid, 1976a; Nevid & Morrison, Note 8) indicate that a growing number of community oriented mental health professionals deny the validity of various medically oriented propositions (e.g., "mental illness is an illness like any other"). It would appear that the polemic criticisms of Szasz (1961, 1970a, 1970b) and others are beginning to have an impact on the attitudes of mental health professionals. However, there appears to be an information lag when one examines the current attitudes of the lay public, and mental patients in particular (Morrison & Nevid, 1976a, 1976b; Morrison, Yablonovitz, Harris & Nevid, 1976).

Seldom do professionals in the field of mental health attempt to inform clients and the public of the confusion which appears to characterize clinical theory and practice. Some community mental health professionals (Morrison, 1976a; Morrison & Nevid, 1976b, 1976c) have advocated "demythologizing" (e.g., "There is no such thing as 'mental illness' ") seminars to educate patients and the public against indiscriminately accepting all mental health services as "therapeutic." However, the philosophy which seems to prevail in the field of mental health is that the public, and especially psychiatric patients, should be shielded from the confusing controversies which are presently typical of the mental health arena. Thus, it would seem that clients are asked to be consumers, but unfortunately consumers of services which are not accepted as ethical or efficacious by many professionals. Unlike other consumers, they are apparently not supposed to be informed that the services they are contracting are unacceptable according to certain standards. Such a "protective" philosophy of course implies that client-consumers are not competent to decide for themselves the services they should have. This implication has long been an implicit, albeit unproven, assumption of mental health professionals.

It is my opinion that most clients do not need to be shielded from the disagreement which characterizes the mental health professions. In fact, I would suggest that, as consumers, it is imperative for clients to have access to the current state of knowledge about the ethics and effectiveness of clinical procedures. Otherwise, clients will never be able to give informed consent to the treatment which they are asked to accept. Not to reveal to clients such information about current treatment would seem tantamount to consumer fraud.

It would appear that the diverse attitudes about the consumer-client derive, in part, from the various theoretical models in vogue at the present time. For example, none of the current variations of the medical model (Blaney, 1975) construe psychiatric patients as persons responsible for their own behavior. On the contrary, the medical model approach to clients fosters a view that the client functions on a sub-normal level of behavior. The client is not seen as responsible for his "aberrant" behavior since, according to this approach, it issues from an illness or disease. Other models of human behavior (e.g., cognitive; social-learning) encourage a different view of clients. In these approaches the assumption is that

clients differ from non-clients in the degree to which they have yet
to resolve certain social/educational/psychological problems in living. By learning certain skills, these problems can be at least
partially resolved. In the cognitive and social-learning approaches,
the psychiatric client is viewed more as similar to, rather than
dissimilar from, the rest of humanity. Through such emphases,
these non-medical models are less prone than the medical model to
foster in the general public the equation that client status is stigma
(Chesno & Kilmann, 1975; Cumming & Cumming, 1965; Lamy,
1966).

The Client as Evaluator of Mental Health Services

Central to the recent reappraisal of mental health professionals' theoretical and operational approach to mental patients
is the proposition that psychiatric clients are appropriate and
knowledgeable evaluators of the services they receive. Mischel
(1968) has brilliantly exposed several problems with projective
testing, suggesting that, if we want to know what a client is thinking or feeling, we should ask the client. Recently, mental health
professionals have been doing just this. A number of studies (Denner & Halprin, 1974; Hart & Bassett, 1975; Ishiyama, 1970; Kotin
& Schur, 1969; Mayer & Rosenblatt, 1974; Powell, Shaw & O'Neal,
1971; Spiegel, Grayson & Spiegel, 1970; Zusman & Slawson, 1972;
Morrison, Pitchford, Dovberg & Smith, note 4) report that clients
can meaningfully evaluate psychiatric services. However, in spite
of such one-shot efforts on the part of some researchers to elicit
evaluative feedback from the psychiatric client, mental health professionals have not taken the next logical step, that of devising a
mechanism whereby clients can regularly and systematically evaluate the services they receive.

Recently I have argued for the creation of client advisory
boards (Morrison, 1976b) so that the real consumers of mental
health services will be able, on a regular basis, to evaluate all
aspects of a mental health service facility. The concept of citizen
advisory boards has certainly been accepted in the mental health
field (Kane, 1975; Meyers, Dorwart, Hutcheson, & Decker, 1974;
Robins & Blackburn, 1974; Rooney, 1968; NASW, Note 7). However, such boards are often wracked with problems (Holton, New,
& Hessler, 1973; Kane, 1975). Moreover, citizen boards are probably largely ineffective because they seldom, if ever, involve
actual consumers of a clinic's services, i.e., the clients. It would

seem reasonable to assume that only a psychiatric facility's clients, not other members of the community, are in the best position to meaningfully evaluate the services of that facility. It is usually a very time consuming process for citizen board members to become sufficiently acquainted with a clinic so that they can suggest important changes in that clinic. A clinic's clients, however, have already experienced the treatment programs of the facility and can thus speak more meaningfully of the changes which are needed.

Some may point out that therapeutic communities already provide adequately for client feedback to clinical staff. Although the basic philosophy of the therapeutic community (Daniels & Rubin, 1968) would at times appear similar to that of the client advisory board, the clients in a therapeutic community actually have no clearly defined power to evaluate a facility's services. And, even though some (e.g., Darley, 1974) have advocated that the clients in therapeutic communities be given more governing power, to date this has not been realized. Furthermore, no one has reported a therapeutic community which actually encourages clients to systematically evaluate the programs and services of that community.

It would seem that to allow clients to have a close look at our services and procedures, and then to encourage them to make appropriate recommendations for change, would help community mental health professionals avoid many of the thorny ethical issues in which we get entangled. For example, if a clinic has an advisory board composed of the consumers, any research which is questionable from an ethical standpoint can be first checked out with the board. Moreover, as a client board periodically evaluates the efficacy of all clinic services, more and more of the ineffective services can be eliminated. Thus, a client advisory board would seem to reflect the general thrust within psychology to safeguard the rights of the consumer (Jacoby, 1975).

Again, I would like to argue that only the client-consumer is in a good position to evaluate the services received. Not to allow this would be tantamount to believing that the automobile manufacturer is the most appropriate person to evaluate the worth of a car, not the buyer or consumer. As strange as this argument sounds, some appear to believe psychologists and psychiatrists are in a better position to judge the effectiveness of psychiatric services than is the client. I would propose that both arguments are illogical in this age of consumer protection.

One way of emphasizing the value of client advisory boards would be to answer objections which some may have against such boards. Those oriented toward the disease model (Osmond, 1970; Siegler & Osmond, 1973) may look with skepticism at efforts to involve a patient in complex evaluative processes. Assumably, patients operate at a deficient level of functioning, and therefore cannot meaningfully evaluate a clinic's services. After all, some may argue, the patients are coming to the clinic precisely because they are not able to resolve their own problems. One might counter this argument by referring to studies (e.g., Klein & Grossman, 1968; Braginsky, Braginsky, & Ring, 1969) which indicate that mental patients are capable of complex and responsible behavior. In fact, as Rosenhan (1973) suggests, mental patients may be at times less subjective and more rational than are mental health professionals.

Others fear that, given the opportunity, clients would be destructive in their negative criticism of a clinic's services. However, a study by Mayer and Rosenblatt (1974) would indicate that patients actually rate a clinic and its services more positively than do clinic personnel.

If clients were to be given more involvement in evaluating a clinic's services, it is not difficult to imagine the fears of administrators that such clients would attempt to take over the management of the clinic; or at least that there would be a continual power struggle between a client board and the administrators of a clinic. Fanning, Deloughery, & Gebbie (1972), however, point out that their survey of psychiatric patients uncovered no desire for such a power struggle.

Mental health professionals are already quite resistant to being evaluated by their peers. It is thus to be expected, that, *a fortiori,* these professionals would resist efforts to create a consumer board which would give clients the opportunity to evaluate staff performance. Nevertheless, where the spirit of evaluation has permeated every transaction of a clinic, the creation of consumer advisory boards wil be viewed by the staff as a logical and desirable step (Morrison, Pitchford, & Smith, note 5). Those who are already putting their clinical practices to empirical test should have little or nothing to fear.

The Consumer as Agent of Change

The preliminary steps necessary to create a client advisory board (CAB) in the community have been described elsewhere (Morrison, 1976b). A demographic study of the CAB (Morrison, note 2), as well as attempts at more empirical evaluation of the effectiveness of such boards (Morrison & Cometa, note 3; Morrison & Yablonovitz, note 6), have already been completed. It may be of interest here to briefly report how a clinic and its services can be improved as the result of CAB recommendations.

In the first six months of the board, the CAB recommended a total of fifty-two changes in the on-going functions and procedures (e.g., programs, treatment, etc.) of the clinic. Of that number, forty-eight or 92.3 percent of these recommendations were implemented by the staff before the end of the six month period (Morrison & Cometa, note 3). Also, as reported in that study, the staff reported very positive attitudes toward the CAB.

In the first six months of the board's operation, the CAB evaluated six clinic programs, the client waiting room, and the family care system. The board sponsored a series of lectures for clients on controversial clinical interventions (e.g., electroshock treatment), so that, if clients elected to undergo such procedures, they would be able to give *informed* consent. The CAB also conducted an in-service training program for staff to educate them to the problematic experience of becoming and remaining a client. Finally, the board began investigating the issue of whether clients were interested in having at least access to what their clinical advisors wrote down in charts. Further details of the client board transactions can be found elsewhere (Morrison, note 2).

There is already some empirical evidence that a client's experience on the board increases awareness of the clinic (e.g., programs, staff roles, etc.), as well as attitudes of independence (Morrison & Yablonovitz, note 6). It is possible that participation in the governing power of a clinic (e.g., by means of being able to evaluate and recommend changes) induces clients to feel less helpless and powerless (Darley, 1974), and have more control over their destiny (Morrison, 1976b). It is likely that such a positive experience can be understood in terms of clients learning to make more positive attributions to themselves, and to thus see less need for dependence on psychiatric services. Such conclusions need to be tested further.

As the present thrust toward a consumer psychology (Jacoby, 1975) continues, more and more professionals will come around to seeing the mental patient not only as the consumer, but also as the rightful evaluator of mental health services. And, as this happens, the rights of clients will be further ensured, and thus psychologists and other mental health professionals will be able to successfully avoid many of the thorny ethical problems involved in clinical and community spheres.

Reference Notes

1. Mancuso, J. C., & Eson, M. E. *Psychologists in the morals marketplace: Endeavor or enterprise.* Unpublished manuscript, State University of New York at Albany, 1973.
2. Morrison, J. K. *A client advisory board: The real consumers evaluate psychiatric services.* Manuscript submitted for publication, 1975.
3. Morrison, J. K., & Cometa, M. S. *The impact of a client advisory board on a community mental health clinic.* Manuscript submitted for publication, 1976.
4. Morrison, J. K., Pitchford, B., Dovberg, N., & Smith, F. J. *Correspondence of staff-client evaluations of discharge readiness and nontreatment therapeutic events.* Manuscript in preparation, 1976.
5. Morrison, J. K., Pitchford, B., & Smith, F. J. *The mental health administrator and evaluative research: Strategies for systematic change.* Manuscript submitted for publication, 1975.
6. Morrison, J. K., & Yablonovitz, H. *Increased clinic awareness and attitudes of independence through client advisory board membership.* Manuscript submitted for publication, 1976.
7. National Association of Social Workers. *Position statement on community mental health.* Unpublished manuscript, National Association of Social Workers, 1968.
8. Nevid, J. S., & Morrison, J. K. *The libertarian mental health ideology scale: Scale validation.* Manuscript in preparation, 1976.

References

American Psychological Association, Committee on Ethical Standards in Psychological Research. *Ethical principles in the conduct of research with human participants.* Washington, D.C.: APA, 1973.

Becker, E. *Revolution in psychiatry.* New York: Fress Press, 1974.

Beit-Hallahmi, B. Salvation and its vicissitudes: Clinical psychology and political values. *American Psychologist,* 1974, *29,* 124–129.

Blaney, P. H. Implications of the medical model and its alternatives. *American Journal of Psychiatry,* 1975, *132,* 911–914.

Braginsky, B. M., & Braginsky, D. D. *Mainstream psychology: A critique.* New York: Holt, Rinehart, & Winston, 1974.

Braginsky, B. M., Braginsky, D. D., & Ring, K. *Methods of madness: The mental hospital as last resort.* New York: Holt, Rinehart, & Winston, 1969.

Breggin, P. R. Psychiatry and psychotherapy as political processes. *American Journal of Psychotherapy,* 1975, *19,* 369–382.

Brown, P. *Radical psychology,* New York: Harper & Row, 1973.

Chesno, F. A., & Kilmann, P. R. Societal labeling and mental illness. *Journal of Community Psychology,* 1975, *3,* 49–52.

Cumming, J., & Cumming, E. On the stigma of mental illness. *Community Mental Health Journal,* 1965, *1,* 135–143.

Daniels, A. K. The captive professional: Bureaucratic limitations in the practice of military psychiatry. *Journal of Health and Social Behavior,* 1969, *10,* 255–265.

Daniels, D., & Rubin, R. S. The community meetings: An analytical study and a theoretical statement. *Archives of General Psychiatry,* 1968, *18,* 60–75.

Darley, P. J. Who shall hold the conch? Some thoughts on community control of mental health programs. *Community Mental Health Journal,* 1974, *10,* 185–191.

Denner, B., & Halprin, F. Measuring consumer satisfaction in a community outpost. *American Journal of Community Psychology,* 1974, *2,* 13–22.

Dohrenwend, B. P., & Dohrenwend, B. S. *Social status and psychological disorder.* New York: Wiley, 1969.

Ennis, B. J. *Prisoners of psychiatry.* New York: Avon Books, 1972.

Ennis, B. J. & Siegel, L. *The rights of mental patients.* New York: Avon Books, 1973.

Fanning, V. L., Deloughery, G. L., & Gebbie, K. M. Patient involvement in planning own care: Staff and patient attitudes. *Journal of Psychiatric Nursing and Mental Health Services,* 1972, *10,* 5–8.

Goffman, E. *Asylums: Essays on the social situation of mental patients and other inmates.* Garden City, N.Y.: Doubleday, 1961.

Haase, W. The role of socioeconomic class in examiner bias. In F. Riessman, J. Cohen, & A. Pearl (Eds.). *Mental health of the poor.* New York: Free Press, 1964.

Halleck, S. L. *The politics of therapy.* New York: Science House, 1971.

Hart, W. T., & Bassett, L. Measuring consumer satisfaction in a mental health center. *Hospital and Community Psychiatry,* 1975, *26,* 512–515.

Holton, W. E., New, P. K., & Hessler, R. M. Citizen participation and conflict. *Administration in Mental Health,* 1973, *2,* 96–103.

Hurvitz, N. Psychotherapy as a means of social control. *Journal of Consulting and Clinical Psychology,* 1973, *40,* 232–239.

Ishiyama, T. The mental hospital patient-consumer as a determinant of services. *Mental Hygiene,* 1970, *54,* 221–229.

Jacoby, J. Consumer psychology as a social psychological sphere of action. *American Psychologist,* 1975, *30,* 977–987.

Joseph, D. I., & Peele, R. Ethical issues in community psychiatry. *Hospital and Community Psychiatry,* 1975, *26,* 295–299.

Kane, T. J. Citizen participation in decision making: Myth or strategy. *Administration in Mental Health,* 1975, *4,* 29–33.

Klein, M. M., & Grossman, S. A. Voting competence and mental illness. *Proceedings, 76th Annual Convention, APA,* 1968, 701–702.

Kotin, J., & Schur, M. Attitudes of discharged mental patients toward their hospital experiences. *Journal of Nervous and Mental Disease,* 1969, *149,* 408–414.

Laing, R. D. *The politics of the family and other essays.* New York: Vintage Books, 1972.

Lamy, R. E. Social consequences of mental illness. *Journal of Consulting Psychology*, 1966, *30*, 450–455.

Levy, M., & Kahn, M. Interpreter bias on the Rorschach test as a function of patients' socioeconomic status. *Journal of Projective Techniques and Personality Assessment*, 1970, *34*, 106–112.

Masling, J., & Harris, S. Sexual aspects of TAT administration. *Journal of Consulting and Clinical Psychology*, 1969, *33*, 166–169.

Mayer, J. E., & Rosenblatt, A. Clash in perspective between mental patients and staff. *American Journal of Orthopsychiatry*, 1974, *44*, 432–441.

Meyers, W. R., Dorwart, R. A., Hutcheson, B. R., & Decker, D. Methods of measuring citizen board accomplishment in mental health and retardation. *Community Mental Health Journal*, 1972, *8*, 311–169.

Miron, N. B. Issues and implications of operant conditioning: The primary ethical considerations. In R. Ulrich, T. Stachnik, & J. Mabry (Eds.), *Control of human behavior*. Vol. II. *From cure to prevention*. Glennview, Ill.: Scott, Foresman, 1970.

Mischel, W. *Personality and assessment*. New York: Wiley, 1968.

Morrison, J. K. Demythologizing mental patients' attitudes toward mental illness: An empirical study. *Journal of Community Psychology*, 1976, *4*, 181–185. (a)

Morrison, J. K. An argument for mental patient advisory boards. *Professional Psychology*, 1976, *7*, 126–131. (b)

Morrison, J. K., & Becker, R. E. Seminar-induced change in a community psychiatric team's reported attitudes toward "mental illness." *Journal of Community Psychology*, 1975, *3*, 281–284.

Morrison, J. K., & Nevid, J. S. The attitudes of mental patients and mental health professionals about mental illness. *Psychological Reports*, 1976, *38*, 565–566. (a)

Morrison, J. K., & Nevid, J. S. Demythologizing the attitudes of family caretakers about "mental illness." *Journal of Family Counseling*, 1976, *4*, 43–49. (b)

Morrison, J. K., & Nevid, J. S. Demythologizing the service explanations of psychiatric patients in the community. *Psychology*, 1976, *13*, 26–29. (c)

Morrison, J. K., Yablonovitz, H., Harris, M., & Nevid, J. S. The attitudes of nursing students and others about mental illness. *Journal of Psychiatric Nursing and Mental Health Services*, 1976, *14*, 17–19.

Osmond, H. The medical model in psychiatry. *Hospital and Community Psychiatry*, 1970, *21*, 275–281.

Powell, B. J., Shaw, D., & O'Neal, C. Client evaluation of a clinic's services. *Hospital and Community Psychiatry*, 1971, *22*, 189–190.

Robins, A. J., & Blackburn, C. Governing boards in mental health: Roles and training needs. *Administration in Mental Health*, 1974, *3*, 37–45.

Robinson, D. N. Harm, offense and nuisance: Some first steps in the establishment of an ethic of treatment. *American Psychologist,* 1974, *29*, 233–238.

Rooney, H. L. Roles and functions of the advisory board. *North Carolina Journal of Mental Health,* 1968, *3*, 33–43.

Rosenhan, D. L. On being sane in insane places. *Science,* 1973, *179*, 250–258.

Sarbin, T. R. The scientific status of the mental illness metaphor. In S. C. Plog and R. B. Edgerton (Eds.), *Changing perspectives in mental illness.* New York: Holt, Rinehart & Winston, 1969.

Sarbin, T. R., & Mancuso, J. C. The failure of a moral enterprise: Attitudes of the public toward mental illness. *Journal of Consulting and Clinical Psychology,* 1970, *35*, 159–173.

Scheff, T. J. *Being mentally ill: A sociological theory.* Chicago: Aldine, 1966.

Schwitzgebel, R. K. Ethical and legal aspects of behavioral instrumentation. In R. L. Schwitzgebel & R. K. Schwitzgebel (Eds.), *Psychotechnology: Electronic control of mind and behavior.* New York: Holt, Rinehart & Winston, 1973.

Siegler, M., & Osmond, H. Schizophrenia and the sick role. *Journal of Orthomolecular Psychiatry,* 1973, *2*, 1–14.

Spiegel, P., Grayson, H., & Spiegel, D. Using the discharge interview to evaluate a psychiatric hospital. *Mental Hygiene,* 1970, *54*, 298–300.

Szasz, T. S. *The myth of mental illness.* New York: Hoeber-Harper, 1961.

Szasz, T. S. *Ideology and insanity.* New York: Hoeber-Harper, 1970. (a)

Szasz, T. S. *The manufacture of madness.* New York: Delta, 1970. (b)

Trachtman, J. P. Socio-economic class bias in Rorschach diagnosis: Contributing psychological attributes of the clinician. *Journal of Projective Techniques and Personality Assessment,* 1971, *35*, 229–240.

Zusman, J., & Slawson, M. R. Service quality profile: Development of a technique for measuring quality of mental health services. *Archives of General Psychiatry,* 1972, *27*, 692–698.

The Role of the Client-Consumer in the Delivery of Psychiatric Services

James K. Morrison and Bernardo P. Gaviria[1]

In recent years, confidence in and respect for psychiatrists[2] seem to have declined amidst trenchant and repeated criticism of psychiatry as a profession and as a sphere of influence, thereby thrusting psychiatrists into what Freedman and Gordon (1973) have aptly described as a "state of siege." To a considerable extent this situation reflects the changed position of the consumer in relation to the providers of psychiatric services. A closer examination of this relationship will illuminate not only some of the conditions necessary for charting a way out of the present dilemma, but also unused client resources for the organization and evaluation of those services.

In the past decade, early critics of psychiatry such as Szasz (1961) and Grinker (1964) have been joined by a swelling chorus of consumer advocates (e.g., Chu and Trotter, 1974), feminists (e.g., Chessler, 1972), attorneys (e.g., Ennis, 1972), sociologists (e.g., Becker, 1974), psychologists (e.g., Sarbin and Mancuso, 1970), historians (e.g., Lasch, 1976), and other psychiatrists (e.g., Breggin, 1975). The morality, legality, as well as the efficacy of a number of clinical interventions have been closely questioned. Many (Goffman, 1961; Braginsky, Braginsky and Ring, 1969) doubt the clin-

14

ical effectiveness of hospitalization in large mental institutions. The negative side effects (e.g., stigma) of psychiatric institutionalization (Cumming and Cumming, 1965; Swanson and Spitzer, 1970) and of other psychiatric treatments are felt by some (Howe, 1972; Straight, Schaffer and Folsom, 1973) to accentuate passive-dependent roles which are alien to the integration of the patients into the community.

Traditional forms of psychotherapy[3] have also long been criticized for their inefficiency and clinical ineffectiveness (Eysenck, 1952; Bergin, 1966; Szasz, 1975). Now others (Breggin, 1975; Brown, 1973; Chessler, 1972; Glenn, 1974; Halleck, 1971; Jones, 1975; Levine, Kamin and Levine, 1974; Tennov, 1975) allege that therapy itself is too often used in discriminatory fashion against certain groups (e.g., poor, blacks, females), thus fostering a preservation of the *status quo*. (Psychiatrists alone cannot be blamed for such alleged discrimination, but often they are an easily identified target.) Furthermore, radical interventions such as psychosurgery are severely criticized as ineffective and immoral (Breggin, 1973; Older, 1974). Even the legality of voluntary hospitalization is being contested in and out of court (Ennis, 1972). The community psychiatry movement, sometimes seen as an answer to some of these problems, has itself come under attack on grounds that it is chaotic and has failed in identifying needs and priorities (Chu and Trotter, 1974; Kirk and Therrien, 1975; Steinhart, 1973).

Perhaps the most publicized polemic against psychiatry has issued from critics (Sarbin and Mancuso, 1970; Szasz, 1961, 1970a, 1970b) who claim that the term "mental illness" is an ineptly applied metaphor which helps psychiatrists to retain administrative and clinical control of the mental health field. Another critic (Torrey, 1974) contends that the concept of mental illness leads straight to "psychiatric fascism" whereby psychiatrists set themselves up as doctors to a sick society and impose all sorts of panaceas in the attempt to cure it. These and other critics also question the appropriateness and utility of certain traditional medical models still strongly embraced, in one form or other (Blaney, 1975), by many psychiatrists.

Possible Reasons for the Critique of Psychiatry

As feelings have become stronger on both sides, criticism, even when cogent, has for many psychiatrists taken on the tone of an attack, and their position one of defense. As tempting as it may have become, it is not enough to simply identify the many possible explanations for this situation. Following an illumination of the reasons for the critique of psychiatry, it will be necessary to move beyond a defensive posture, and ultimately to improve performance in those areas where psychiatric interventions appear warranted.

Undoubtedly, the power, status, and income of psychiatrists make them prone to attack by those who see these as advantages based on tradition and privilege, rather than on accomplishment. However, such an explanation is naively reductionistic, since it explains away the present attack on psychiatry as just another attack on the establishment. Simplistic, single-cause explanations do not penetrate to the core of the problem.

Looking dispassionately at the last twenty-five years, it is difficult not to recognize that much of society's dissatisfaction with psychiatry stems from the profession's failure to deliver on its promises. This inability in turn may have partly resulted from the overinvolvement of psychiatry in too many areas. For Rome (1968) to define psychiatry's catchment area as "the world," seems not only grandiosely vague, but also dangerously optimistic. Such calls to "save the world" from its ills lead others (e.g., Lasch, 1976) to categorize psychiatry as a new religion. The false expectations that psychiatry can cure the ills of the world have undoubtedly encouraged psychiatrists to become involved with a mélange of moral, legal, religious, and political problems, and even to claim a certain expertise in those areas.

Not only have psychiatrists claimed the treatment of abnormal behavior as their domain, they have also in the past assumed that they possess, by virtue of their psychiatric training, special skills in personnel counseling, management, and budgeting. Similar claims of relevant skills by psychiatrists have been made in education, government, and the courtroom. In 1964, to the embarrassment of many of their colleagues, many psychiatrists produced on demand a psychiatric evaluation of Senator Goldwater's fitness for the presidency of the United States. Instead of learning a lesson from episodes such as this, psychiatrists have marched on, advocating that they have specialized skills in educational planning, and that they should screen both presidents of the United States (Hutschnecker, 1973) and judges (Kuvin and Saxe, 1975). Some psychiatrists, as Freedman and Gordon (1973) explain it, seem to have borrowed the public trust given to professionals to sanction their private political preferences. Perhaps it is no surprise then that the two groups now under the most severe attack from the public are politicians and psychiatrists (Brown, 1976). And, according to recent opinion polls, the general public expresses only a small degree of confidence in the psychiatric profession (Lasch, 1976).

Is it any wonder that professionals of many other disciplines have begun to look with concern at this redefinition of life's problems in terms of psychiatric concepts? Many psychiatrists themselves oppose their profession's overextension into so many areas of concern, especially since this situation has placed unwanted burdens on psychiatrists. Certainly, many psychiatrists do not cherish their legal responsibility for the involuntary commitment of certain persons to mental hospitals. However, the psychiatric profession has become saddled with such tasks by its own resistance to sharing such responsibilities. No single profession can be faulted for the limited success of such overambitious programs as the nationwide community mental health center movement or the mixed results of the massive placement of hospital patients in unprepared communities, but psychiatrists have borne the brunt of public unhappiness because of the apparent unwillingness on the part of some to allow other professionals to play a more powerful role in the field of mental health.

Adding to the self-damaging results of such possessiveness is the aloofness from everyday public concerns which seems to characterize much psychiatric theorizing. At the same time that psychiatrists expound on such ambitious goals as primary prevention, critics point out that psychiatrists have failed to identify the psychiatric needs of the poor and severely disabled. This is reflected in the continuing trend of psychiatrists to spend more than twice as much time treating private patients (seldom the poor or the massively disabled) than they do caring for patients in public settings (Chu and Trotter, 174).

A result of armchair speculation unrestrained by reality is the rush to unrestricted intervention in areas where psychiatry has only limited relevance. For example, Caplan (1964) suggests that mental health specialists convince unwed mothers to marry. Setting oneself up as an arbiter of morality, even if presented in the context of sexual counseling, is construed by many as an unwarranted intrusion into the sphere of expertise more appropriately claimed by moral theologians and moral philosophers. Similar incursions into the ethics of abortion or capital punishment, carried out in the name of psychiatric expertise, can only breed hostility among those who have long been suspicious of psychiatrists.

Insularity and claims to universality are not the only undesirable features in the psychiatric profession's image. Unfortunately, Ralph Nader's consumer group has charged psychiatry
with self-righteousness and elitism, sardonically characterizing
psychiatrists as "the field's ruling elite" (Chu and Trotter, 1974).
Others such as Lasch (1976) categorize psychiatrists in elitist
terms when they call the psychiatric profession the equivalent of
a priesthood which discharges priestly functions without the social structure of a church. Even in trying to establish reasonable
limits to psychiatric intervention, some psychiatrists appear to
cloak themselves with more than a little self-righteousness. At one
moment, a psychiatrist soundly advises psychiatrists against being
caught in the legal controversy over what is "insanity," and then
at another, proceeds to lecture the world on punishment and sin. In
an analogous situation, while another psychiatrist questions the
deprivation by the state of mental patients' civil rights, at other
times he seems to slip into the position of advising the legal profession on drafting the "best" mental health legislation. The temptation to extend psychiatric expertise to areas of influence where
it is often uninvited and unwelcome seems irresistible.

Justifiably or not, psychiatrists are now facing a new task,
that of defending what they do. In assuming this new task, psychiatrists may find less time to fulfill their professional responsibilities. Regardless of the ultimate role psychiatry assumes in
society, it is necessary for members of that profession to listen to
the expectations, wishes, and concerns of those who use their
services. The psychiatric profession will have to chart the nature
of its tasks and the scope of its goals. And they might well share
this effort, at all levels, with their clients.

A Responsible Resolution to the Conflict

It would be presumptuous as well as futile to try to formulate
a simple solution to such complex problems. Ultimate solutions and
panaceas will never emerge in the field of human behavior; any
improvements will necessarily be gradual and incomplete. Nonetheless, it is possible to describe some necessary preconditions or
requirements for mapping the proper sphere of influence for
psychiatry and for defining the rights and obligations of psychiatrists related to individuals or institutions.

Three general requirements or preconditions become clear.
First, psychiatrists will have to renounce any claimed expertise in

moral, legal, religious, and educational matters. This pre-condition, discussed and emphasized for a number of years, has not yet been fully accepted by a substantial number of psychiatrists. Secondly, psychiatrists must identify and chart those areas where, on the basis of an organized body of knowledge and proved technical skill, the profession can legitimately make its contribution to society. Again, this pre-condition has long been proposed, but not yet translated into any substantial redefinition of the role of psychiatry. Unlike these two pre-conditions, a third one has received less attention. It is that the psychiatrists must return to the patient much, if not most, of the responsibility for treatment decisions. If this requirement can be converted into a common feature of psychiatric practice, much of the current criticism against psychiatrists may be effectively countered. Following is a discussion of some of the contributions clients can make, not only to their own treatment, but to the planning, organization, and evaluation of services. We believe this is a sensible approach based on results which have been most encouraging.

Consumerism and Client Responsibility for Treatment

This may well be the era in which the client will not only be the consumer of mental health services, but the rightful evaluator of those services as well (Morrison, 1977a). If indeed psychiatric clients, as any other consumers, should have some voice in the final judgment of any service, then it is logical to more actively involve the client-consumer from the outset in the delivery of mental health services. (To some extent, Jones [1953] has led the way with the concept of the therapeutic community.) It would also follow, in the spirit of client consumerism, that psychiatric clients must assume more responsibility for the success or failure of the services which they contract (Morrison, 1976a; 1977a).

Although one could argue that the traditional medical model[4] is not very conducive to giving clients the right to evaluate services, or to giving clients more responsibility for the effectiveness of services contracted, still good medical practice has always emphasized the active cooperation of the client in treatment. Thus, despite research evidence (Morrison, Bushell, Hanson, Fentiman, and Holdridge-Crane, 1976) that passive-dependent attitudes of psychiatric clients correlate (.61) significantly with medical-model attitudes, psychiatrists who have actively involved their clients in treatment (whether psychoanalysis or psychotropic agents) have often found such interventions more effective than treatment in which the clients remained only passively involved.

It makes no logical sense to ask nonmedical persons or clients to cure a disease when such a cure requires unique skills which clients lack. And it makes no sense to ask for their active participation in treatment if such participation is totally unnecessary. These considerations, valid when interpreting a laboratory report or performing surgery, seldom apply to the planning and delivery of psychiatric services. In such cases, it makes a great deal of sense to ask clients to expend time and energy in the resolution of their *problems*. Here no clients are unskilled, having spent much of their lives learning and practicing a vast array of interpersonal and social techniques. And here active participation is indispensable in carrying out any plan, including that of drug administration. Furthermore, if psychiatrists and other mental health professionals would emphasize the active role of the client in treatment, then they might more easily convince the client that he has the primary responsibility for resolving problems.

Client Interest in Increased Responsibility

At this point, we need to answer two questions. First, are clients *willing* to accept at least some responsibility for their success or failure in problem resolution? Second, will such an acceptance of responsibility accrue *benefits* to clients? In answer to the first question, there is evidence that at least some clients not only accept that responsibility, but even welcome it. Two studies (Morrison, 1976b; Morrison and Nevid, 1976) indicated that clients were interested in attending "demythologizing" seminars which expose various myths (e.g., "Psychiatrists can usually cure mental illness") about psychiatric clients and psychopathology. One could argue that such seminars help clients adopt more responsible, active roles in their own treatment (Morrison, 1976b). A study of a client advisory board (Morrison and Cometa, 1976a) suggests that a large percentage (25 percent) of a client population is interested in participating (and actually does participate) in a board which takes an active and responsible role in a clinic. Furthermore, a telephone survey (Morrison and Dvelis, 1975) of a group of psychiatric outpatients indicated that 83 percent were interested in seeing their records to better understand, and more actively participate in, their treatment. Another study (Nevid, Morrison,

Gaviria and Rathus, 1976)) suggested that clients willingly accept some responsibility for the definition and planning of the resolution of their problems by participating with individual clinicians in joint problem definition and problem resolution evaluation. In conclusion, there is some evidence that clients are interested in becoming more active in their treatment.

Client Advisory Boards, Contracts, and Educational Seminars

Even if it should be generally true that psychiatric clients are willing to assume a larger role in their treatment process, this does not mean that, *de facto*, they are capable of doing so. Nevertheless, there is some evidence that client participation in the treatment process can facilitate treatment effectiveness. Participation in a client advisory board, a mechanism established to ensure systematic evaluation by clients of clinic programs, appeared to significantly increase those clients' attitudes of independence as well as their awareness of clinic staff and programs (Morrison and Yablonovitz, 1977). Thus, by comparison with a matched group of client controls, client board members appeared to be able to assume more responsibility for treatment. Furthermore, another study (Morrison and Cometa, 1976a) indicated that in a twelve month period, client advisory board members were 85 percent effective in inducing clinic staff to implement their recommendations for changes in the programs, procedures, and physical environment of a clinic, changes which the psychiatric staff judged would eventually lead to more effective client services.

Schwitzgebel (1975) has recommended the use of contracts with psychiatric clients to ensure quality of treatment. Such contracts allow clients to sue for breach of contract in those cases where clinical staff are grossly negligent in fulfilling the conditions of the contract. More importantly, the active involvement of clients in the contracting process may counter the frequent expectation of clients that they are coming to a hospital or clinic "to have something done to them," that is, "to be cured." Such increased involvement on the part of the client may well lead to more energetic attempts by the client to resolve his problems.

Nevid and Morrison (1976) describe a contract with one very paranoid patient who was terrified that should she engage in certain behaviors (e.g., arguing with her mother), she would be arbi-

trarily committed to a mental hospital. The contract clearly specified which behaviors would and would not necessitate psychiatric
hospitalization. This contract appeared to dramatically change the
client's behavior so that she could become a more responsible and
less troubled citizen in the community. Another use of the contract,
protecting clients in group psychotherapy from having confidential
information revealed to others by fellow group members, seemed
to facilitate increased self-disclosure by clients as well as increased
group trust (Morrison, Federico, and Rosenthal, 1975). Such contracting procedures allow clients a more active role in determining
the course of their treatment, and protect therapists from unwarranted claims of mistreatment. Specified contracts with clients
about individual therapy may also help in the treatment process
by defining treatment goals and by protecting the therapist from
lawsuits (Morrison and Cometa, 1976b; Strupp, 1975).

There is some limited evidence that educational seminars,
geared toward establishing more realistic client expectations of
service, increase client responsibility for problem resolution and
subsequently reduce the need for psychiatric hospitalization (Morrison, 1976b; Morrison and Nevid, 1976). In one study (Morrison,
Fasano, Becker and Nevid, 1976), clinicians found that if they
drastically reduced their telephone time with more "manipulative-
dependent" outpatients, these clients actually reported feeling more positive about themselves. Thus, it would appear that as
clinicians induce clients to become more independent, and to thus
resolve problems on their own, some of these clients may actually
benefit therapeutically from this approach. Increased client responsibility, at least in some cases, may lead to increased problem
resolution. The implications for clinical practice become clear.
Those psychiatrists and other mental health professionals who may
have slipped into a somewhat paternalistic stance may thereby inadvertently discourage clients from doing more on their own to
resolve their problems.

The Client as Evaluator

There are numerous studies (e.g., Denner and Halprin, 1974;
Hart and Bassett, 1975; Powell, Shaw and O'Neal, 1971; Zusman
and Slawson, 1972) which suggest the advantages of involving
psychiatric clients in evaluating their treatment. Such evaluations
again give more responsibility to clients, since the implication is

that client-consumers are capable and intelligent enough to participate. The message is also clear that the opinions of such consumers
are important. Not only may such participation in evaluating treatment effectiveness benefit those who wish to assume more responsibility in electing a treatment regimen, but again such client
involvement would seem to preclude the clinical *faux pas* of continuing to offer consumers the same old treatment regardless of its
effectiveness or ineffectiveness.

Psychiatrists and other clinical professionals might also consider the possibility of having consumers, through a client advisory
board or other mechanism, carry out their own evaluations separately from those of researchers and other staff (Morrison,
1977b). In other words, clients themselves can solicit the judgments of other clients about treatment effectiveness. Denner and
Halprin (1974) have suggested that when staff solicit
client opinion of treatment effectiveness, the responses are inflated
in a positive direction. As described elsewhere (Morrison, 1976a;
Morrison and Cometa, 1976a), anonymous client evaluations of
other patients may add another valuable dimension to staff evaluations of treatment effectiveness. If we are really serious about
consumer rights, then we will always entertain the possibility that
staff judgments of service effectiveness may be less than accurate.

Goal Definition and Service Selection

Perhaps psychiatrists can involve clients more in the precise
definition of goal attainment or problem resolution (Nevid, Morrison, Gaviria and Rathus, 1976). Using procedures such as the
problem-oriented medical record, we can share with clients more
responsibility for the planning of treatment. Without such client
involvement, there is the danger that clients will continue to construe treatment as something defined, planned, and evaluated *for*
them, rather than as something for which they assume at least
partial responsibility.

Other possibilities also become apparent. Recently, in one
satellite clinic, during initial screening for possible admission, we
have begun to give potential clients booklets describing all our
therapeutic programs so that they will have more choice in selecting their treatment regimen. Clients discuss with their therapists
the particular advantage of each program. Eventually, a mutual
decision by client and clinician is reached as to the most effective

treatment regimen. Such participation in treatment decisions would seem to provide psychiatrists and other professionals with a responsible way to deal with some of the thorny ethical issues which are part of today's mental health movement. For example, if a client, well informed as to any risks involved in ECT, still elects the treatment and signs a statement to that effect, there is less likelihood that this procedure can be judged immoral or illegal.

Benefits of Client Consumerism to Psychiatrists

We have attempted to outline some of the benefits of increased client responsibility or client consumerism. Although it is still too early to conclude with complete confidence that increased client responsibility generally leads to therapeutic effects, our research evidence allows us to conclude that out consumer approach is more than a modest effort. Hopefully, this approach will offer some promise for the future. Now we must ask whether it is realistic to expect that psychiatrists and other mental health professionals will welcome or at least accept the position of client-consumerism outlined above? In other words, what will psychiatrists and other professionals gain from a consumer approach which will attract them to change their approach to clients? First, giving more responsibility to clients may save psychiatrists and other professionals much time, time which could be valuably used in the evaluation of existing programs, or in the development of new ones. Research (Morrison, Fasano and Becker, 1976; Morrison, Fasano, Becker and Nevid, 1976) has demonstrated that inducing psychiatric clients to accept more responsibility for those problems they could handle themselves saved clinicians time which was then devoted to more relevant clinical work.

Second, a step in the direction of client consumerism assists the psychiatrist in following a responsible path through a maze of ethical and legal problems. To actively involve clients usually means that psychiatrists will be in close touch with what attorneys and moral philosophers have been recommending. Criticism and lawsuits related to clinical interventions will decrease, as they should, simply because we are taking seriously the rights of the individual.

Another problem remains unresolved. Even if psychiatrists begin to give clients more responsibility for their treatment, is there not a danger that some psychiatrists, for a variety of reasons (e.g., time demands, unwillingness to work with certain classes of clients, and so on), might use the concept of increased client responsibility as a pseudo rationale for discharging certain unwanted clients? One could well imagine the overworked psychiatrists telling a client: "You've got to accept responsibility for your problems and whether they get resolved or not. I've done my best. If you can't take it from here, then you had better find another psychiatrist." Although at times such an approach might be appropriate (e.g., with the manipulative, passive-dependent client), there are likely to be abuses within this approach, abuses which obstruct the true spirit of client consumerism. Some of us might be tempted to use client responsibility as an excuse to get rid of clients whom we do not like. For example, client-consumerism could easily become a disguise for discrimination on the basis of color, sex, religion, or social class.

Perhaps the real test of client-consumerism is how consistently we relate the message of client responsibility to the clients we would like to keep, because therapy with them is interesting and rewarding. Perhaps this type of client is the one who can accept and benefit most from an active participation in the treatment process.

Client consumerism will only take hold in the field of psychiatry if psychiatrists can become excited about the opportunities this approach can provide. If clients can be engaged actively in treatment evaluation, and if they can become less dependent on psychiatrists, to give two examples, then psychiatrists will have more time to spend on clinical interventions. And the lack of time for personal interaction between psychiatrist and client is, after all, what many psychiatrists and consumers have been complaining about.

Some Conclusions

We have examined the critique of psychiatry and concluded that, at least in part, current criticism of the profession has increased due to the overambitious attempts by psychiatrists and others to resolve a myriad of social/education/moral problems. Focusing on one partial solution to the present attack on psychiatry, we suggest that psychiatrists move in the direction of client consumerism. By actively involving clients in the entire treatment process, we thereby give part of the responsibility for treatment back to clients. Psychiatrists can benefit from this new thrust toward client responsibility because they will be able to find more time to devote to their primary task, that of assisting clients in problem resolution.

Notes

1. The authors would like to acknowledge the constructive comments of Bernard Berkowitz, M.D., during the preparation of this manuscript.
2. Although present criticism focuses most often on psychiatrists, similar critique can be or has been applied to other mental health professionals.
3. Although today psychotherapy is practiced by a wide variety of professionals and non-professionals, psychiatrists have traditionally been identified as the ones who do psychotherapy.
4. What we refer to as the "traditional medical model," Blaney (1975) refers to as models 1 and 3.

References

Becker, E. *Revolution in Psychiatry;* Free Press, 1974.

Bergin, A. E. "Some Implications of Psychotherapy Research for Therapeutic Practice." *Journal of Abnormal Psychology* (1966) 71:235–246.

Blaney, P. H. "Implications of the Medical Model and Its Alternatives." *American Journal of Psychiatry* (1975) 132:911–914.

Braginsky, B. M., Braginsky, D. D., and Ring, K. *Methods of Madness: The Mental Hospital as Last Resort;* Holt, Rinehart and Winston, 1969.

Breggin, P. R. "Reply to 'Lobotomies Defended.'" *American Journal of Psychiatry* (1973) 130:608.

Breggin, P. R. "Psychiatry and Psychotherapy as Political Processes." *American Journal of Psychotherapy* (1975) 19:369–382.

Brown, B. S. "The Life of Psychiatry." *American Journal of Psychiatry* (1976) 133:489–495.

Brown, P. *Radical Psychology;* Harper and Row, 1973.

Caplan, G. *Principles of Preventive Psychiatry;* Basic Books, 1964.

Chessler, P. *Women and Madness;* Doubleday, 1972.

Chu, F. D., and Trotter, S. *The Madness Establishment;* Grossman, 1974.

Cumming, J., and Cumming, E. "On the Stigma of Mental Illness." *Community Mental Health Journal* (1965) 1:135–143.

Denner, B., and Halprin, F. "Measuring Consumer Satisfaction in a Community Outpost." *American Journal of Community Psychology* (1974) 2:13–22.

Ennis, B. J. *Prisoners of Psychiatry;* Avon Books, 1972.

Eysenck, H. J. "The Effects of Psychotherapy: An Evaluation." *Journal of Consulting Psychology* (1952) 16:319–324.

Freedman, D. X. and Gordon, R. P. "Psychiatry Under Siege: Attacks from Without." *Psychiatric Annals* (1973) 3:10–34.

Glenn, M. (Ed.) *Voices from the Asylum;* Harper and Row, 1974.

Goffman, E. *Asylums: Essays on the Social Situation of Mental Patients and Other Inmates;* Doubleday, 1961.

Grinker, R. R. "Psychiatry Rides Madly in All Directions." *Archives of General Psychiatry* (1964) 10:228–237.

Halleck, S. L. *The Politics of Therapy;* Science House, 1971.

Hart, W. T. and Bassett, L. "Measuring Consumer Satisfaction in a Mental Health Center." *Hospital and Community Psychiatry* (1975) 26:512–515.

Howe, L. "The Concept of Community." In A. Biegel and A. I. Levenson (Eds.), *The Community Mental Health Center;* Basic Books, 1972.

Hutschnecker, A. A. "The Stigma of Seeing a Psychiatrist." *New York Times,* November 19, 1973.

Jones, E. "Psychotherapists Shortchange the Poor." *Psychology Today* (1975) 8 (April): 24–28.

Jones, M. *The Therapeutic Community;* Basic Books, 1953.

Kirk, S. A., and Therrien, M. E. "Community Mental Health Myths and the Fate of Former Hospitalized Patients." *Psychiatry* (1975) 38: 209–217.

Kuvin, S. F., and Saxe, D. B. "Psychiatric Examination of Judges." *New York Times,* December 12, 1975.

Lasch, C. "Sacrificing Freud." *New York Times Magazine* (1976) (February 22):11–12; 70–72.

Levine, S. V., Kamin, L. E., and Levine, E. L. "Sexism and Psychiatry." *American Journal of Orthopsychiatry* (1974) 44:327–336.

Morrison, J. K. "An Argument for Mental Patient Advisory Boards." *Professional Psychology* (1976a) 7:127–131.

Morrison, J. K. "Demythologizing Mental Patients' Attitudes Toward Mental Illness: An Empirical Study." *Journal of Community Psychology* (1976) 4:181–185.

Morrison, J. K. "The Client as Consumer and Evaluator of Community Mental Health Services." *American Journal of Community Psychology* (1977a) in press.

Morrison, J. K. (Ed.) *A Consumer Approach to Community Psychology;* Nelson-Hall, 1977b, in press.

Morrison, J. K., Bushell, J., Hanson, G., Fentiman, J., and Holdridge-Crane, S. "A Correlational Study of Client Dependence and Attitudes Toward Mental Illness." Manuscript submitted for publication, 1976.

Morrison, J. K., and Cometa, M. S. "The Impact of a Client Advisory Board on a Community Mental Health Clinic" (1976a). Manuscript submitted for publication.

Morrison, J. K., and Cometa, M. S. "The Effect of Emotive-Reconstructive Therapy on Client Problems Resolution: Early Empirical Findings" (1976b). Manuscript submitted for publication.

Morrison, J. K., and Dvelis, R. "A Survey of Psychiatric Patients' Interest in Their Records" (1975). Unpublished manuscript.

Morrison, J. K., Fasano, B. L., and Becker, R. E. "Systematic Reduction of a Community Mental Health Team's Telephone Time with Patients," *Psychology* (1976), 4:3–6.

Morrison, J. K., Fasano, B. L., Becker, R. E., and Nevid, J. S. "Changing the 'Manipulative-Dependent' Role Performance of Psychiatric Patients in the Community," *Journal of Community Psychology* (1976) 4:246–252.

Morrison, J. K., Federico, M., and Rosenthal, H. J. "Contracting Confidentiality in Group Psychotherapy," *Journal of Forensic Psychology* (1975) 7:1–6.

Morrison, J. K., and Nevid, J. S. "Demythologizing the Service Expectations of Psychiatric Patients in the Community," *Psychology* (1976) 13:26–29.

Morrison, J. K., and Yablonovitz, H. "Increased Clinic Awareness and Attitudes of Client Independence Through Client Advisory Board Membership," *American Journal of Community Psychology* (1977), in press.

Nevid, J. S., and Morrison, J. K. "Preventing Involuntary Hospitalization: A Family Contracting Approach," *Journal of Family Counseling* (1976), 4: 27–31.

Nevid, J. S., Morrison, J. K., Gaviria, B., and Rathus, S. "The Problem-Oriented Goal Attainment Scaling System: A Method of Case Centered Evaluation," In R. Hammer, G. Landsberg, and W. Neigher, *Program Evaluation in Community Mental Health Centers: A Manual;* D and O Press, 1976.

Older, J. "Psychosurgery: Ethical Issues and a Proposal for Control," *American Journal of Orthopsychiatry* (1974) 44:661–674.

Osmond, H. "The Crisis Within," *Psychiatric Annals* (1973) 3:59–81.

Powell, B. J., Shaw, D., and O'Neal, C. "Client Evaluation of a Clinic's Services," *Hospital and Community Psychiatry* (1971) 22:45–46.

Rome, H. P. "Psychiatry and Foreign Affairs: The Expanding Competency of Psychiatry," *American Journal of Psychiatry* (1968) 125: 729.

Sarbin, T. R., and Mancuso, J. C. "The Failure of a Moral Enterprise: Attitudes of the Public Toward Mental Illness," *Journal of Consulting and Clinical Psychology* (1970) 35:159–173.

Schwitzgebel, R. K. "A Contractual Model for the Protection of the Rights of Institutionalized Mental Patients," *American Psychologist* (1975) 30:815–820.

Steinhart, M. "The Selling of Community Mental Health," *Psychiatric Quarterly* (1973) 47:325–340.

Straight, E. M., Schaffer, R. C., and Folsom, J. C. "Patient Self-Care: Its Impact on Psychiatric Hospital Staff," *Psychiatric Quarterly* (1973) 47:377–385.

Strupp, H. H. "On Failing One's Patient," *Psychotherapy: Theory, Research and Practice* (1975) 12:39–41.

Swanson, R. M., and Spitzer, S. P. "Stigma and the Psychiatric Patient Career," *Journal of Health and Social Behavior* (1970) 21:44–51.

Szasz, T. S. *The Myth of Mental Illness;* Hoeber-Harper, 1961.

Szasz, T. S. *The Manufacture of Madness;* Delta, 1970a.

Szasz, T. S. *Ideology and Insanity;* Doubleday, 1970b.

Szasz, T. S. "The Myth of Psychotherapy," *American Journal of Psychotherapy* (1975) 18:517–525.

Tennov, D. *Psychotherapy: The Hazardous Cure;* Abelard-Schuman, 1975.

Torrey, E. F. *The Death of Psychiatry;* Chilton Book Co., 1974.

Zusman, J. and Slawson, M. R. "Service Quality Profile: Development of a Technique for Measuring Quality of Mental Health Services," *Archives of General Psychiatry* (1972) 27:692–698.

2
Attitudes of Client-Consumers and Others toward Mental Illness

Overview

IN RECENT YEARS there has emerged a growing interest on the part of mental health professionals in the attitudes of psychiatric clients toward "mental illness." It is assumed, and quite logically, that such attitudes are of some importance in determining the role of clients within the psychiatric milieu.

In spite of interest in such attitudes, researchers have failed to focus on whether mental health professionals and psychiatric clients may differ in the degree to which they accept or reject the most influential paradigm of "abnormal" behavior, that of the medical model. The implications for "treatment" are substantial in our question as to the possible differences between the attitudes of clients and mental health professionals. Thus, if the attitude of clients in one clinic generally reflect an acceptance of a traditional medical approach to their problems, their expectations for service may cause frustrations for their clinicians who may have attitudes more characteristic of proponents of an anti-medical model. The three modest studies in this chapter are attempts to determine attitude differences among client-consumers and service-providers.

The first two articles in this chapter indicate that psychologists appear to endorse the anti-medical model position more than any other group of mental health professionals. Psychiatric clients tend to be much less accepting of this position, and their attitudes toward mental illness are similar to those of psychiatrists and psychiatric nurses. In comparing the tables in the first two articles it becomes evident that students in three disciplines (psychology, nursing, psychiatry) are more accepting of the anti-medical model position than are the trained professionals in these same disciplines. The attitude measure used in these two studies is the CAQ-A (see Appendices).

In the final article of this chapter, a later version of the CAQ-A, the CAQ-B (see Appendices), was used in a pilot study to explore whether agency affiliation might influence acceptance or rejection of an anti-medical model. The data suggests that such affiliation indeed does appear to have an effect on how much one professes to adopt controversial mental health opinions. Mental health professionals (multidisciplinary) appear to be more accepting of this position than are public health agencies whose orientation is understandably more oriented toward the medical model. The attitudes of psychiatric nursing students and social agency staff were similar in being more oriented to the medical model than the attitudes of mental health professionals. Such divergent theoretical orientations among caregivers can assumably on occasion lead to interagency confusion, with the client-consumer caught in the middle.

These three articles suggest that a number of problems may arise in delivering mental health services to clients because some professionals (e.g., psychologists, social workers) apparently have very different views of psychiatric ideology and practice than do the clients. To protect the client-consumer from being victimized by interdisciplinary (and interagency) disputes over treatment approaches, educative seminars, such as those described in Chapter 3 may be necessary for both clients and staff of various agencies. Such seminars may increase communication between professionals, clients, and agencies and thus make client service less confusing for all concerned.

The Attitudes of Mental Health Professionals and Client-Consumers about Mental Illness*

James K. Morrison and Jeffrey S. Nevid

IN REVIEWING THE present state of research on attitudes toward mental illness, Rabkin (1972) concludes that existing attitude measures are inadequate. Admittedly, a number of studies (Appleby, Ellis, Rogers, and Zimmerman, 1961; Baker and Schulberg, 1967; Cohen and Struening, 1962, 1964, 1965; Reznikoff, 1963; Reznikoff, Gynther, Toomey, and Fishman, 1964; Williams and Williams, 1961; Wright and Klein, 1966) have demonstrated differences between some mental health professionals' (mostly nurses and aides) attitudes about mental illness. However, none of the attitude measures employed in these studies take into consideration that current approach to psychiatric ideology and practice which might be termed the controversial psycho-social approach (Laing, 1972; Sarbin, and Mancuso, 1970; Szasz, 1960, 1970a, 1970b).

*Reprinted in expanded form from the original with permission of publisher from: Morrison, J. K., and Nevid, J. S. Attitudes of mental patients and mental health professionals about mental illness. *Psychological Reports*, 1976, *38*, 565–566.

A further problem with the present state of research is that few reported studies (Imre, 1962; Imre, and Wolf, 1962; Manis, Houts, and Blaker, 1963; Toomey, Reznikoff, Brady, and Schumann, 1961) attempt to compare the attitudes of various mental health professionals with those of client-consumers. Perhaps one reason for this paucity of studies is that most of the existing attitude measures are too complex in both terminology and response mode to be adequately understood by mental patients, especially those who have resided for years in mental institutions. Even in the few reported studies comparing attitudes of patients with those of mental health professionals, the measures used cannot adequately measure attitudes about some of the issues raised by Szasz and others. In summary, there appears to be a need for an easily understood attitude measure which can determine a respondent's endorsement of the controversial psychosocial approach to psychiatric ideology and practice.

The measure employed in our study, the Client Attitude Questionnaire (CAQ-A), represents an initial attempt to overcome the above-mentioned problems on measuring attitudes toward mental illness. The CAQ-A was designed to be easily understood by both patients and mental health professionals, and to include items (e.g., "There is no such thing as mental illness") representative of the controversial psychosocial approach to psychiatric ideology and practice.

In this study, further evidence of construct validity was sought. Lower scores (hence, less acceptance of the psycho-social position) were predicted for professionals (nurses, psychiatrists) in disciplines involving extensive training within medical model approaches than for professionals (psychologists, social workers) more oriented toward non-medical, social learning approaches. Second, since previously hospitalized psychiatric outpatients would have more than likely been exposed (while in a mental hospital) to a medical model orientation toward mental illness, their attitudes, as given by questionnaire scores, were expected to be less oriented to the psychosocial position than the attitudes of psychologists, social workers, and psychiatric out-patients never hospitalized for psychiatric reasons.

Method

Subjects. All mental health professionals employed by two community facilities (a small community mental health center and a local medical center) in a particular city were canvassed. Fifty-six percent of the psychologists solicited had earned a Ph.D. Sixty-eight percent of the solicited social workers had obtained an M.S.W. All nurses were licensed, and all psychiatrists were certified. The sample consisted of 20 psychiatrists, 23 psychiatric nurses, 16 psychologists, and 25 social workers.

The first patient sample consisted of 41 outpatients, all with a history of previous psychiatric hospitalization. These patients were living in the community and receiving after-care services from a community mental health center satellite clinic. The second patient sample consisted of 20 outpatients, none of whom had a history of previous psychiatric hospitalization. All of these patients were receiving individual and/or group psychotherapy from the same community mental health center satellite clinic.

No further demographic information on the sample respondents was available since the anonymity of the respondents was considered of greater importance in obtaining unbiased attitude statements than demographic data. Anonymity was considered particularly important since the senior author was personally known to most of the professionals solicited in this sample.

Attitude measure. The Client Attitude Questionnaire (CAQ-A), a highly reliable (Morrison and Becker, 1975) twenty-item rating scale, is a measure of a respondent's degree of endorsement of the controversial psychosocial approach to psychiatric ideology and practice, identified with the writings of Szasz (1970), and Sarbin and Mancuso (1970), among others. To avoid possible response bias, the scale items were positively and negatively keyed. The scale was constructed in a three point format, with provision for the respondent to answer either true, not sure, or false for each item. These three response categories were scored 3, 2, and 1, respectively, for items positively keyed to the controversial psychosocial or anti-medical view of mental illness (e.g., "Mental hospitals should be abolished."). Reversal scoring was used for negatively keyed items.

Procedure. Attitude questionnaires were mailed to all psychologists, psychiatrists, social workers, and psychiatric nurses listed by the personnel offices of both facilities. Only professional identification was requested from each respondent. Both the previously hospitalized ($n = 41$) and nonhospitalized ($n = 20$) patients were randomly selected from a sample of 82 outpatients receiving psychiatric services from the same community mental health center satellite clinic. Clients filled out the questionnaire anonymously and all were returned to the author by way of a third party. The only discrimination asked for was whether the patient had ever been hospitalized for psychiatric reasons or not, noted by the patient on his questionnaire.

The return rate of questionnaires among professionals ranged from 89 percent for nurses and psychologists to 91 percent and 96 percent for psychiatrists and social workers, respectively. Due to this extremely high return rate, the respondent sample can be considered representative of the local mental health community.

Results

The means and standard deviations of the groups are presented in Table 1. Comparisons by *t*-tests showed, as expected, that psychologists' reported attitudes were more oriented to the psycho-social or anti-medical position than the attitudes of social

Table 1
Means and Standard Deviations For Client Attitude Questionnaire Scores Across Subjects

Subjects	N	M	SD
Psychologists	16	49.25	5.24
Social workers	25	45.76	4.67
Psychiatric nurses	23	42.87	4.30
Psychiatrists	20	42.80	5.15
Mental patients Previously nonhospitalized	20	42.75	5.33
Previously hospitalized	40	40.71	5.17

workers ($t = 2.17$, df $= 39$, $p < .05$), nurses ($t = 4.17$, $df = 37$, $p < .001$), psychiatrists ($t = 3.80$, $df = 35$, $p < .001$), and previously hospitalized patients ($t = 3.80$, $df = 55$, $p < .001$). Second, the attitudes of the sampled social workers were more consistent with the psychosocial position than the reported attitudes of nurses ($t = 2.23$, $df = 46$, $p < .025$), psychiatrists ($t = 2.06$, $df = 44$, $p < .025$), and previously hospitalized patients ($t = 3.99$, $df = 64$, $p < .001$). The results indicated a nonsignificant trend ($p < .10$) for the attitudes of previously hospitalized patients to be less oriented to the psychosocial approach than previously nonhospitalized patients.

Discussion

The results attest to the construct validity of the Client Attitude Questionnaire and suggest that the variety of attitudes toward mental illness may often lead to divergent staff-client expectations for service. For example, if our local sample accurately reflects the attitudes of psychologists and mental patients toward mental illness, then psychologists may need to spend some time with new clients discussing attitude differences since divergent expectations for services often derive from different attitudes about psychiatric ideology and practice. Orientation seminars (Morrison, 1976) focusing on these differences may at least partially resolve this problem.

The failure to attain significant differences between the attitudes of hospitalized and nonhospitalized patients may suggest that a medical model orientation is not learned only from a hospital setting but also from the popular media, e.g., "Mental illness is an illness like any other," and the traditional orientation of state-supported outpatient clinics. Further research on such patients may illuminate any differences in attitudes.

In conclusion, the evidence from this study supports the existence of differences among mental health professionals and psychiatric outpatients regarding their respective attitudes toward current psychiatric ideology and practice. Psychologists clearly endorse the psychosocial model more than all the other professional and patient respondents. Social workers are more inclined to support the psychosocial position than are psychiatrists, nurses, and patients. This finding would tend to indicate that, related to attitudes toward mental illness, social workers occupy a more moderate position among psychiatric professionals.

References

Appleby, L., Ellis, N.C., Rogers, G.W., & Zimmerman, W.A. A psychological contribution to the study of hospital structure. *Clinical Psychology*, 1961, *17*, 390–393.

Baker, F., & Schulberg, H.C. The development of a community mental health ideology scale. *Community Mental Health Journal*, 1967, *3*, 216–225.

Cohen, J., & Struening, E.L. Opinions about mental illness in the personnel of two large mental hospitals. *Journal of Abnormal Social Psychology*, 1962, *64*, 349–360.

Cohen, J., & Struening, E.L. Opinions about mental illness: Hospital social atmosphere profiles and their relevance to effectiveness. *Journal of Consulting Psychology*, 1964, *28*, 291–298.

Cohen, J., & Struening, E.L. Opinions about mental illness: Hospital differences in attitude for eight occupational groups. *Psychological Reports*, 1965, *17*, 25–26.

Imre, P. Attitudes of volunteers toward mental hospitals compared to patients and personnel. *Journal of Clinical Psychology*, 1962, *18*, 516.

Imre, P., & Wolf, S. Attitudes of patients and personnel toward mental hospitals. *Journal of Clinical Psychology*, 1962, *18*, 232–234.

Laing, R.D. *The politics of the family and other essays*. New York: Vintage Books, 1972.

Manis, M., Houts, P.S., & Blaker, J.B. Beliefs about mental illness as a function of psychiatric status and psychiatric hospitalization. *Journal of Abnormal Psychology*, 1963, *67*, 226–233.

Morrison, J.K. Demythologizing mental patients' attitudes toward mental illness: An empirical study. *Journal of Community Psychology*, 1976, *4*, 181–185.

Morrison, J.K., & Becker, R. Seminar-induced change in a community psychiatric team's reported attitudes toward "mental illness." *Journal of Community Psychology*, 1975, *3*, 281–284.

Rabkin, J.G. Opinions about mental illness: A review of the literature. *Psychological Bulletin*, 1972, *77*, 153–171.

Reznikoff, M. Attitudes of psychiatric nurses and aides toward psychiatric treatment and hospitals. *Mental Hygiene*, 1963, *47*, 354–360.

Reznikoff, M., Gynther, M.D., Toomey, L.C., & Fishman, M. Attitudes toward the psychiatric milieu: An interhospital comparison of nursing personnel attitudes. *Nursing Research*, 1964, *13*, 71–72.

Sarbin, T.R., & Mancuso, J.C. Failure of a moral enterprise: Attitudes of the public toward mental illness. *Journal of Consulting and Clinical Psychology*, 1970, *35*, 159–173.

Szasz, T. *The myth of mental illness*. New York: Hoeber-Harper, 1961.

Szasz, T. *The manufacture of madness*. New York: Delta, 1970a.

Szasz, T. *Ideology and insanity*. New York: Doubleday, 1970b.

Toomey, L.C., Reznikoff, M., Brady, J.P., & Schumann, D.W. Some relationships between the attitudes of nursing students toward psychiatry and success in psychiatric affiliation. *Nursing Research*, 1961, *10*, 165–169.

Williams, J., & Williams, H.M. Attitudes toward mental illness, anomia and authoritarianism among state hospital nursing students and attendants. *Mental Hygiene*, 1961, *45*, 418–424.

Wright, F.H., & Klein, R.A. Attitudes of hospital personnel and the community regarding mental illness. *Journal of Counseling Psychology*, 1966, *13*, 106–107.

The Attitudes of Nursing Students and Others about Mental Illness*

James K. Morrison, Harold Yablonovitz, Michael R. Harris, and Jeffrey S. Nevid

THE ATTITUDES OF student nurses toward mental illness have been frequently studied.[1-6] However, according to Rabkin,[7] the type of attitude measures used in these studies appear inadequate to the task of determining current attitudes toward mental illness. That is, none of the existing attitude measures contain items which specifically reflect the current "revolution" in psychiatric ideology and practice, the radical psychosocial approach.[8-13]

Recently the senior author and his associates have begun to employ a newly developed attitude measure, the Client Attitude Questionnaire (CAQ), to determine attitudes toward mental illness.[14-17] This instrument allows respondents to report a wide range of attitudes toward mental illness, ranging from conservative (e.g., "Mental illness is a disease") to radical (e.g., "Mental illness is a myth"). In the present study, the attitudes of student nurses about mental illness are compared with the attitudes of psychiatric nurses and students in psychology, psychiatry, and education. It was pre-

*This article was originally published in the *Journal of Psychiatric Nursing and Mental Health Services*, 1976, 14, 17–19. Reprinted by permission.

dicted that student nurses (more oriented to the medical model) would be significantly less radical than psychology students (more oriented to the psychosocial model), similar in attitudes to psychiatric residents and nurses (also oriented to the medical model approach), and more radical than teacher-students in the field of education, who normally reflect the more conservative views of the general public.

Description of the Study

The attitude instrument employed in this study was the highly reliable Client Attitude Questionnaire (CAQ), developed by the senior author, and proven to have excellent construct and predictive validity.[14-17] This measure consists of 20 items, positively and negatively keyed, with a response scale constructed in a simplified three point format (true, not sure, false) so that the measure could be more easily used with a wide variety of respondents at different educational levels. Items include those which tap a radical psychosocial view of mental illness (e.g., "People have been duped or fooled into believing that there is such a thing as mental illness;" "Mental hospitals should be abolished").

The student nurse sample ($n = 35$) consisted of senior nursing students completing their studies at a local university. These students were gaining clinical field experience in a community public health setting. All of the students were females in their early twenties.

The psychology student sample ($n = 15$)was composed of students (7 second-year graduate psychology students on "practicum," and 8 senior undergraduates majoring in psychology and engaging in independent studies in the field) gaining clinical experience at a community mental health satellite clinic. This sample consisted of 10 males and 5 females, ranging in age from 21 to 29 years.

The psychiatric residents ($n = 13$) were students at a relatively small local medical school. These residents were from all years of residency training. Eleven of the 13 residents were male, and the total sample ranged in age from 26 to 34 years.

The sample of teacher-students consisted of 16 certified teachers in secondary education taking a graduate course toward a further degree. The teacher-students were primarily female, and ranged in age from 23 to 39.

The remaining sample consisted of local psychiatric registered nurses ($n = 23$) whose CAQ scores were obtained in a related study.[16]

The CAQ questionnaires were distributed to all of the sample respondents. Names were not requested in order to facilitate a reporting of the respondents' true attitudes.

Results and Discussion

Table 1 presents the means and standard deviations for each sample. Analysis of variance for groups revealed significant intergroup differences ($F = 24.44$, $df = 4/97$, $p < .001$). The Newman Keuls analysis for paired comparisons indicated, as expected, that student nurses reported significantly ($p < .05$) less radical attitudes on the CAQ than did psychology students, but significantly ($p < .05$) more radical attitudes than teacher-students. Also, as predicted, the attitudes toward mental illness held by nursing students did not significantly differ from those of psychiatric residents. Contrary to prediction, student nurses were significantly ($p < .05$) more radical in their attitudes than were psychiatric nurses.

Table 2
Means and Standard Deviations for CAQ Responses by Sample

Sample	Mean	Standard Deviation
Psychology students ($n = 15$)	54.13	3.60
Student nurses ($n = 35$)	46.43	4.53
Psychiatric residents ($n = 13$)	44.31	5.17
Psychiatric nurses ($n = 23$)	42.87	4.30
Teacher-students in education ($n = 16$)	40.06	3.45

The results of this study would suggest that student nurses maintain somewhat moderate attitudes toward mental illness, at least by contrast with the more radical psychology students and the more conservative teacher-students in education. It had been correctly hypothesized that student nurses, educationally oriented toward the medical model, would be more similar to psychiatric residents (also oriented to the same model) than to psychology students trained in psychosocial approaches. These student nurses were less conservative than teacher-students in the field of education, who usually tend to reflect the attitudes of the general public.

The student nurses' responses on the CAQ indicated that they strongly maintain the following attitudes: (1) Psychological tests cannot determine mental illness; (2) Psychiatrists and psychologists cannot usually distinguish the "mentally ill" from the "normal"; (3) Mental problems are not usually caused by brain pathology; (4) The general public has not been duped into believing in mental illness. Student nurses, as a group, appeared to be undecided as to whether mental hospitals should be abolished, and as to whether mental illness is a myth or not.

An unexpected result of this study was that student nurses tended to be significantly more radical in their attitudes about mental illness than the sample of psychiatric nurses. Student nurses tended to be less rejecting than psychiatric nurses of the following radical positions: the abolishment of mental hospitals, the myth of mental illness, removal of locked wards for treating mental patients, and the unreliability of psychiatric diagnoses. This greater tendency away from the more conservative position held by psychiatric nurses would suggest that student nurses had received greater exposure to the more current criticisms of the "medical model" positions.[8-13] Indeed, it was learned that these student nurses had taken some psychology courses at the university's psychology department, a department known for its psychosocial orientation.

Conclusions

Student nurses tend to report somewhat moderate attitudes toward mental illness in that they appear to be less radical than psychology students, but less conservative than teacher-students in education. Their attitudes are similar to those of psychiatric residents but more radical than those of psychiatric nurses.

References

1. Canter, F. M. The relationship between authoritarianism, attitudes toward mental hospital patients, and effectiveness in clinical work with mental hospital patients. *J Clin. Psychol.* 19: 124, 1963.

2. Gelfand, S. & Ullman, L. P. Change in attitudes about mental illness associated with psychiatric clerkship training. *Int. J. Soc. Psychiat.* 7:292, 1961

3. Hicks, H. M. & Spaner, F. E. Attitude change as a function of mental hospital experience. *J. Abnorm. Soc. Psychol.* 65:112, 1962.

4. Johannsen, W. J., Redel, M. C., & Engel, R. G. Personality and attitudinal changes during psychiatric nursing affiliation. *Nurs. Res.* 13:343, 1964.

5. Lewis, I. L. & Cleveland, S. E. Nursing students' attitudinal changes following a psychiatric affiliation. *J. Psychiat. Nurs.* 4:223, 1966.

6. Williams, J. & Williams, H. M. Attitudes toward mental illness, anomia, and authoritarianism among state hospital nursing students and attendants. *Ment. Hyg.* 45:418, 1961.

7. Rabkin, J. G. Public attitudes toward mental illness: A review of the literature. *Schiz. Bull.* 10:9, 1974.

8. Braginsky, B., Braginsky, D., & Ring, K. *Methods in madness.* New York: Holt, Rinehart and Winston, 1969.

9. Laing, R. D. *The politics of the family and other essays.* New York: Vintage Books, 1972.

10. Sarbin, T. R. & Mancuso, J. C. Failure of a moral enterprise: Attitudes of the public toward mental illness. *J. Consult. Clin. Psychol.* 35:159, 1970.

11. Szasz, T. *The Myth of Mental Illness.* New York: Hoeber-Harper, 1961.

12. Szasz, T. *The Manufacture of Madness.* New York: Delta, 1970.

13. Szasz, T. *Ideology and Insanity.* New York: Doubleday, 1970.

14. Morrison, J. K. & Becker, R. E. Seminar-induced change in a community psychiatric team's reported attitudes toward "mental illness." *J. Commun. Psychol.* 3:281, 1975.

15. Morrison, J. K. Demythologizing mental patients' attitudes toward mental illness. *P. Commun. Psychol.* (in press), 1976.

16. Morrison, J. K., & Nevid, J. S. The attitudes of mental patients and mental health professionals about mental illness. *Psychol. Rep.* (in press), 1976.

17. Morrison, J. K. & Nevid, J. S. Demythologizing the attitudes of family caretakers about "mental illness." *J. Fam. Counsel.* (in press), 1976.

Differential Attitudes of Community Agencies toward Mental Illness: A New Dilemma for the Psychiatric Nurse*

James K. Morrison, Michelle P. Schwartz, and
Susan Holdridge-Crane

ALTHOUGH RABKIN,[1] IN her review of relevant studies, concludes that attitudes toward mental illness are at least partly a function of one's professional identification, no research is presently available which addresses the question of whether such attitudes are also partly a function of agency identification. If one's educational training as a professional influences one's attitudes toward mental illness, as seems to be the case,[2-3] then it is also reasonable to assume that one's practical experience within a particular agency would also influence those attitudes. Thus, for example, if one works for a county health clinic, it should not be surprising if such a person's attitudes toward mental illness are strongly influenced by the medical model. By way of contrast, professionals working for social service agencies may find their attitudes toward mental illness increasingly molded by psychosocial assumptions (e.g., social-learning theory).

*This article was originally published in the *Journal of Psychiatric Nursing and Mental Health Services*, 1977, *15*, 25–29. Reprinted by permission.

Because student nurses often gain their psychiatric nursing experience in some relationship with community mental health centers, they are faced, in doing advocacy work with clients, with the complex problem of relating to a number of health, mental health and social agencies in order to arrange medical, educational, social, vocational, and psychological services for clients. Often the lack of contact and communication betweeen such agencies leads to confusion and misunderstanding. Few agencies appear to clearly understand the role and task of any one agency, and thus agencies often make inappropriate referrals, and frequently have difficulty arranging for their clients' ancillary services from other agencies. Ultimately, it is the client-consumer who suffers from such inter-agency confusion.

Much of the contact between community agencies is of a superficial nature. Either the contacts are informal, or, even when centered around inter-agency consultation, they do not usually lead to any real definition or clarification of each agency's attitudes toward mental illness. Thus, student nurses working in community settings may at times face the dilemma of having to relate to a variety of different agencies with divergent attitudes toward mental illness. This position can be uncomfortable for the student nurses because divergent attitudes can lead to inter-agency conflicts. For example, if a social worker with the county department of social services rejects the recommendation by a nursing student's supervisor (a psychiatrist with a mental health clinic) that the mutual client of both agencies be psychiatrically hospitalized, the student, along with the client, may feel the crush of conflict.

The purpose of the present study was to determine whether attitudes toward mental illness do in fact differ, in part, as a function of an employee's agency affiliation; and also how in one community the attitudes of student nurses toward mental illness compare with attitudes of the employees of several community agencies. In order to understand attitude divergence within the context of inter-agency communication and contact, the authors also attempted to study the degree and type of contact between the community mental health center satellite clinic and other community agencies (categorized as "social" or "health" agencies).

Description of the Study

The attitude measure employed in this study was the Client Attitude Questionnaire (CAQ-B). This instrument consists of

20 items, positively and negatively keyed, to which respondents answer, "true," "false," or "not sure." This simplified three point response format was developed so that the measure could be more easily used with a wide variety of respondents of varying educational backgrounds. Responses appear to distinguish respondents' orientation either toward a "radical psychosocial" view of mental illness (e.g., "Mental hospitals should be abolished"), or toward the traditional medical model (e.g., "Mental problems are quite often caused by some disorder of the body"). The minimum score is 20, the maximum 60. (The CAQ-B is a revised version of the CAQ-A.[2])

A second questionnaire (Agency Relationship Questionnaire or ARQ) was developed for the study in order to determine the type of relationship which characterizes the interaction between a psychiatric agency and other community agencies. This instrument consists of eleven items, including "subjective" questions which focused on opinions (e.g., "How beneficial do you feel the psychiatric agency is?") and "objective" questions which centered on facts (e.g., "Have you ever referred a client to the psychiatric agency?"). The ARQ allowed a variety of response modes: multiple choice, "yes" and "no" and open-ended responses.

The social agency sample consisted of personnel ($n = 20$) from a variety of non-medical, community service agencies, i.e., Department of Social Services, Cooperative Extention, Inc., Human Services, Intake and Referral, Youth Employment, Legal Aid, and Neighborhood Youth Corps. The agency personnel included social workers, lawyers and a variety of non-professional outreach workers.

The health agency sample consisted of personnel ($n = 7$) from the county health department and a medically-oriented alcoholic rehabilitation program. The personnel surveyed included rehabilitation counselors, public health nurses, and other health department personnel.

The sample of mental health workers ($n = 14$) consisted of the clinicians and interns on a multidisciplinary community mental health satellite team.

The student nurse sample ($n = 18$) consisted of senior nursing students completing their studies at a local university. The students were gaining clinical field experience in a community public health setting. They shared an office corridor with the personnel of a community mental health agency, and worked in the same building with the personnel of the social and health agencies surveyed in this study. The student nurses often collaborated with the personnel of the other agencies, especially the mental health workers from the psychiatric agency.

The CAQ-B and ARQ were distributed to all the health and social agency sample respondents. Names were not requested in order to facilitate an honest reporting of responses. These persons were asked only to identify the agency with which they were affiliated. Seventy-three percent of the questionnaire-packets were returned. The CAQ-B alone was distributed to, and returned by, all of the student nurses and psychiatric staff.

Results

Table 1 presents the means and standard deviations for the CAQ-B responses of each sample. Analysis of variance performed on the data supplied by all samples indicated significant between-group differences on the CAQ-B, F (3.54) $= 22.26$, $p < .01$. Further analysis by means of t-tests indicates that the attitudes of the community mental health team toward mental illness were significantly more oriented toward a radical psychosocial model (and away from the medical model) than were the attitudes of the other three samples: nursing students ($t = 5.69$, $df = 30$, $p < .001$), social agencies ($t = 6.56$, $df = 31$, $p < .001$), and health agencies ($t = 6.65$, $df = 19$, $p < .001$). The attitudes of health agency personnel were significantly more oriented toward the medical model (and away from the radical psychosocial model) than were those of nursing students ($t = 2.33$, $df = 23$, $p < .05$), social agency personnel ($t = 2.13$, $df = 24$, $p < .05$), and psychiatric staff (see above). The attitudes toward mental illness reported by nursing students and social agencies did not significantly differ from each other.

Table 1
Means and Standard Deviations for CAQ-B Responses By Sample

Sample	n	Mean	SD
Mental Health Team Personnel	14	53.14	6.57
Nursing Students	18	39.83	6.19
Social Agency Personnel	20	38.90	5.28
Health Agency Personnel	7	34.28	3.95

The information supplied by the ARQ allows further understanding of the type of relationship which health and social agency personnel ($n = 27$) have with the psychiatric agency. The majority (81 percent) of social and health agency personnel had at least one contact with psychiatric agency staff in the past year. The type of contacts appeared to be evenly distributed between formal (e.g., referring clients) and informal (e.g., parties, lunch) contacts. Most contacts were made by telephone, sometimes combined with personal contacts and written memoranda. The usual amount of time spent by the majority of health and social agency personnel in any one contact with the psychiatric agency was 5–15 minutes. A large percentage (65 percent) of agency personnel had referred at least one of their clients to the mental health agency in question.

When asked to rate how beneficial social and health agency personnel felt the psychiatric agency was to the community, 69 percent responded "much" or "very much." However, a rather large percentage (31 percent) were "not sure" of any community benefits. No one responded that the mental health agency was of "little" or "very little" benefit to the community. Overall, the mean "benefit" rating was 4.0 ($n = 26$), indicating that, as a group, agency personnel felt positively about the psychiatric agency's effect on the community. It is interesting to note that the social agency personnel ($n = 20$) rated the psychiatric agency significantly ($t = 1.83$, $df = 24$, $p < .05$) more positively ($M = 4.15$) than did the six (one person did not rate) health agency personnel ($M = 3.50$).

Respondents were also asked to describe the type of clients for whom the psychiatric agency provides service. (Such clients are primarily female, middle-aged, with a history of psychosis and psychiatric hospitalization.) Half (50 percent) of the respondents provided reasonably accurate descriptions; the rest were either unsure, or wrote down a description which was at least partially inaccurate (e.g., "The clients are persons with any emotional problems").

When asked to describe the programs (e.g., social club, adult basic education) and services (e.g., medication, group therapy) offered by the clinic, respondents mentioned a mean of 3.5 programs. Sixty-seven percent of the sample mentioned three or more of the sixteen services and/or programs provided by the clinic.

The majority (58 percent) of respondents correctly estimated the number of employees ($n = 8$), excluding students and interns, who worked at the psychiatric agency. Eighty-five percent of the health and social agency personnel indicated interest in attending a seminar on mental health, and 88 percent indicated it would be helpful to have more information about the psychiatric agency.

Discussion

The analysis of the data supplied by the CAQ-B indicates that one's attitudes toward mental illness may indeed be a function, at least in part, of one's agency affiliation. It would appear from our samples that as we progress from health to social to mental health agencies, we find a decrease of medical model orientation, and a corresponding increase of a psychosocial orientation. (It should be mentioned that the staff of this community mental health team viewed themselves as being non-traditional in their theoretical and operational approach to clients.) Nursing students, doing field work in the community, appear to be more similar, in their orientation, to personnel of social agencies than to personnel of health or mental health agencies. Such differences in orientation suggest that nursing students may be in a position of some potential difficulty. Thus, if one's orientation (as reflected in attitudes toward mental illness) influences the treatment offered to clients, there may be occasional disagreements between the personnel of agencies providing different services to the same client. In the community involved in this study, divergence of attitudes toward mental illness among the personnel of various agencies points out the need for nursing students to understand a variety of theoretical positions if they are to properly understand and relate to a variety of agencies.

Considering the data supplied by the ARQ and the CAQ-B, we find that the contact of social/health agencies with a mental health agency is not sufficient to lead to a strong mutual influence on their attitudes toward mental illness. Social/health agency contact with this psychiatric agency tends to be brief, and quite superficial, in spite of the fact that all these agencies share the same building. This type of minimal contact may partially explain the apparent discrepancy in the attitudes toward mental illness on the part of health, social, and mental health agencies. A further reflection of the somewhat superficial relationship between the psychiatric agency personnel and staff of the other agencies is the high percentage (50 percent) of social and health agency personnel who could not accurately describe the typical kind of clients frequenting the mental health clinic. Such high degree of misinformation can lead to inappropriate referrals to the psychiatric agency.

It is also important to note evidence which suggests that perhaps an agency's attitudes toward mental illness may influence that agency's perception of a mental health agency's effectiveness in the community. Interestingly, those agencies (i.e., health agencies) which maintained attitudes toward mental illness most divergent from those of the mental health agency are also the agencies which were the most uncertain about the effectiveness of the mental health agency in the community. Social agencies, however, who gave the mental health agency a higher effectiveness rating, maintained attitudes toward mental illness more similar to those of the psychiatric agency's staff.

The results of our study point to the need for further research on the relationship between an agency's attitudes toward mental illness, amount of inter-agency communication, and perception of other agencies. Furthermore, in order to clearly establish that attitudes toward mental illness are a function, in part, of agency affiliation, a research design is needed which studies the attitudes of professionals of the same discipline (e.g., nursing) and training, but with different agency affiliation (e.g., Mental Hospital vs. Community Mental Health Center). Thus, the present study must be considered as a pilot study, and the results somewhat inconclusive.

It is at least encouraging that the vast majority of personnel from health and social agencies are interested in gaining more information about the psychiatric agency. Perhaps it is here that the student-nurse can find another useful role. Student-nurses could organize educative seminars[4] which provide the staff of all agencies with the opportunity to discuss their theoretical positions, and thus to come to a better understanding of each other's attitudes toward mental illness. By facilitating more substantial inter-agency contact, student-nurses would ultimately be facilitating the optimal delivery of services to clients.

Conclusions

Considering the differences in attitudes toward mental illness among one group of social, health and mental health agencies, it would appear useful for the student-nurse working with all these agencies to be cognizant of the need to facilitate a greater exchange of information between these agencies. Through educative seminars the personnel of each agency can learn to work with personnel of differing attitudes. The client-consumers should benefit immeasurably from a service-agency network within which there is a high level of communication.

References

1. Rabkin, J G: Opinions about mental illness: A review of the literature. *Psychol. Bulletin,* 77: 153, 1972.
2. Morrison, J K, Nevid, J S: The attitudes of mental patients and mental health professionals about mental illness. *Psychol. Rep.* 38: 565, 1976.
3. Morrison, J K, Yablonovitz, H, Harris, M R, Nevid, J S: The attitudes of nursing students and others about mental illness. *J. Psychiat. Nurs. Ment. Health Serv.,* 14: 17, 1976.
4. Morrison, J K, Becker, R E: Seminar-induced change in a community psychiatric team's reported attitudes toward "mental illness." *J. Commun. Psychol.,* 3: 281, 1975.

3
Changing the Attitudes of Client-Consumers and Service Providers

Overview

FOLLOWING DELINEATION OF the attitudes of client-consumers and others toward mental illness in Chapter 2, it is now appropriate to focus on how such attitudes can be effectively altered.

The first article describes in detail the "demythologizing approach" to community education. What I consider as myths about psychiatric ideology and practice are specified, and references given so that the interested reader can become more thoroughly immersed in the evidence marshalled in favor of declaring that certain attitudes are based on myths.

The second article argues in favor of rejecting the medical model approach to clients, at least in community psychology. Only by changing current attitudes of clients toward mental illness can we make inroads toward changing their attitudes so that they begin to see themselves as more competent, self-sufficient, and independent of caregivers. Not every client can reach high levels of independence. However, I believe most can reach *higher* levels of independence than is now the case.

In the third article, "Seminar-induced Change in a Community Psychiatric Team's Reported Attitudes toward 'Mental Illness,'" Roy Becker and I demonstrate how the attitudes of mental health professionals can be "demythologized." It is important in a total consumer approach to spend some time educating the service providers in the client-consumer philosophy. A client-consumer approach may actually imply a rejection of the traditional medical model. Thus, if a person is a "patient" with a "mental illness," it makes no sense to speak of that person's responsibility for "curing" himself. However, if a person is a "client" who has multiple "problems" which must be "resolved" then the client can take some of the responsibility for the successful resolution of the problem. Because much of our professional training has inbred in us the medical-model approach, educative seminars can help reshape our constructs of the client. This article describes the effectiveness of a demythologizing seminar in changing the attitudes of mental health professionals. Such attitude change appeared to be stable, in the last posttest, as long as eight months after the seminar had been held.

In the fourth article, "Demythologizing the Attitudes of Family Caretakers about Mental Illness," Jeffrey Nevid and I describe a similar attempt at demythologizing, in this case changing the attitudes of family caretakers. Family caretakers are persons who try to provide a substitute family and home for clients, discharged from mental hospitals, who do not have suitable living situations. We have found such caretakers to entertain many attitudes based on misinformation and fear. This fourth article shows that family caretakers, before the seminar, as oriented toward a traditional medical model as psychiatrists, nurses and mental patients, became much less accepting of this model in their post-seminar attitudes. The attitude change was so large that we must conclude that the demythologizing approach can be most persuasive. I have constantly observed that most people find a consumer-oriented approach a logical and forceful one.

In the fifth article, "Demythologizing Mental Patients' Attitudes toward Mental Illness: An Empirical Study," the clients themselves are afforded the opportunity of hearing of another approach. Long inbred with the self-constructs shaped by the medical model philosophy of mental hospitals and clinics, clients hear that some mental health professionals maintain a different view, a view which many clients find less anxiety-arousing. (To view oneself as prone to a mental illness does not exactly bolster a client's sense of responsibility, confidence, and independence.)

The sixth article indicates that the demythologizing approach can substantially change the attributions of psychiatric clients. Using the Semantic Differential as a measure of clients' image of the typical mental patient, the study demonstrates that clients' pretest negative image of the mental patient can be changed in a positive direction by means of a demythologizing approach.

In the final article in this chapter another group of client-consumers are "demythologized" so that their expectations of service at our clinic might become more realistic and in tune with the staff's overall consumer philosophy. Both open-ended interviews and repeated self-report measures of attitudes indicated that the seminars succeeded in inducing significant attitude change toward an anti-medical model position.

Attitude change does not by itself constitute a revolutionary change. The test of real change is of course when both mental health professionals and clients begin to relate to one another differently. I believe that subsequent chapters will convince many readers that concrete, productive changes took place in our clinic when clients changed their attitudes toward mental illness.

It should be noted that the attitude measure referred to in the studies as the CAQ is the CAQ-A (see Appendixes).

Demythologizing Approach to
Community Education

James K. Morrison

IN THE PAST, many community mental health teams have approached the community with the intention of educating it to accept the position that "mental illness is like any other illness." Sarbin and Mancuso (1970), in reviewing studies of the public's attitudes toward "mental illness," conclude that the illness metaphor has not been widely accepted by the public. They also contend that the public tends to be more tolerant of deviant conduct when it is not described with mental illness labels.

If the use of a metaphor such as "mental illness" actually produces negative social consequences for those so labeled (Chesno and Kilmann, 1975; Lamy, 1966; Phillips, 1963, 1964), and if the general public does not accept the validity of the illness metaphor (Sarbin and Mancuso, 1970), then it may be time to cease promoting the shibboleth that mental illness is like any other illness. Rabkin (1974), after reviewing the literature on attitudes toward mental illness and efforts to sell the illness metaphor to the public, concludes that a psychosocial approach, emphasizing the importance of social and psychological factors in the development and maintenance of problematic behavior, offers more explanatory value to the public. However, Rabkin adds, prevailing educational efforts still follow the traditional format. I believe it is time for a radically different educational approach to the community—a "demythologizing" approach. In this approach, the community is introduced not to concepts of "mental illness," but rather to the myths surrounding psychiatric ideology and practice. Proponents of a radical psychosocial approach such as Szasz (1961; 1970a; 1970b), Sarbin and Mancuso (1970), and Laing (1972), emphasize the myth of mental illness; the unwarranted legal, social and moral power of the psychiatric profession; the inadequacies of the diagnostic process; and the social injustices within large mental hospital systems. The thrust of the demythologizing approach is to warn the consumers and potential consumers of services of charlatans and incompetents. This is often done by defining the limitations of present mental health ideology and practice.

It is not surprising that mental health professionals have not taken a demythologizing approach to the community, since, like most established professionals, they are too frequently resistant to change (Berlin, 1969). Often the resistance to new approaches, according to Berlin, issues from fear that the status, financial return, work satisfaction, and feelings of competency of professionals will be diminished. At one time or another all of us fear that we might be found incompetent or poorly informed. Little wonder then that many mental health professionals—perhaps many who have already fallen prey to the Peter Principle—are afraid to reveal to the community their limitations in clinical theory and practice.

Hirschowitz (1971) has cautioned that, in attempting to change a community's psychiatric ideology, values must be promoted that are attractive and acceptable to most people. Otherwise, according to Hirschowitz, one ends up engaging in ideological warfare. It has been my experience that demythologizing seminars restore long-lost integrity to mental health professionals. On numerous occasions I have heard those attending such seminars remark that it was a refreshing experience to hear such professional honesty and candor. People have long suspected many of the theoretical propositions maintained by mental health professionals, and the public has lost some of its confidence in the effectiveness of psychiatric treatment (Sarbin and Mancuso, 1970). Perhaps the innumerable "shrink" jokes, as well as the movie and television image of the "shrink" as an incompetent, ineffectual boob, have long reflected the public's real feelings about mental health professionals. Fortunately, writers such as Szasz, Sarbin, Mancuso, and Laing have had the courage to speak out. Perhaps the community will still be able to respect the mental health professions if we make efforts to be honest about our limitations and inadequacies.

The Demythologizing Approach

What is the demythologizing approach in practice? What psychiatric tenets are considered myths?

In light of the theoretical stance of the psychosocial theorists, precisely how does one present such an approach to the community? My associates and I have found the most effective way of presenting this approach is in relatively small (12 to 15 people) seminars, allowing a didactic presentation as well as ample discussion of the issues. If such small seminars are not possible, it is still possible to present this approach in a lecture form to large groups.

During the seminar or lectures, the discussant presents the following series of psychiatric *myths* (the books and articles in parenthesis present *counter*-evidence to the myths listed) for the consideration of those attending the seminars:

1. *Mental illness is like any other illness* (Szasz, 1961, 1970a, 1970b, 1974).
2. *Mental patients are more dangerous than the average citizen* (Ennis, 1972; Steadman, 1973; Steadman and Cocozza, 1975).
3. *Mental illness strikes people regardless of social class, race, or sex* (Braginsky and Braginsky, 1974; Chessler, 1972; Dohren-wend and Dohrenwend, 1969; Ennis, 1972; Foucault, 1965; Glenn, 1974; Haase, 1964; Jones, 1975; Levy and Kahn, 1970; Masling and Harris, 1969; Tennov, 1976; Trachtman, 1973).
4. *Mental hospitals are usually therapeutic* (Berke, 1971; Braginsky and Braginsky, 1973; Braginsky and Braginsky, 1974; Braginsky, Braginsky, and Ring, 1969; Ennis, 1972; Glenn, 1974; Goffman, 1961).
5. *Mental patients are strange, bizarre and ineffectual "non-persons"* (Braginsky, Braginsky, and Ring, 1969; Chesno and Kilmann, 1975; Morrison, Becker, Fasano, and Nevid, 1976; Sarbin, 1969; Sarbin and Mancuso, 1970; Shean, 1973).
6. *Psychiatrists and psychologists can tell what kind of mental illness a patient has by giving him various projective tests* (Braginsky, Braginsky, and Ring, 1967; Mischel, 1968; Soskin, 1954).
7. *Psychiatrists and psychologists can distinguish a "mentally ill" from a "normal" person* (Braginsky and Braginsky, 1973;

Braginsky and Braginsky, 1974; Braginsky, Braginsky, and Ring, 1969; Jones, 1975; Rosenhan, 1973).

8. *Mental patients have the same rights in society as do any other group* (Ennis, 1972; Ennis and Siegel, 1973; Medvedev and Medvedev, 1971; Szasz, 1970b).

9. *A person just goes "crazy"* (Laing, 1972; Laing and Esterson, 1964; Szasz, 1961; 1970a; 1970b).

Although a growing number of mental health professionals would agree that many of the above statements are myths, or at least inaccurate in some respects, few of those professionals seem to be doing anything about dispelling the community's myths. It is important to stress that we are *not* necessarily suggesting that mental health administrators adopt a radical psychosocial model, and then propagandize the community. Rather, we recommend that mental health administrators have an obligation to honestly inform citizens of the wide disagreement among clinicians related to psychiatric ideology and practice. With more professional honesty on the part of mental health workers, the community might reduce some of its hostility toward the mental health professions.

It is reasonable to believe that proponents of the medical model can present their ideology in such a fashion as to also earn the respect of the public. One could certainly argue, as have Siegler and Osmond (1973) and Blaney (1975), that the medical model can be therapeutic to patients who are incapacitated and feel guilty. But, at this point in time, a medical model may have to be presented in such a way as to also admit that many proponents of this model have often assumed a mantle of arrogance by prematurely declaring their limited knowledge of human behavior as dogma.

References

Berke, J. Anti-Psychiatry: An interview with Dr. Joseph Berke. In R. Boyers and R. Orvill (Eds.), *R. D. Laing and anti-psychiatry.* New York: Harper and Row, 1971.

Berlin, I. N. Resistance to change in mental health professionals. *American Journal of Orthopsychiatry*, 1969, *39*, 109–115.

Blaney, P. H. Implications of the medical model and its alternatives. *American Journal of Psychiatry*, 1975, *132*, 911–914.

Braginsky, B., and Braginsky, D. Schizophrenic patients in the psychiatric interview: An experimental study of their effectiveness at manipulation. *Journal of Consulting Psychology*, 1967, *31*, 543–547.

Braginsky, B., and Braginsky, D. Mental hospitals as resorts. *Psychology Today*, 1973, *6*, 22–34; 100.

Braginsky, B., and Braginsky, D. *Mainstream psychology: A critique*. New York: Holt, Rinehart, and Winston, 1974.

Braginsky, B., Braginsky, D., and Ring, K. *Methods of madness*. New York: Holt, Rinehart and Winston, 1969.

Chesno, F. A., and Kilmann, P. R. Societal labeling and mental illness. *Journal of Consulting Psychology*, 1975, *3*, 49–52.

Chessler, P. *Women and madness*. Garden City, N.Y.: Doubleday, 1972.

Dohrenwend, B. P., and Dohrenwend, B. S. *Social status and psychological disorder*. New York: Wiley, 1969.

Ennis, B. J. *Prisoners of psychiatry*. New York: Avon Books, 1972.

Ennis, B. J., and Siegel, L. *The rights of mental patients*. New York: Avon Books, 1973.

Foucault, M. *Madness and civilization*. New York: Pantheon, 1965.

Glenn, M. (Ed.) *Voices from the asylum*. New York: Harper and Row, 1974.

Goffman, E. *Asylums: Essays on the social situation of mental patients and other inmates*. Garden City, New York: Doubleday, 1961.

Haase, W. The role of socioeconomic class in examiner bias. In F. Riessman, J. Cohen, & A. Pearl (Eds.), *Mental health of the poor*. New York: Free Press, 1964, 241–247.

Hirschowitz, R. G. Dilemmas of leadership in community mental health. *Psychiatric Quarterly*, 1971, *45*, 102–116.

Jones, E. Psychotherapists shortchange the poor. *Psychology Today*, April 1975, pp. 24–28.

Laing, R. D. *The politics of the family and other essays*. New York: Vintage Books, 1972.

Laing, R. D., and Esterson, A. *Sanity, madness and the family*. Baltimore, Md.: Penguin Books, 1972.

Lamy, R. E. Social consequences of mental illness. *Journal of Consulting Psychology*, 1966, *30*, 450–455.

Levine, S. V., Kamin, L. E., and Levine, E. L. Sexism and Psychiatry. *American Journal of Orthopsychiatry*, 1974, *44*, 327–335.

Levy, M., and Kahn, M. Interpreter bias on the Rorschach test as a function of patients' socioeconomic status. *Journal of Projective Techniques and Personality Assessment*, 1970, *34*, 106–112.

Masling, J., and Harris, S. Sexual aspects of TAT administration. *Journal of Consulting and Clinical Psychology*, 1969, *33*, 166–169.

Medvedev, Z., and Medvedev, R. *A question of madness*. New York: Vintage Books, 1972.

Mischel, W. *Personality and assessment*. New York: Wiley, 1968.

Morrison, J. K., Fasano, B. L., Becker, R. E., and Nevid, J. S. Changing the "manipulative-dependent" role performance of psychiatric patients in the community. *Journal of Community Psychology*, 1976, *4*, 246–252.

Phillips, D. L. Rejection: A possible consequence of seeking help for mental disorders. *American Sociological Review*, 1963, *28*, 963–972.

Phillips, D. L. Rejection of the mentally ill: The influence of behavior and sex. *American Sociological Review*, 1964, *29*, 679–686.

Rabkin, J. G. Public attitudes toward mental illness: A review of the literature. *Schizophrenia Bulletin*, 1974, *10*, 9–33.

Rosenhan, D. L. On being sane in insane places. *Science*, 1973, *179*, 250–258.

Sarbin, T. The scientific status of the mental illness metaphor. In S. C. Plog and R. B. Edgerton (Eds.), *Changing perspectives in mental illness*. New York: Holt, Rinehart and Winston, 1969.

Sarbin, T., and Mancuso, J. The failure of a moral enterprise: Attitudes of the public toward mental illness. *Journal of Consulting and Clinical Psychology*, 1970, *35*, 159–173.

Shean, G. Perceptual conformity and responsiveness to social reinforcement in chronic schizophrenics. *Journal of Abnormal Psychology*, 1973, *82*, 174–177.

Siegler, M., and Osmond, H. Schizophrenia and the sick role. *Journal of Orthomolecular Psychiatry*, 1973, *2*, 1–14.

Siegler, M., and Osmond, H. Models of madness: Mental illness is not romantic. *Psychology Today*, 1974, *8*, 70–78.

Soskin, W. F. Bias in postdiction from projective tests. *Journal of Abnormal and Social Psychology*, 1954, *49*, 69–74.

Steadman, H. J. Some evidence on the inadequacy of the concept and determination of dangerousness in law and psychiatry. *The Journal of Psychiatry and Law*, 1973, 409–426.

Steadman, H. J., and Cocozza, J. J. We can't predict who is dangerous. *Psychology Today*, 1975, *8*, 32–35; 84.

Szasz, T. S. *The myth of mental illness*. New York: Hoeber-Harper, 1961.

Szasz, T. S. *Ideology and insanity*. New York: Doubleday, 1970a.

Szasz, T. S. *The manufacture of madness*. New York: Delta, 1970b.

Tennov, D. *Psychotherapy: The hazardous cure*. New York: Anchor, 1975.

An Argument for a Paradigm Which Fosters Client Independence

James K. Morrison

ALTHOUGH ONE COULD cogently argue that the medical model may enhance the treatment of patients in mental hospitals, conversely one could make a strong case that this same approach retards the independent functioning of psychiatric outpatients in the community. Despite my general lack of enthusiasm for the medical paradigm of psychopathology, I would have to agree that there are some advantages of this model (Siegler and Osmond, 1974). And, I believe, in mental hospitals or psychiatric wards of general hospitals one finds patients in such a state of crisis that they often need, at least during their first few days or weeks, an approach which leads to feelings of security. Such feelings are often experienced when a patient can depend on his doctor, nurse, or other advisor for most of his needs. It must also be comforting to patients with severe thought disorders to know that psychotropic agents (e.g., Mellaril, Haldol, and so on) will relieve much of their anxiety. Thus, what appears to be at least an implicit assumption of the medical model (i.e., that a patient with a "mental illness" needs the assistance of a trained physician to "cure" this illness) may, on the one hand, facilitate the treatment of the patient in the hospital, while, on the other hand, it may lead to such excessive dependence on psychiatric staff that, upon discharge from the hospital, such clients find it virtually impossible to function independently in the community.

Psychiatric institutionalization and other medical interventions are judged by some (Howe, 1972; Straight, Schaffer, and Folsom, 1973) to induce patients into passive-dependent roles in the community. Precisely how can the medical model approach lead to client dependence? As suggested earlier, those patients hospitalized in time of crisis really need the secure and responsibility-free atmosphere which the medical model encourages. A client under severe stress in the community cannot be expected to handle much responsibility while in the hospital, at least for a while. However, a drastic mistake is made, in my opinion, when the hospital either discharges a patient in such a state of dependence, or when community psychiatric service deliverers continue to approach the discharged client from a similar medical perspective. In the community the primary goal of community psychology is to encourage the independent functioning of the client so that eventually that client can be fully integrated into the community.

A series of clinical interventions, usually more associated with the medical model than with any other, may lead aftercare patients in the community to construe themselves as patients with an illness to be treated and cured (by medical practitioners), rather than as clients with problems to be resolved (at least partially through their own efforts). For example, when clients are given tranquilizers (and other medications) or ECT, they get the message that their treatment will be characterized by their passive acceptance of curative agents. Even the client assumption that "one goes to the clinic to be cured," although fitting nicely within certain medical paradigms, leads clients to construe themselves as dependent, passive, and nonresponsible.

Thus, by continuing the medical-model approach in the community, we make the community a microcosm of the mental hospital. The setting seems different, but the philosophy is the same. Instead of patients sitting passively around the hospital ward watching television, now they sit around family-care homes, halfway houses, and hostels, or their own apartments. Passivity and dependence continue to characterize the clients in the community, thus retarding their integration into the community. They *receive* welfare, *receive* medication, *receive* home visits, and wait. They wait for a cure, and then seem hostile when it does not happen.

Research on the Medical Model and Dependence

A recent study (Morrison, Fasano, Becker, and Nevid, 1976) describes an attempt by a small community mental health team to reduce nonrelevant, "manipulative-dependent" telephone calls from psychiatric clients. Although not mentioned, this study began as an attempt to study the effectiveness of a new team approach (social-learning model), after the medical model had, in the opinion of the clinicians, inadvertently reinforced passive-aggressive, limit-testing, manipulative-dependent behavior on the part of some clients. The research study suggested that a straight-forward, no-nonsense approach to such calls significantly reduced their frequency and duration and led to more positive attitudes of clients toward themselves and the clinical staff.

What this study suggests is that inducing clients to accept more responsibility for the resolution of their problems actually leads to an improved self-image and less hostility toward psychiatric staff. After all, if clients are induced by staff to discover that they are not helpless, incompetent, and irresponsible citizens, they not only feel better about themselves, they also lose some of their frustration with staff since they can no longer blame staff for their own failure to resolve problems. Now they realize that their success or failure at problem resolution depends, at least in part, on their own efforts. By giving clients the message (e.g., by quickly terminating nonrelevant telephone calls) that they can "do it themselves," clinicians actually communicate another message—that clients are reasonably competent and sufficiently responsible. The message of the medical approach to clients is often the converse, that clients are not competent or responsible and clinicians will "do it for them." While the latter may reduce stress, excessive anxiety and guilt in the hospital, the same message can work against the client's independent role functioning in the community.

Another research study (Morrison, Bushell, Hanson, Fentiman, and Holdridge-Crane, in press) establishes this relationship between attitudes reflecting the adoption of a medical paradigm and attitudes of dependence (e.g., "I will just have to wait for a real cure for whatever is bothering me"; see *Client Independence Questionnaire* in Appendixes for other items). On the other hand, clients reporting nonmedical model attitudes on the *Client Attitude Questionnaire* tend to report attitudes of independence on the *Client Independence Questionnaire* (Morrison, and Yablonovitz, in press).

Other studies (Morrison, 1976b; Morrison, and Nevid, 1976) indicate that when clients are demythologized of the medical model perspective, they are hospitalized for psychiatric reasons fewer times than a matched group of controls. This seminar approach focused on the clients' need to construe themselves as reasonably competent to resolve many of their own problems. Another study (Morrison, 1977) indicated that demythologizing seminars made significantly more positive the attributions which clients made on the Semantic Differential to the "mental patient," and that these changes were stable as long as three months later on followup.

When a client advisory board (Morrison & Yablonovitz, in press) was established, those clients who participated in this board during a three month period reported significantly more attitudes of independence than a matched group of controls. Since the board spent most of its time evaluating the effectiveness or ineffectiveness of clinic programs and of other staff interventions, it would seem that these changes in board members resulted mostly from the message from staff to clients that they were competent enough to judge clinic functioning, a very responsible role indeed. The implicit message, probably not missed by some board members, was that if they were partially responsible for the functioning of an entire clinic, they must be at least partially responsible for their own functioning.

The process of making a person dependent can be also seen within the context of labeling, as when a parent begins to construe her child, diagnosed as "autistic," differently (Morrison, 1974). In this case study, the parent had to be educated or demythologized to see her child as really quite responsible before the child would give up his passive-aggressive, manipulative-dependent behavior.

A More Productive Community Approach

If the medical approach to clients in the community is less than productive, which approach may be more effective? A number of other nonmedical paradigms (e.g., cognitive theory, social-learning theory, and so on) may suffice, as long as the clinicians adopting these theoretical approaches construe the client as a person with problems to be resolved, at least in part through his/her own efforts. Adopting such an approach does not necessarily prohibit the use of psychotropic medications. However, it does abrogate the use of such medications exclusively or unnecessarily (e.g., without "drug holidays"), or indefinitely (e.g., for years without a "holiday").

The nonmedical community approach also implies, if not demands, that we encourage client advisory boards (Morrison, 1976b), client-consumer follow-up studies, client participation in collecting evaluative data, skill-training (e.g., problem-solving skills; social skills, and so on) programs, client participation in goal-setting and goal attainment evaluation (Nevid, Morrison, and Gaviria, in press), active client involvement in determining treatment regimens, and special client contracts (Nevid and Morrison, 1976; Morrison, Federico, and Rosenthal, 1975).

A non-medical approach to primary prevention will perhaps be more productive than an approach which focuses on preventing "mental illness." To view primary prevention as teaching social and intellectual skills to potentially retarded children, or teaching coping skills to the recently divorced, may be of more heuristic value. Such a nonmedical paradigm leads to tighter and more research-oriented operational definitions of problems to be resolved than do medical paradigms.

In my opinion, nonmedical approaches also lead to better cooperation with the many nonmedical professionals (vocational rehabilitation counselors, attorneys, social workers, and so on), whose services are needed by clients. For example, viewing a vocational rehabilitation counselor as another professional who teaches specialized skills to the psychiatric client seems conducive to having that professional see himself as a peer in a joint educational effort (Connelly, Harris, and Morrison, in press). Such paradigms take some of the mystique away from mental health interventions, thus diluting some of the fear and suspicion which the community sometimes experiences related to what psychiatric professionals do.

Hopefully, if a nonmedical paradigm is universally adopted within the community, by physicians and nonphysicians, the attitudes of the general public may also reflect a more favorable view of mental patients and psychiatric professionals. If we demythologize or expose the myths about "mental illness" to the general public, they may construe psychiatric clients as less bizarre, dangerous, and unpredictable and as more normal, safe and predictable (Morrison, and Teta, in press). Such public attitudes should allow clients discharged from mental hospitals to more easily mix with other citizens, and thus to become better integrated into the community. If this happens it should encourage clients to give up the dependent roles that the community often insists they adopt and maintain.

Conclusions

Because of the differences in goals for clients in the hospital and those in the community, I have argued for a nonmedical approach to client-consumers who are attempting to function independently in the community. A number of research studies suggest that when staff and clients adopt a nonmedical paradigm (as reflected in attitudes toward so-called mental illness), a number of benefits (e.g., increased independence, improved self-image, more realistic expectations for service) accrue to clients. Although I favor a cognitive paradigm, certain social-learning models also seem to promote client independence.

References

Connelly, J. J., Harris, M. R., & Morrison, J. K. A client newsletter: The message becomes the medium. In J. K. Morrison (Ed.), *A consumer approach to community psychology,* Chicago: Nelson-Hall.

Howe, L. The concept of community. In A. Biegel and A. I. Levenson (Eds.), *The community mental health center.* New York: Basic Books, 1972.

Morrison, J. K. Labeling: A study of an "autistic" child. *Journal of Family Counseling,* 1974, *2,* 71–80.

Morrison, J. K. An argument for mental patient advisory boards. *Professional Psychology,* 1976, *7,* 127–131. (a)

Morrison, J. K. Demythologizing mental patients' attitudes toward mental illness: An empirical study. *Journal of Community Psychology,* 1976, *4,* 181–185. (b)

Morrison, J. K. Changing negative attributions to mental patients by means of demythologizing seminars. *Journal of Clinical Psychology,* 1977, *33,* 549–551.

Morrison, J. K., Bushell, J. D., Hanson, G. D., Fentiman, J. R. & Holdridge-Crane, S. Relationship between psychiatric patients' attitudes toward mental illness and attitudes of dependence. In J. K. Morrison (Ed.), *A consumer approach to community psychology,* Chicago: Nelson-Hall.

Morrison, J. K., Fasano, B. L., Becker, R. E., & Nevid, J. S. Changing the "manipulative-dependent" role performance of psychiatric patients in the community. *Journal of Community Psychology,* 1976, *4,* 246–252.

Morrison, J. K., Federico, M., & Rosenthal, H. J. Contracting confidentiality in group psychotherapy. *Journal of Forensic Psychology*, 1975, *7*, 1–6.

Morrison, J. K., & Nevid, J. S. Demythologizing the service expectations of psychiatric patients in the community. *Psychology*, 1976, *13*, 26–29.

Morrison, J. K., & Teta, D. Increase of positive self-attributions by means of demythologizing seminars. *Journal of Clinical Psychology*, in press.

Morrison, J. K., & Yablonovitz, H. Increased clinic awareness and attitudes of client independence through client advisory board membership. *American Journal of Community Psychology*, in press.

Morrison, J. K., Yablonovitz, H., Harris, M., & Nevid, J. The attitudes of nursing students and others about mental illness. *Journal of Psychiatric Nursing and Mental Health Services*, 1976, *14*, 17–19.

Nevid, J. S., & Morrison, J. K. Preventing involuntary hospitalization: A family contracting approach. *Journal of Family Counseling*, 1976, *4*, 27–31.

Nevid, J. S., Morrison, J. K. & Gaviria, B. Problem-oriented goal attainment scaling on a satellite community mental health team. In J. K. Morrison (Ed.), *A consumer approach to community psychology*, Chicago: Nelson-Hall

Siegler, M., & Osmond, H. Models of madness: Mental illness is not romantic. *Psychology Today*, 1974, *8*, 70–78.

Straight, E. M., Schaffer, R. C., & Folsom, J. C. Patient self-care: Its impact on psychiatric hospital staff. *Psychiatric Quarterly*, 1973, *47*, 377–385.

Seminar-Induced Change in a Community Psychiatric Team's Reported Attitudes toward "Mental Illness"[*]

James K. Morrison and Roy E. Becker[**]

ALTHOUGH RESEARCHERS[3-7, 10, 16] HAVE already provided empirical evidence that didactic presentations can be effective in altering the attitudes toward "mental illness" held by some mental health professionals (mostly nurses) and students, no one has attempted to empirically change such attitudes among a wide variety of psychiatric professionals on a community-based after-care team. The present researchers attempted to reduce team members' "medical model"[8] orientation, with its emphasis on hospitalization and psychotropic medication of patients, and to induce these mental health professionals to adopt a social learning theory[11, 12, 13] approach to clients, with its emphasis on the learning of problem-solving skills. Also incorporated in this latter approach were postulates best defined as those deriving from "radical psychology"[2] and including theoretical propositions by Braginsky, Braginsky and Ring,[1] Laing,[9] Sarbin and Mancuso,[17] Scheff,[18] and Szasz.[19,20]

*This article was originally published in the *Journal of Community Psychology*, 1975, *3*, 281–284. Reprinted by permission.
**The authors would like to thank Mrs. Beverly Fasano for her assistance in preparing this manuscript.

Method

Subjects. Ss were thirteen psychiatric team members, five male and eight female, with professional training in different fields (e.g., psychology, psychiatry, social work, nursing). The clinicians provide a wide range of psychiatric services primarily for patients discharged from state mental hospitals.

Measure. The Client Attitude Questionnaire[*1] (CAQ) was originally developed by the first author as a twenty item measure to determine mental patients' attitude change toward mental illness following didactic seminars. This instrument indicated the degree to which a person accepts or rejects the "medical model" orientation. Responses (true, false, not sure) are scored in such a way as to indicate how strongly the S has accepted a social learning approach to the problems of so-called mental patients. Examples of the twenty items are: No. 14, "Mental hospitals should be abolished." No. 18, "Mental patients are not able to fool a psychiatrist."

Procedure. At the beginning of the four hour seminar the first author distributed booklets containing his own theoretical and operational approach to mental patients. The team members were asked, before reading the booklet, to first outline briefly their own theoretical orientations as a way of having each person define more clearly his approach to clients. Then the clinicians were administered the CAQ (pretest) before the first author's presentation and subsequent discussion. At the end of the seminar the Ss were again administered the CAQ (posttest I). Nine weeks after the seminar the clinicians were given the CAQ a third time (posttest II) to determine the stability of training effects.

Approximately eight months after posttest II the six clinicians (three male and three female), whose scores had changed by four or more points from pretest to either posttest, were interviewed by an independent researcher. The interviews were based on eight open-ended discussion items (e.g., "What would you say are common causes of mental health problems?" and "How do you feel about mental hospitals?"). Each item was derived from those CAQ questions on which at least two persons had evidenced change. Each item included an inquiry concerning whether the particular attitude or perception had changed and, if so, when.

Following the interviews the CAQ was again administered (posttest III) to the twelve clinicians who could be located to determine the long time stability of reported attitude change.

---

1. Test-retest reliability coefficient of .81, $p < .001$, N = 13 over three months.

Results

Table 1 presents the means and *SD*s on the CAQ for clinicians over the four test phases of the study. Data analysis employing *t*-tests indicated that clinicians' attitudes toward "mental illness" changed significantly from pretest to posttest I ($t = 3.43$, $p <$ .01), and from pretest to both posttest II ($t = 3.87$, $p < .01$) and posttest III ($t = 2.85$, $p < .01$) in the predicted direction, that of "radical psychology." The clinicians' attitudes, as reflected in the CAQ responses, did not significantly change from posttest I to either of the follow-up posttest (II, 9 weeks; III, 8 months). Thus,

Table 1
Means and Standard Deviations on the CAQ For Clinicians
(N = 13) Over Test Phases

Test Phase							
Pretest		Posttest I		Posttest II		Posttest III	
$\overline{X}$	SD	$\overline{X}$	SD	$\overline{X}$	SD	$\overline{X}$	SD
49.92	6.33	52.77	4.53	53.31	4.59	52.42*	4.34

*N = 12

the training effects appeared to be comparatively stable over time. The coefficient of reliability for the CAQ over 9 weeks (posttest I to posttest II), with thirteen clinicians, was .93; and for twelve clinicians, over 8 months (posttest I to posttest III), was .90.

The follow-up interviews, which averaged an hour and twenty minutes in length, were noticeably lacking in psychiatric jargon and interpretations. Only one clinician (a social worker) used the word "schizophrenic" and that was in the context of identifying genetic causality for some mental problems. All those interviewed stressed social, environmental and familial factors as influentially relevant to persons being labeled "mentally ill." There was a noticeable hesitancy to use this term and, when used, a marked tendency for the clinicians to qualify this concept.

The six interviewed clinicians seemed unanimous in the identification of mental illness as a socially defined and frequently misapplied label, and not as an "illness" detectable through psychiatric tests. Most of those interviewed felt that hospitals contributed to the depersonalization and dehumanization of patients. Clinicians clearly felt that institutions were more frequently dysfunctional than helpful in solving problems. Many of the responses indicated that the staff members did not maintain a single perspective on mental patients, even though, in general, their open-ended responses reflected a social learning approach.

All those interviewed were asked whether their attitudes on these issues had ever differed from what they were at the time of the interview. While the change at times was occasionally identified as having occurred, in part, previous to the seminar in question, there were several references to the demythologizing seminar. Four of the six persons interviewed spontaneously mentioned either the seminar leader, the items in the interview as related to questions they answered as part of the seminar, or theoreticians and ideas discussed in the seminar.

Discussion

The results indicate the effectiveness of a didactic seminar in altering the attitudes of an outpatient team toward "mental illness." Item analysis of the CAQ scores on pretest and posttest I indicated that, in general, clinicians changed their attitudes in a direction reflecting the following: (1) Mental problems are not usually caused by brain pathology; (2) Psychiatrists and psychologists cannot determine what kind of "mental illness" a person has by giving him certain psychological tests; (3) Most people in mental hospitals are among society's poor and unwanted; (4) Psychiatrists and psychologists cannot really distinguish between the "mentally ill" and the "normal" person; (5) People with psychiatric problems should have a nice comfortable place to go for a rest or vacation, not mental hospitals with locked wards; (6) Mental hospitals should be abolished; (7) "Mental illness" can best be understood as a learned reaction, usually to one's family.

Five of the thirteen clinicians involved in the seminar had made CAQ responses on pretest which indicated that they held attitudes strongly indicative of a "medical model" orientation. On posttest I, however, all five of these seminar members apparently changed their attitudes as suggested by their CAQ scores. These scores were no longer in a range which could be interpreted as reflective of a "medical model" approach to the psychiatric milieu.[15] On the CAQ those five clinicians accounted for 62.2 percent of the total attitude response change from pretest to posttest I. Five of the other eight seminar members, whose scores on pretest already suggested a more radical approach to "mental illness," on testing immediately after the seminar reported further amplification of their attitudes in a direction even further away from the "medical model" approach. All of the above mentioned attitude changes and amplifications appeared not to undergo substantial alteration during the eight month follow-up period.

When interviewed eight months after the seminar, the psychiatrist, nurse, and social workers who accounted for most of the reported attitude change, evidenced a high level of doubt concerning the "medical model," and a strong tendency toward accepting the postulates of "radical psychology" and of social learning theory. These results correspond with the data provided by another study,[14] including a control group, in which the reported attitudes of a different sample (mental patients) toward "mental illness," also changed in a "radical psychology" direction by means of an approach similar to that used in this study.

Summary

A study attempting seminar-induced change in attitudes toward "mental illness" held by thirteen members of a community psychiatric team indicated that such attitudes could be effectively changed in a direction away from the more traditional "medical model." A nine week and an eight month follow-up indicated the reported attitude changes were stable.

References

1. Braginsky, B., Braginsky, D., & Ring, K. *Methods of Madness.* New York: Holt, Rinehart and Winston, 1969.
2. Brown, P. *Radical Psychology.* New York: Harper and Row, 1973.
3. Costin, F., & Kerr, W. D. The effects of an abnormal psychology course on students' attitudes toward mental illness. *J. Educ. Psychol.,* 1962, *53,* 214–218.
4. Dixon, C. R. Courses on psychology and students' attitudes toward mental illness. *Psychol. Rep.,* 1967, *29,* 50.
5. Graham, C., Jr. Effects of introductory and abnormal psychology courses on students' attitudes toward mental illness. *Psychol. Rep.,* 1968, *22,* 448.
6. Gulo, E. V., & Fraser, W. Student attitudes toward mental illness. *College Student Survey,* 1967, *3,* 61–63.
7. Hicks, J. M., & Spaner, F. E. Attitude change as a function of mental hospital experience. *J. abn. soc. Psychol.,* 1962, *65,* 112–120.
8. Joint Commission on Mental Illness and Health. *Action For Mental Health.* New York: Basic Books, 1961.

9. Laing, R. D. *The Politics of the Family and Other Essays.* New York: Vintage Books, 1972.
10. Long, R. S. Changing attitudes through "remotivation." *J. clin. Psychol.,* 1963, *19,* 338–341.
11. Kanfer, F. H., & Phillips, J. S. *Learning Foundations of Behavior Therapy.* New York: Wiley, 1970.
12. Mischel, W. *Personality and Assessment.* New York: Wiley, 1968.
13. Mischel, W. On the empirical dilemmas of psychodynamic approaches: Issues and alternatives. *J. abn. Psychol.,* 1973, *82,* 335–344.
14. Morrison, J. K. Demythologizing mental patients' attitudes toward mental illness: An empirical study, 1975, in preparation.
15. Morrison, J. K., & Nevid, J. S. The attitudes of mental patients and mental health professionals about mental illness, 1975, in preparation.
16. Quay, L. C., Bartlett, C. J., Wrightsman, L. S., Jr., & Catron, D. Attitude change in attendant employees. *J. soc. Psychiat.,* 1961, *55,* 27–31.
17. Sarbin, T. R., & Mancuso, J. C. Failure of a moral enterprise: Attitudes of the public towards mental illness. *J. consult. clin. Psychol.,* 1970, *35,* 157–173.
18. Scheff, T. J. *Being Mentally Ill: A Sociological Theory.* Chicago: Aldine, 1966.
19. Szasz, T. *The Myth of Mental Illness.* New York: Hoeber-Harper, 1961.
20. Szasz, T. *The Manufacture of Madness.* New York: Delta, 1971.

Demythologizing the Attitudes of Family Caretakers about "Mental Illness"*

James K. Morrison and Jeffrey S. Nevid

THE ATTITUDES OF family and substitute families (e.g., family caretakers) about "mental illness" appear to affect the relationship with the psychiatric patient. By the time hospitalization occurs, most families have begun to construe their "deviant" members as "mentally ill" (Kriesman and Joy, 1974). In spite of the limited and somewhat contradictory literature on this topic, there is some evidence (Alivisatos and Lyketsos, 1964; Cumming and Cumming, 1957; Hollingshead and Redlich, 1958; Myers and Bean, 1968; Rawnsley, Loudon, and Miles, 1962; Rose, 1959) that the negative attitudes toward a family member who has become hospitalized—perhaps due to the newly assigned stigma of "mental illness" (Goffman, 1963)—often hinders the reintegration of that member into the family and the community.

It is because of family resistance to the reintegration of the patient into the family, especially in lower class families (cf. Hollingshead and Redlich, 1958; Myers and Bean, 1968), that a system of state supported family care homes has been established. The

---

*This article was originally published in the *Journal of Family Counseling*, 1976, *4*, 43–49. Reprinted by permission.

caretakers of these homes attempt to provide the disenfranchised patient with a substitute family atmosphere. However, at times, such caretakers find themselves reinforcing the same role of docile, passive, and helpless "patient" demanded of the client by his family and the hospital system. For example, family caretakers in one area, all women, became very "maternal" in their approach to patients under their care and began treating their adult patient-residents as children. Silberstein (1969) found that caretakers encouraged residents to be docile, non-demanding and to shun the responsibilities for daily living.

There is evidence (Lamb and Geortzel, 1971) that when caretakers in after-care environments reinforce independence and responsibility, community tenure and instrumental, job oriented performance are increased. There is also evidence (Fairweather et al., 1969; Richmond, 1969) that high expectation environments break the cycle of passivity and dependency so characteristic of patient behavior in the mental hospital (Barton, 1959). The emphasis in the high expectation, sociologically oriented halfway house lies in its stress on a resident's self-initiative and autonomy through leadership tasks and responsibilities within the house setting (Richmond, 1969). In contrast, house environments which are more consistent with the "medical model" are characterized, according to Richmond (1969), by involvement in extensive psychotherapy, a concentration on intra-psychic dynamics in the treatment of "mental illness," and a closer affiliation with psychiatric hospitals. If, as the literature apparently demonstrates (Fairweather et al., 1969; Lamb and Geortzel, 1971; Richmond, 1969), a sociological approach to the reintegration of the mental patient is more facilitative of therapeutic progress our concern should be directed toward reeducating family caretakers within the psychosocial model. The family caretaker must take on the important role of engineering a social environment in which the mental patient gradually regains participatory citizenship.

It is the contention of this study that the family care system should encourage more than the mere continuation of the passive and docile role which both the original family, as well as the hospital system (Goffman, 1961), appear to demand of the patient. As a first step the reeducation of the caretakers appears necessary. The first purpose of this study is to examine the effectiveness of a brief training program in introducing family caretakers to the utility of accepting an alternative approach to the traditional medical model. This alternative view can be described as the "de-

mythologizing" or radical psychosocial position (e.g., "Mental illness is a myth") identified with such writers as Szasz (1961,
1970a, 1970b), Sarbin and Mancuso (1970), Laing (1972), and
Braginsky, et al. (1969). The senior author and his associates have
already successfully demonstrated that the attitudes of mental
patients (Morrison, 1976; Morrison and Nevid, 1975b) and mental
health professionals (Morrison and Becker, 1975) about so-called
"mental illness" can be significantly changed, following demythologizing seminars. However, this approach has not yet been attempted with family caretakers. It is the second goal of this study
to compare the attitudes of family caretakers about "mental illness" with the attitudes of four major groups of mental health
professionals (nurses, psychiatrists, psychologists, social workers),
and of previously hospitalized mental patients. It was predicted
that, as previous research (Richmond, 1969) has suggested, the
preseminar attitudes of caretakers would be more consistent with
those of professionals (psychiatrists and nurses) and patients
(previously hospitalized) more influenced by the "medical model"
than with attitudes of professionals (psychologists, social workers)
whose training generally emphasizes a psychosocial, non-medical
approach. Following demythologizing it was expected that family
caretakers would demonstrate attitudes similar to those of psychologists and social workers.

Method

Subjects. Seventeen family caretakers (14 females, 3 males),
attending a series of weekly training seminars for proprietors of
family care homes, served as subjects. Family caretakers provide
food, lodging, and support services to psychiatric patients discharged from mental hospitals. The experience of the caretakers
in working with mental patients ranged from approximately two
months to five years.

The samples of professionals and mental patients, with whom
the caretakers were compared, were obtained in another study
(Morrison and Nevid, 1975a). These groups consisted of 25 social
workers, 23 psychiatric nurses, 20 psychiatrists, 16 psychologists,
and 41 previously hospitalized mental patients. The attitudes of
all of these groups were solicited anonymously so as to ensure a
reporting of the most honest attitudes of those professionals and
patients who make up a relatively small community mental health

center. More details about this sample can be found elsewhere (Morrison and Nevid, 1975a).

Attitude Measure. The *Client Attitude Questionnaire* (CAQ) is a 20 item, highly reliable (Morrison and Becker, 1975) measure developed by the senior author (Morrison, 1976) to determine a respondent's acceptance of the radical psychosocial position. To avoid possible response bias, the scale items were positively and negatively keyed. The scale was constructed in a three point format, with provision for the respondent to answer either "true," "not sure," or "false" for each item. These three response categories were scored 3, 2, and 1, respectively, for items positively keyed in terms of a radical psychosocial position (e.g., "There is no such thing as mental illness"). Reversal scoring was used for negatively keyed items.

Procedure. All family caretakers sponsored by a state psychiatric agency were invited to attend a series of five weekly three hour seminars for purposes of training the caretakers in modalities of family-centered residential treatment. The second seminar centered on a radical, demythologizing view of "mental illness." The three hour seminar focused on providing counter-evidence to a number of popularly held attitudes (e.g., mental patients have a mental illness, mental health professionals can distinguish the "mentally ill" from the "normal," etc.) which the radical psycho-social proponents maintain are myths. The leader made it clear that the majority of mental health professionals would not necessarily endorse his demythologizing orientation. The participants in the seminar were encouraged to express their own views.

Subjects were administered the CAQ both before and after the seminar. They were also asked to fill out the questionnaire anonymously. At both pre and post testing, the subjects were instructed that whatever their responses, their attitudes would find support within one or more of the mental health professions. The caretakers were urged to report their real attitudes, not simply responses which the caretakers might feel the seminar leader would like to hear.

Results

Pre and post treatment means and standard deviations for subjects' scale scores on the CAQ are provided in Table 1. The data were analyzed by means of paired *t*-test comparisons. As predicted,

Table 1
Pre and Post Treatment Means and Standard Deviations for Subjects'
(n = 17) Scores on The CAQ

Test Phase	X	SD
Pretest	41.06	3.78
Posttest	52.18	5.21

following demythologizing the subjects reported attitudes which were significantly ($t = 8.12$, $df = 16$, $p < .0001$) changed in the direction of a radical psychosocial approach.

Table 2 presents the means and standard deviations for family caretakers, psychologists, social workers, nurses, psychiatrists, and previously hospitalized mental patients. Analysis of inter-

Table 2
Means and Standard Deviations for CAQ Scores Across Subjects

Subjects	X	SD
Family caretakers ($n = 17$)	41.06*	3.78
	52.18**	5.21
Psychologists ($n = 16$)	49.25	5.24
Social workers ($n = 25$)	45.76	4.67
Psychiatric nurses ($n = 23$)	42.87	4.30
Psychiatrists ($n = 20$)	42.80	5.15
Mental Patients ($n = 41$)	40.71	5.17

*Pretest Score.
**Posttest Score.

group differences on the CAQ by means of multiple t-tests revealed that before the seminar the attitudes of family caretakers were significantly less radical than those of psychologists ($t = 5.18$, $df = 31$, $p < .0001$), but not significantly different from attitudes of psychiatrists, nurses or mental patients. By way of contrast, following the seminar, caretakers reported attitudes which were now significantly more radical than those of nurses ($t = 6.19$, df - 38, $p < .001$), psychiatrists ($t = 5.49$, $df = 35$, $p < .001$), previously hospitalized mental patients ($t = 7.68$, $df = 56$, $p < .001$), and social workers ($t = 4.17$, $df = 40$, $p < .001$), but not significantly different from the attitudes of psychologists.

Discussion

Data analyses indicated that family caretakers, following demythologizing, reported a significant attitude change in the direction of a radical psychosocial position. Apparently the attitudes of family caretakers were not deeply entrenched in sound theoretical foundations and were susceptible to change. Item analysis clarified how the family caretakers, following the seminar, had changed their views on "mental illness." On posttest the caretakers clearly reported construing mental patients and the psychiatric milieu in the following manner: (1) The dysfunctional behavior, which some call "mental illness," is actually behavior learned primarily within a family context; (2) Mental illness is a myth, sold to the general public by mental health professionals; (3) The process of psychiatric diagnosis (testing, labeling) is not only unreliable, but also dangerous for the patient; (4) Mental hospitals, as they exist, should be abolished; (5) Mental patients are not unaware of their environment and are able to use "impression management" to attain self-established goals; (6) Being labeled "mentally ill" depends partially on one's sex and economic status; and (7) The "mentally ill" are often deprived of their civil rights in our society.

One might question whether the attitude change was in reality more than superficial response change. However, a number of studies (Morrison and Becker, 1975; Morrison, 1976; Morrison and Nevid, 1975b) have corroborated, with various groups (mental patients, different mental health professionals), the validity and stability of this seminar induced change. In those studies, the genuineness of attitude change was determined by means of open-ended interviews, as well as by repetitive administrations of the CAQ as much as nine months after demythologizing. When one considers that before the seminar the caretakers had had little training in psychiatric ideology and practice, it is not that unreasonable that the caretakers would be open to counter-arguments to the "medical model."

In comparing the attitudes of family caretakers with four groups of mental health professionals, it would appear, as predicted, that before demythologizing the former were more similar in their attitudes to psychiatrists, psychiatric nurses, and espe-

cially previously hospitalized mental patients, than to social workers or psychologists. However, following the demythologizing
process, these same caretakers appeared to be more similar in their
attitudes to psychologists. These comparative data support the
previous conclusion that the seminar was effective in changing
caretakers' attitudes away from the medical model approach.

It is curious that caretakers' pre-seminar attitudes were most
similar to those of previously hospitalized mental patients. Perhaps, since family caretakers have traditionally received such little
formal training in psychiatric ideology, they tend (in their attitudes about "mental illness") to be positively influenced by the
attitudes of their patient-residents who have been discharged from
a system usually oriented toward the medical model.

This study was not an attempt to answer the more important
question, i.e., whether a demythologized approach on the part of
family caretakers would facilitate caretakers in the adoption of a
role which promotes the independent functioning of patients.
Future research will have to establish whether such an approach
can lead to higher patient role performance, as previously mentioned studies would suggest.

The authors take the position that adherence to the disease
metaphor ("mental illness") for explaining behavioral disorders
may undermine attempts at reintegration of the mental patient
into family and community. Therapeutic change is often hampered
by the clients' attribution of their personal problems to an inherent
disease process. Psychiatric patients, who are exposed to a medical
model orientation by psychiatric caregivers, may begin to construe
their behavior as an inexorable consequence of their inferred
pathology. Secondly, if the family caretakers adopt a medical model
approach, they may minimize the therapeutic influence of the psychosocial environment, and expect that their job is solely to make
the patients "comfortable" (and helpless), while the "real" therapy
goes on elsewhere. However, the authors expect that if caregivers
(family caretakers or the immediate family) adopt a psychosocial
approach, emphasizing the development of problem solving skills
and the exercise of personal responsibility within a high expectation environment, reintegration of the client may be facilitated.
The authors intend to examine, in future research, whether a
didactic approach may be effective in changing the medical model
orientation of the patient's family. Morrison (1974) has suggested
how with one family such an approach can not only be effective in
changing a family's attitudes toward "mental illness," but also in

positively changing the patient's behavior within that family context.

References

Alvisatos, G., and Lyketsos, G. "A Preliminary Report of Research Concerning the Attitude of the Families of Hospitalized Mental Patients," *International Journal of Social Psychiatry,* 10 (1964), 37–44.

Barton, R. *Institutional Neurosis.* Bristol, England: John Wright & Sons, Ltd., 1959.

Braginsky, B. et al. *Methods in Madness.* New York: Holt, Rinehart, and Winston, 1969.

Cumming, E., and Cumming, J. *Closed Ranks: An Experiment in Mental Health Education.* Cambridge, Mass.: Harvard University Press, 1957.

Fairweather, G. W., et al. *Community Life For the Mentally Ill: An alternative to Institutional Care.* Chicago: Aldine, 1969.

Goffman, E. *Stigma: Notes on the Management of a Spoiled Identity.* Englewood Cliffs, N.J.: Prentice-Hall, 1963.

Goffman, E. Asylums: Essays on the Social Situation of Mental Patients and Other Inmates. New York: Anchor Books, 1961.

Hollingshead, A., and Redlich, F. *Social Class and Mental Illness.* New York: John Wiley, 1958.

Kreisman, D. E., and Joy, V. D. "Family Response to the Mental Illness of a Relative." *Schizophrenia Bulletin, 10* (1974), 34–57.

Laing, R. D. *The Politics of the Family and Other Essays.* New York: Vintage Books, 1972.

Lamb, H. R. and Goertzel, V. "Discharged Mental Patients—Are They Really in the Community?" *Archives of General Psychiatry, 24* (1971), 29–34.

Morrison, J. K. "Labeling: A Study of an 'Autistic' Child." *Journal of Family Counseling, 2*:2 (1974), 71–80.

————. "Demythologizing Mental Patients' Attitudes Toward Mental Illness: An Empirical Study." *Journal of Community Psychology,* in press, 1976.

Morrison, J. K. and Becker, R. "Seminar Induced Change in a Community Psychiatric Team's Reported Attitudes Toward 'Mental Illness.'" *Journal of Community Psychology, 3*:3 (1975), 281–284.

Morrison, J. K. and Nevid, J. S. "The Attitudes of Mental Patients and Mental Health Professionals About Mental Illness." In preparation. 1975a.

————. "Demythologizing the Service Expectations of Psychiatric Patients in the Community." In preparation. 1975b.

Myers, J. and Bean, L. *A Decade Later: A Follow-up of Social Class and Mental Illness.* New York: John Wiley & Sons, 1968.

Rawnsley, K. et al. "Attitudes of Relatives to Patients in Mental Hospitals." *British Journal of Preventive and Social Medicine. 16,* 1–15.

Richmond, C. "Transitional Houses." In Lamb, H. R., Heath, D., Downing, J. J. (Eds.) *Handbook of Community Mental Health Practice.* San Francisco: Jossey-Bass, 1969.

Rose, C. "Relatives' Attitudes and Mental Hospitalization." *Mental Hygiene, 43* (1959), 194–203.

Silberstein, S. O. "A Survey of the Mental Health Functions of the System of Residential Care for the Mentally Ill and Retarded in the Sacramento Area." Unpublished Paper, 1969.

Sarbin, T. R. and Mancuso, J. C. "Failure of a Moral Enterprise: Attitudes of the Public toward Mental Illness." *Journal of Consulting and Clinical Psychology, 35* (1970), 159–173.

Szasz, T. *The Myth of Mental Illness.* New York: Hoeber-Harper, 1961.

————. *The Manufacture of Madness:* New York: Delta, 1970. a

————. *Ideology and Insanity.* New York: Doubleday, 1970. b

Demythologizing Mental Patients' Attitudes toward Mental Illness: An Empirical Study*

James K. Morrison**

ALTHOUGH THE ATTITUDES of mental patients about mental illness have been frequently studied (Johannsen, 1969; Rabkin, 1972, 1974; Sarbin & Mancuso, 1970), available instruments cannot adequately (Rabkin, 1974) measure current attitudes concerning psychiatric ideology and practice. Thus, existing attitude measures cannot determine a respondent's degree of endorsement of the controversial "psychosocial" approach (Becker, 1964; Braginsky, Braginsky & Ring, 1969; Laing, 1972; Sarbin & Mancuso, 1970; Szasz, 1961, 1970a, 1970b) to so-called mental illness, an approach quite different from the traditional medical model.

It has not yet become common practice for mental health professionals to focus on the attitudes of psychiatric patients about mental illness. This may be unfortunate, especially for community mental health professionals who must provide services to patients discharged from state mental hospitals. These patients often come

---

*This article was originally published in the *Journal of Community Psychology*, 1976, *4*, 181–185. Reprinted by permission.

**The author would like to thank the following for their assistance in this study: Roy Becker, David Doty, Beverly Fasano, Irv Hassenfeld, Al Israel, James Mancuso, and Fred Smith. Requests for reprints should be sent to James Morrison, C.D.P.C., 169 Mohawk St., Cohoes, N.Y. 12047.

to community mental health centers with attitudes toward mental illness quite divergent from those of the center's clinicians. Unrealistic expectations of clinical service are not uncommon among such clients. For example, a patient may expect psychotropic medication, as the main thrust of treatment, whereas the center's professional staff expect the client to become involved in social, educational, and behavioral change programs. Such divergence of expectations derives partly from a difference in staff-client attitudes about mental illness. These attitudes are, of course, partly shaped by the prevailing ideological model of the setting in which staff and clients have found themselves. Thus, for example, at the state mental hospital a staff's medical model approach reinforces patients' attitudes that their problems are an "illness," whereas in certain community settings the staff's psychosocial approach influences clients to construe themselves as having social/educational/psychological "problems in living."

There is ample empirical evidence that the attitudes of nonpatients (students and some mental health professionals) toward mental illness can be altered by means of didactic presentations (Rabkin, 1972). Morrison (1974) has described how an educational approach can be effective in changing the attitudes of a patient's family about mental illness. However, no studies have reported systematic attempts to change the attitudes of mental patients. There is evidence that the specific didactic approach (a "demythologizing" approach), employed in the present study with mental patients, is an effective means of changing the attitudes of certain groups (e.g., mental health professionals) about mental illness (Morrison & Becker, 1975).

The main purposes of the present study are: (1) To determine mental patients' degree of endorsement of the controversial psychosocial model; and, (2) To empirically change those attitudes in a direction more congruent with the psychosocial approach of the clinicians providing service to those patients.

Method

Subjects. The 26 psychiatric outpatients who acted as subjects tended to be primarily unmarried (19 unmarried, 7 married), not well educated ($M = 11.30$ years of formal education) females ($n = 19$) in their late thirties ($M = 37.0$ years), oriented toward the medical model (as reflected in their pretest attitude scores) and primarily diagnosed as psychotic ($n = 22$). These patients, 21 of whom had a history of previous psychiatric hospitalization, were assigned either to an experimental group (demythologizing seminars) or to a non-treatment control group.

Instruments. Two attitude measures were employed in this study: (1) *Patient Attitude Test* (PAT) ; a shorter 30 item version of the PAT developed by Braginsky, Braginsky, and Ring (1969), employing only those items which, in the opinion of the author, permit responses indicative of the controversial psychosocial model; and only those items relevant to psychiatric patients living in the community. A six point scale was used to measure the extent of patient agreement with the items. Responses reflecting a psychosocial approach to psychiatric theory and practice were scored as "positive." For example, strong agreement to item 28 ("Most patients in a state hospital are not mentally ill") was scored as the most "positive" or "radical" response. (2) *Client Attitude Questionnaire* (CAQ) ; a 20 item, highly reliable (Morrison & Becker, 1975) measure, developed by the author to determine a respondent's acceptance of the psychosocial position. To avoid possible response bias, the scale items were positively and negatively keyed. The scale was constructed in a three point format, with provision for the respondent to answer either "true," "not sure," or "false" for each item. These three response categories were scored 3, 2, and 1, respectively, for items positively keyed in terms of a controversial psychosocial model (e.g., "Mental hospitals should be abolished"). Reversal scoring was used for negatively keyed items. This measure was developed as a more easily understood test of patient attitudes than the more complex PAT, and one which would enable subjects to express more radical views than the PAT items allow.*

Procedure. Before the first seminar the patients of a community based psychiatric team were notified of a 12 week "psychology course" offered one evening a week for one hour. Thirteen patients, or 30 percent of the 44 clients followed by the team, attended a mean of 9.2 sessions. These subjects were then matched with 13 controls** on age, sex, marital status, years of formal education, psychotropic medication, diagnosis, and their pretest scores on both attitude measures.

The 12 seminars consisted of didactic "demythologizing"

---

*The pretest correlation (.59) of the PAT and CAQ scores of 26 subjects reached significance ($p < .01$).

**All 13 controls were interested in attending the seminars, but were unable to for a variety of reasons.

presentations on the inaccuracy of certain diagnostic tests (e.g., Rorschach), the deleterious effects of psychiatric hospitalization, the unjust deprivation of patients' civil rights in society, the myth of "mental illness," the stigma of psychiatric diagnoses, the determinants of mental patients' problems (a social-learning approach), and the ability of patients to solve many of their own problems independently of psychiatric professionals. Five clinical psychologists and one psychiatrist, all oriented toward the psychosocial approach, attended different sessions and presented their views. A great deal of time during the seminars was spent in discussion of the issues. (Some patients actively disagreed with some of the views presented.) It was emphasized to the clients that they were free to maintain their pre-seminar attitudes since many mental health professionals would agree with such attitudes.

Both experimental and control subjects were tested on the PAT and CAQ before and after the 12 week period. Finally, the CAQ and PAT were again administered in a three month follow-up. (Two control subjects did not complete their attitude measures on the three month follow-up.)

Results

Table 1 presents the means and standard deviations for both test measures by group and test phase. One way analyses of variance, with repeated measures, of the data provided by the two attitude measures indicated the following: (1) Condition main effects reached significance in the predicted direction for both PAT, $F (1,70) = 16.77, p < .001$, and CAQ, $F (1,70) = 18.76, p <$

Table 1
Means and Standard Deviations for Both Measures
by Condition and Test Phase

		Test				Phase	
		Pretest		Posttest I		Posttest II	
Measure	Condition	M	SD	M	SD	M	SD
PAT	Exper	138.69	15.66	147.54	19.74	148.15	21.46
	Contr	130.69	11.73	126.46	20.16	125.82[a]	18.80
CAQ	Exper	42.31	3.47	49.31	6.13	48.92	6.81
	Contr	40.77	5.10	41.15	7.34	40.73[a]	6.33

[a]$n = 11$

.001. (2) The test phase main effect did not reach significance for either of these two attitude measures. (3) None of the interaction effects attained significance for either of the measures. In summary, the differences between conditions, presumably induced by the experimental manipulation, appeared to account for most of the variation of test scores.

Analyses employing t-tests were performed on the PAT and CAQ data to determine whether the data conformed to the hypotheses. (Neither the PAT nor CAQ yielded significant between-group differences on pretest.) Analysis of the data provided by both measures indicated the following: (1) PAT: Subjects in the experimental and control conditions differed significantly from each other in the predicted direction on both posttest I, immediately after the seminars, t (22) = 2.69, p <.01, and posttest II, three months later, t (22) = 2.76, p <.01. (2) CAQ: Subjects in both conditions again differed significantly from each other in the expected direction on both posttest I, t (23) = 3.08, p <.005, and posttest II, t (22) = 3.05, p <.01. Apparently, the experimental manipulation was effective in producing the predicted between-group differences on posttest I on both of the attitude measures. These differences were maintained three months later on posttest II.

Analysis of within-group change, as reflected in the data provided by this study's instruments, revealed the following: (1) PAT: As predicted, only the experimental subjects significantly increased their scores in the predicted direction from pretest to posttest I, t (12) = 2.43, p <.025. In comparing pretest and posttest II scores on the PAT, again only the experimental subjects' attitudes significantly changed in the expected direction from pretest to posttest II, t (12) = 2.28, p <.025. Neither the experimental nor the control subjects significantly changed in their attitudes on the PAT from posttest I to posttest II. (2) CAQ: As expected, the control subjects did not change significantly in test scores on any of the three test phase comparisons. As predicted, the experimental subjects' attitudes significantly changed in the expected direction from pretest to posttest I, t (12) = 4.80, p <.0005, and from pretest to posttest II, t (12) = 3.91, p <.005; but not from posttest I to II.

In summary, the control subjects did not change significantly over test phases on either of the measures. As predicted, the experimental subjects reported attitudes as significantly changed in the psychosocial direction on the two attitude measures from pretest to posttest I. The experimental subjects did not continue to change significantly in their attitudes on these instruments from pretest I to II, once the experimental manipulation (didactic seminars) was withdrawn. Comparisons of test scores on pretest and posttest II for the experimental subjects indicated that the experimentally produced attitude changes on posttest I were maintained three months later on posttest II.

Discussion

The results of this study indicate that didactic demythologizing seminars can effectively alter the reported attitudes of psychiatric outpatients toward mental illness. In comparison with pretest-equated controls, experimental subjects reported greater acceptance of the more controversial psychosocial approach to mental illness following the seminars.

Before the demythologizing seminars both the experimental as well as the control subjects reported attitudes more characteristic of mental health professionals (psychiatrists, psychiatric nurses) educated in a medical model approach (Morrison & Nevid, note 1). These attitudes are not surprising since most of the patients had been previously hospitalized in a state mental institution known for its medical model approach.

Following the demythologizing seminars, the experimental subjects reported attitudes more typical of mental health professionals (psychologists) more influenced by a psychosocial approach (Morrison & Nevid, Note 1), as well as of the community team providing services to these clients (Morrison & Becker, 1975). Thus, the attitudes of the team and of the patients about mental illness apparently became more congruent.

It is legitimate to ask whether the attitude change reported by the experimental subjects was really anything more than superficial response change due to "impression management"? In other words, did the seminar patients have reason to respond on the attitude measures in such a way as to ingratiate the seminar leaders? In response, it should be mentioned that attempts were made before each administration of the measures to impress upon the clients the importance of expressing their true attitudes. It was explained that there is a great deal of disagreement among mental health professionals related to the attitude statements listed on the measures, and that, for any of their responses, they could find strong support. It is quite unlikely that the type of patients (mostly "chronic," formerly hospitalized patients with limited education and social skills) who were involved in the seminars would be that adept at remembering so consistently the psychosocial responses on two different measures a full three months after the presentations were over, unless these responses issued from genuine attitude change. A recent replication study (Morrison & Nevid, note 2) indicated that most patients who are "demythologized" are able to explain and justify their attitude change in open-ended interviews.

The focus of the present study was on the feasibility of altering patients' attitudes about so-called mental illness. Further research is presently underway to determine the effect of attitude change on patients' behavior, the attitudes of staff toward clients, and the course of a patient's treatment. Even though the effect of attitude change on clients' behaviors must be more systematically studied, it can be noted that in the six months of this study psychiatric hospitalizations were less frequent among "demythologized" clients than among controls (1 vs. 4 hospitalizations).

Reference Notes

1. Morrison, J. K., & Nevid, J. S. *The attitudes of mental patients and mental health professionals about "mental illness."* Manuscript submitted for publication, 1975.
2. Morrison, J. K., & Nevid, J. S. *Demythologizing the service expectations of psychiatric patients in the community.* Unpublished manuscript, 1975.

References

Becker, E. *Revolution in psychiatry.* Glencoe, Ill.: Free Press, 1964.

Braginsky, B., Braginsky, D., & Ring, K. *Methods of madness.* New York: Holt, Rinehart & Winston, 1969.

Johannsen, W. Attitudes toward mental patients: A review of empirical research. *Mental Hygiene,* 1969, *53,* 218–225.

Laing, R. D. *The politics of the family.* New York: Random House, 1972.

Morrison, J. K. Labeling: A study of an "autistic" child. *Journal of Family Counseling,* 1974, *2,* 71–80.

Morrison, J. K., & Becker, R. Seminar-induced change in a community psychiatric team's reported attitudes toward "mental illness." *Journal of Community Psychology,* 1975, *3,* 281–284.

Rabkin, J. G. Opinions about mental illness: A review of the literature. *Psychological Bulletin,* 1972, *77,* 153–171.

Rabkin, J. G. Public attitudes toward mental illness: A review of the literature. *Schizophrenia Bulletin,* 1973, *10,* 9–33.

Sarbin, T. R., & Mancuso, J. C. Failure of a moral enterprise: Attitudes of the public towards mental illness. *Journal of Consulting and Clinical Psychology,* 1970, *35,* 157–73.

Szasz, T. S. *The myth of mental illness.* New York: Hoeber-Harper, 1961.

Szasz, T. S. *Ideology and insanity.* New York: Doubleday, 1970a.

Szasz, T. S. *The manufacture of madness.* New York: Delta, 1970b.

Changing Negative Attributions to Mental Patients by Means of Demythologizing Seminars*

James K. Morrison

ALTHOUGH RESEARCH HAS indicated that psychiatric clients view the "mental patient" in very negative terms, no research has been conducted to determine whether such constructs can be changed in a positive direction by means of educative seminars. Studies (Crumpton, Weinstein, Acker, & Annis, 1967; Giovannoni & Ullman, 1963) have indicated that psychiatric patients tend to construe the "mental patient" and the "insane man" very negatively (e.g., weak, excitable, unpredictable). Such attributions by mental patients toward those similarly categorized resemble those of the general public about such patients in that attributions of both are highly negative (Giovannoni & Ullman, 1963).

Recent studies (Morrison, 1976; Morrison & Nevid, 1976) indicate that a series of demythologizing seminars, focusing on various myths (e.g., of "mental illness") concerning psychiatric ideology and practice effectively change mental patients' attitudes toward so-called mental illness. Such attitude change appeared to

*This article was originally published in the *Journal of Clinical Psychology*, 1977, *33*, 549–551. Reprinted by permission.

be stable, as determined by 3-month follow-up measures and open-ended interviews.

In the present study the semantic differential was used as a measure of the effect of demythologizing seminars on the negative attributions of mental patients toward the mental patient. It was predicted that seminars that focus on psychiatric clients as persons with problems in living, rather than as patients with a mental illness, would help those clients to construe mental patients as more normal and subsequently to make more positive attributions to such persons.

Method

Subjects. The 26 psychiatric outpatients who were Ss tended to be unmarried ($N = 19$), not well educated ($\overline{X} = 11.3$ years of formal education), females ($N = 19$) in their late thirties ($\overline{X} = 37.0$ years), and primarily diagnosed as psychotic ($N = 22$). The patients, 21 of whom had been hospitalized previously for psychiatric reasons, were assigned either to an experimental group (demythologizing seminars) or to a nontreatment control group (no seminars).

Instrument. The study employed the Semantic Differential (SD), a 30-item, 7-point scale that allows a respondent to rate the mental patient on a series of bipolar dimensions (e.g., predictable-unpredictable; excitable-calm; happy-sad). Ratings on positive dimensions were scored as 5, 6 and 7, ratings on the negative dimensions as 1, 2, and 3, and ratings on the neutral dimension as 4. Thus, the maximum possible total score was 210; the minimum was 30.

Procedure. Before the demythologizing seminars began the patients of a community-based psychiatric team were informed of a 12-week "psychology course" offered one evening a week for 1 hour. Thirteen patients, or 30 percent of the 44 clients followed by the team, attended a mean of 9.2 seminars. These patients were matched with 13 controls* on age, sex, years of formal education, marital status, psychotropic medication, diagnosis, and their pretest scores on the semantic differential.

The 12 seminars consisted of didactic demythologizing presen-

---

*All 13 controls were interested in attending the seminars, but were unable to do so for a variety of reasons (e.g., sickness, out of town, etc.).

tations of data that suggest that mental illness is a myth, that psychiatric diagnoses unjustly stigmatize the psychiatric client, that mental patients are not weak, unaware and ineffectual persons, and, finally, that mental patients do not "just go crazy," but rather develop various psychological/social/medical problems due to a host of understandable causes. Information sharing and discussion also centered on the inaccuracy of diagnosis, the inequities of treatment (e.g., for the poor, blacks, females, etc.), and the inadequacy of projective testing. It also was emphasized that clients can solve many of their problems independently of psychiatric professionals and mental health agencies.

One psychiatrist and five clinical psychologists, all oriented toward a psychosocial approach to mental illness, presented their views on the above topics. A great deal of seminar time was spent in discussion of the issues. It was emphasized to patients that they were free to hold their preseminar attitudes because many mental health professionals would agree with such attitudes.

Experimental and control Ss were administered the SD before (pretest) and after (posttest I) the 12-week period. Finally, the SD was administered again in a 3-month follow-up (posttest II). (Two control Ss did not complete their attitude measures on the 3-month follow-up.)

Results

Table 1 presents the means and standard deviations derived from responses to the SD. t-test analysis of the respondents' total scores indicated that the control Ss did not experience significant change in their attributions during the 6-month period of the study. As predicted, experimental Ss made significantly more positive attributions in describing the mental patient after the demytho-

Table 1
Means and Standard Deviation on Semantic Differential
by Condition and Test Phase

| | Test Phase | | | | | |
| | Pretest | | Posttest I | | Posttest II | |
Condition	X	SD	X	SD	X	SD
Experimental	115.85	23.40	127.62	22.08	124.85	22.63
Control	120.00	23.39	113.39	26.95	114.09[a]	30.41

[a]$N = 11$

logizing seminars (posttest I, $t = 2.62$, $p < .025$). The stability of this change is indicated by the significantly more positive attributions made by the experimental Ss on posttest II (3-month follow-up) than on pretest, $t = 1.79$, $p < .05$. There appeared to be no significant attribution change from posttest I to posttest II.

Discussion

The data derived from the semantic differential indicate that demythologizing seminars that deemphasize the differences between mental patients and nonmental patients are effective to induce psychiatric clients to make more positive attributions in describing the mental patient. Such attribution change apparently is rather stable, as indicated by the 3-month follow-up data.

Item analysis indicated that subsequent to the seminars the patients in the experimental condition construed the mental patient as *more* understandable, fair, brave, strong, and familiar, and as *less* remote, constrained, delicate, defensive, tense, slow, passive, and sad. On only one item was the mental patient construed slightly more negatively, i.e., "more insincere," by the demythologizing clients subsequent to the seminars. Perhaps such change occurred because during the seminars some clients had related how they had lied to psychiatrists and nurses in order to obtain release from mental hospitals.

Although it is legitimate to question whether the change experienced in this study was really more than superficial response change due to impression management, evidence from other attitude change studies (Morrison, 1976; Morrison & Nevid, 1976) suggests that the effect of demythologizing seminars is stable and genuine. Further research will be necessary to determine whether a positive change of clients' attributions toward the mental patient has a specific therapeutic effect on the behavior of those clients.

References

Crumption, E., Weinstein, A. D., Acker, C. W., & Annis, A. P. How patients and normals see the mental patient. *Journal of Clinical Psychology*, 1967, *23*, 46–49.

Giovannoni, J. M., & Ullman, L. P. Conceptions of mental health held by psychiatric patients. *Journal of Clinical Psychology*, 1963, *19*, 398–400.

Morrison, J. K. Demythologizing mental patients' attitudes toward mental illness: An empirical study. *Journal of Community Psychology*, 1976, *4*, 181–185.

Morrison, J. K., & Nevid, J. S. Demythologizing the service expectations of psychiatric patients in the community. *Psychology*, 1976, *13*, 26–29.

Demythologizing the Service Expectations of Psychiatric Patients in the Community*

James K. Morrison and Jeffrey S. Nevid

ALTHOUGH MENTAL PATIENTS often approach psychiatric facilities with attitudes toward mental illness quite divergent from those of the clinical staff, little attention has been paid to such differences (Morrison, 1976). It is reasonable to assume that if a psychiatric client attributes his personal difficulties to an underlying disease process ("mental illness"), his expectations of psychiatric service from mental health professionals oriented to a more radical psychosocial model (Sarbin and Mancuso, 1970; Szasz, 1970) may be very unrealistic.

Irrespective of the problems in delivering effective service to clients with divergent expectations (Bent, Putnam, Kiesler, and Nowicki, 1975; Hart and Basset, 1975), only one study (Morrison, 1976) has been reported which attempts to determine whether the attitudes, and hence expectations, of more medical-model-minded clients can be changed in the direction of the non-medical approach of the professional staff. Although apparently successful, the results of this study did not rule out the possibility that the attitude changes on posttest may have been primarily a function of client

*This article was orginally published in *Psychology*, 1976, *13*, 26–29. Reprinted by permission.

efforts at "impression management." A further issue raised by the author concerned the feasibility of shortening the "demythologizing" process from 12 one hour seminars to 4 one and one half-hour seminars. The present study then was an attempt to determine through open-ended interviews, as well as a self report measure, the authenticity of client attitude change following demythologizing. Secondly, it was the purpose of the present study to evaluate the effectiveness of an abbreviated demythologizing procedure in inducing client attitude change.

Method

Subjects. Thirty-two psychiatric outpatients were assigned either to an experimental group (1–4 demythologizing seminars) or to a no treatment control group. Subjects in the experimental ($n = 16$) and control ($n = 16$) conditions were equated for age, sex, type of psychotherapy received, years of formal education, antipsychotic medication, diagnosis, number and duration of previous psychiatric hospitalizations, length of time between pre and post testing, and pretest scores on the *Client Attitude Questionnaire*. Experimental and control subjects represented a mixed group of male and female, previously hospitalized and non-hospitalized clients, with a mean reported age of 33 and 36.6 years, and mean educational level of 12.4 and 12.1 years, respectively.

Instrument. The *Client Attitude Questionnaire* (CAQ) is a 20 item, highly reliable measure, developed by the senior author (Morrison and Becker, 1975) to determine a respondent's acceptance of the radical psychosocial position within psychiatry; the position identified with such writers as Szasz (1970), Sarbin and Mancuso (1970), and Morrison (1976). To avoid possible response bias, the scale items were positively and negatively keyed. The scale was constructed in a three point format, with provision for the respondent to answer either "true," "not sure," or "false" for each item. These three response categories were scored 3, 2, and 1, respectively, for items positively keyed in terms of a radical demythologizing view of the psychiatric milieu (e.g., "There is no such thing as mental illness"). Reversal scoring was used for negatively keyed items.

Procedure. All clients followed by the community team were invited to attend a "psychology course." Clients attending at least one of four 1½ hour demythologizing seminars ($n = 16$) were included in the experimental group. A matched group of clinic clients, not participating in the course, were selected to serve as controls. The four seminars focused on exposing several popular myths about psychiatric services (e.g., mental patients are dangerous; projective tests are reliable and valid; mental illness is like physical illness; etc.). The authors who conducted the seminars made it clear that their approach to psychiatric ideology and practice was not the view held by all professionals in the field, and that the clients should adopt attitudes which made the most sense to them. The clients in the experimental group participated in a mean number of 2.25 sessions.

Control and experimental subjects were administered the CAQ immediately preceding, and following, the four seminars. In the two weeks following the final seminar, open-ended interviews were conducted by the authors with experimental "high-change" clients ($n = 9$) who, according to a predetermined decision, had increased five or more points on their CAQ scores from pre to post testing.

Results

The means and standard deviations for pre and post treatment testing on the CAQ for experimental and control subjects appear in Table 1. A t-test comparison of these groups revealed nonsignificant pretest differences. Pre and post treatment scores were ana-

Table 1
Mean CAQ Scores and Standard Deviations on Pre and Post Testing
for Experimental and Control Subjects

Subjects	Pretest		Posttest	
	M	SD	M	SD
Experimental	42.19	5.01	49.13	6.94
Control	40.38	6.94	41.13	7.06

lyzed by means of a 2×2 analysis of variance with repeated measures on the last factor (trials). As expected, a significant effect was found for groups ($F = 5.30$, $df = 1/30$, $p < .05$), demonstrating a more positive orientation toward the radical psychosocial position for experimental subjects. However, since the main effect for groups was derived by summing across pre and post treatment testing, its significance is attenuated. Likewise, although the trials effect showed a significant change in the direction of increased radicalism on posttesting ($F = 23.71$, $df = 1/30$, $p < .01$), it is confounded since it is derived from summation across experimental and control subjects. The term of particular significance is the Groups X Trials interaction, which shows, as expected, a significant differential response across trials by experimental subjects in the direction of increased radicalism, as compared with control subjects ($F = 15.36$, $df = 1/30$, $p < .01$).

A further within-groups analysis was conducted through the use of paired t-tests. As predicted, the experimental subjects showed an increase in radicalism from pre to post treatment ($t = 4.18$, $df = 15$, $p < .001$). No significant differences in radical orientation between pre and post treatment testing were found for control subjects.

None of the Pearson product-moment correlations* or pre-post treatment attitude change scores with certain client demographic variables (sex, years of formal education, number of psychiatric hospitalizations, number of months psychiatrically hospitalized, membership in psychotic-nonpsychotic diagnostic categories) reached significance. These correlations ranged from $-.19$ to $+.38$.

In the open-ended interviews, 8 of the 9 "high-change" subjects demonstrated, in the judgment of the interviewers, that they had understood the basic content of the seminars they had attended. Six clients were cognizant that their attitudes toward the psychiatric milieu had changed in a radical psychosocial direction. Only one client clearly was aware of any substantial behavior change as a function of seminar attendance.

Discussion

In support of previous findings (Morrison, 1976), the psychiatric clients who attended didactic demythologizing seminars about psychiatric ideology and practice demonstrated significant attitude change in a direction consistent with seminar orientation. Compared with untreated, matched controls, the experimental subjects in this study showed significantly greater attitude change toward greater acceptance of a non-disease oriented, psychosocial view of mental health ideology and practice.

The results from the open-ended interviews corroborate the

---

*Specific information about these correlations can be obtained from the senior author upon request.

authenticity of the attitude change, as demonstrated on the CAQ. "High-change" subjects appeared to have integrated the content of the seminars such that most were now aware that their attitudes had changed in a radical direction. Consistent with previous studies (Wicker, 1969), this attitude change was not related to significant behavioral changes, as reported by "high-change" subjects.

Although the evidence provided by the open-ended interviews adds more strength to the argument in favor of *genuine* attitude change on the part of psychiatric clients following demythologizing, one cannot with complete confidence exclude the possibility that the clients in the present study may have engaged in some limited impression management. However, when one considers that some non-patient groups (family caretakers; Morrison and Becker, 1975) also reported similar attitude changes after demythologizing, and that such changes have been shown to remain stable as long as three (Morrison, 1976) and nine months (Morrison and Becker, 1975) after the seminars, the case for substantial and genuine attitude change is strengthened still further.

Apparently, psychiatric clients, many of whom have long psychiatric "careers," are receptive to an "unorthodox" position about psychiatric ideology and practice. Furthermore, this attitude change can be obtained quickly and appears to be genuine. Attitude change was found to be relatively independent of such client variables as sex, educational level, number of previous hospitalizations, number of months of previous hospitalizations, and psychotic vs. non-psychotic group membership.

The authors will direct their future efforts toward investigating whether changed attitudes about psychiatric ideology and practice reflect changes in the client's attitudes about himself and his problems, as well as whether such attitude change facilitates therapeutic change in behavior.

References

Bent, R. J., Putnam, D. G., Kiesler, D. J., and Nowicki, Jr. S. Expectancies and characteristics of outpatient clients applying for services at a community mental health facility. *Journal of Consulting and Clinical Psychology*, 1975, *43*, 280.

Hart, W. T. and Basset, L. Measuring consumer satisfaction in a mental health center. *Hospital and Community Psychiatry*, 1975, *26*, 512–515.

Morrison, J. K. Demythologizing mental patients' attitudes toward mental illness: An empirical study. *Journal of Community Psychology*, 1976, in press.

Morrison, J. K. and Becker, R. Seminar-induced change in a community psychiatric team's reported attitudes toward "mental illness." *Journal of Community Psychology*, 1975, *3*, 281–284.

Morrison, J. K. and Nevid, J. S. Demythologizing the attitudes of family caretakers about "mental illness." *Journal of Family Counseling*, 1976, in press.

Sarbin, T. R. and Mancuso, J. C. Failure of a moral enterprise: Attitudes of the public towards mental illness. *Journal of Consulting and Clinical Psychology*, 1970, *35*, 157–173.

Szasz, T. S. *Ideology and insanity*. New York: Doubleday, 1970.

Wicker, A. W. Attitudes versus actions: The relationship of verbal and overt behavioral responses to attitude objects. *Journal of Social Issues*, 1969, *25*, 41–75.

4
Client Advisory Boards for Consumer Protection

Overview

A CONSUMER APPROACH to community psychology finds its fruition in the concept of a client advisory board. The client advisory board described in the three articles of this chapter is, to my knowledge, the first of its kind.

In the first article an argument is made for the establishment of client advisory boards. In the second and third articles of Chapter 4 my colleagues and I attempt to demonstrate the utility and effectiveness of client advisory boards.

By way of client boards the consumers of community mental health services have a voice in what services are offered. Without such boards there is always the possibility that some mental health professionals might offer the same therapeutic modalities over and over to clients regardless of their ineffectiveness. But if clients are given the responsibility of thoroughly evaluating the effectiveness of all the services offered to clients, it is less likely that psychiatric staff will be able to thrust unwanted and ineffective services on consumers.

Perhaps the most promising aspect of client boards lies in the direct benefits which accrue to those client-consumers who become board members. As indicated by this chapter's third article, clients who become board members tend to adopt more independent attitudes related to the clinic and its staff. Such attitude change reflects the willingness of clients, following their experience on the board, to construe themselves as more responsible and self-reliant. Such independence is the kind of mental-set which clients need in order to survive in the community. In my opinion, a client board may be one way to ensure that community psychology can really work.

An Argument for Mental Patient Advisory Boards*

James K. Morrison

ALTHOUGH COGENT ARGUMENTS have been presented for the creation of citizen community mental health boards (Robins & Blackburn, 1974; Rooney, 1968; National Association of Social Workers, note 1), no one has yet advocated advisory boards composed of the actual consumers, that is, the psychiatric clients. Perhaps this parochialism in thinking derives in part from the traditional construing of the mental patient as somewhat bizarre and ineffectual (Arieti, 1959; Bellak, 1958; Joint Commission on Mental Illness and Health, 1961; Schooler & Parkel, 1966; Searles, 1965). In fact, according to Sarbin (1969), the mental patient, especially the "psychotic," is often viewed as a "non-person." If this perception of the mental patient is common in the field of mental health, it is not surprising that professionals in the field have not seriously considered establishing advisory boards composed of such patients.

It is the contention of proponents of a radical psychosocial model (Braginsky, Braginsky, & Ring, 1969; Laing, 1972; Sarbin

---

*This article was originally published in *Professional Psychology*, 1976, 7, 127–131. Copyright © 1976 by American Psychological Association. Reprinted by permission.

& Mancuso, 1970; Szasz, 1961, 1970a, 1970b) that mental patients are persons with "problems in living," who, despite the stigma attached to the patient "sick role" (Parsons, 1951; Petroni, 1972), are capable of social sensitivity in their intelligent use of impression management to attain desired goals. Patients' perception of and evaluation of others are at times surprisingly more accurate than that of psychiatric professionals (cf. Rosenhan, 1973). The disenfranchisement of mental patients from society is often based on the false assumption that they are incompetent in all areas of human activity. However, studies such as the one by Klein and Grossman (1968) indicate that patients are competent in at least certain areas (e.g., voting) of functioning.

If mental patients are actually quite capable persons, why are they so seldom consulted? It is true that therapeutic communities (Daniels & Rubin, 1968; Mardikian & Glick, 1969) have informally solicited patients' opinions at community meetings. However, in such settings clients have no clear authority to formally evaluate treatment programs, the staff, or the clinic setting in general. In spite of the hypothesized risks involved in giving patients more control over their treatment, Darley (1974) and Weitz (1972) have argued that this type of patient involvement would foster the kind of independent role functioning that mental health professionals hope to encourage in clients. The case for client advisory boards is actually a logical extension of this type of reasoning.

But if patients are to become advisory board members and if they are then to act more maturely and more responsibly, they must be viewed and treated as reasonably intelligent persons capable of such behavior. If being a mental patient is, at least in part, a learned role (Becker, 1962; Erikson, 1957; Goffman, 1961; Lemert, 1962; Scheff, 1966; Szasz, 1970a, 1970b), then such a negatively valued role can be unlearned (Morrison, 1974; Morrison, Fasano, Becker & Nevid, note 2) and more positively valued roles (e.g., an evaluator of treatment, a spokesman for fellow clients, etc.) learned. But such learning will not take place in an atmosphere in which the expectations of behavior change are minimal. And certainly, client boards will not be effective in facilities in which the staff have not begun to view clients as capable of higher level functioning.

It has already been argued that one of the obstacles to the establishment of client advisory boards is the outmoded traditional view of the client as incompetent, strange, and irresponsible. Another obstacle to the creation of such boards is the fear on the part

of many mental health professionals that patients would uni-
laterally evaluate a facility's programs in a very negative fashion
if given the opportunity to evaluate those programs. However, a
study by Mayer and Rosenblatt (1974) suggests that when given
the opportunity, mental patients express a more positive view of
a mental health facility's programs than do the mental health professionals who work there. Other professionals may fear that
clients will attempt to take over the running of the clinic. But one
study (Fanning, Deloughery & Gebbie, 1972) of patient attitudes
has suggested that patients have no real desire to take over the control of mental health facilities.

The following suggestions for the establishment of a client
advisory board derive from the author's experience in establishing
such a board. Because the specific structure of this board was designed for its appropriateness to a relatively small community
mental health team (8 staff members, 70 psychiatric aftercare
patients), the suggestions that follow are general so as not to
exclude their application to a variety of settings.*

Preliminary Meetings

Before establishing a client board, it is useful to call five or six
preliminary meetings of staff and clients in order to solicit the
opinions of staff, and especially of clients, about the optimal structure and composition of such a board. Both staff and clients can be
rotated through such meetings until all of the staff and a representative sample of patients have had the opportunity to voice their
opinions. These preliminary meetings will introduce many clients
to the concept of client responsibility for treatment. For many
patients it will be for the first time they have been asked for their
opinions about the services they receive. This kind of experience
offers clients a better idea of what an advisory board will be like
and thus should facilitate a decision on the part of patients as to
whether they should become involved in such a board in the future.

Initial Proposal for an Advisory Board

After soliciting ideas from at least 15 percent of the client
population, a proposal for the structure and composition of the

---

*Specific details related to the client advisory board created by the author and
his staff can be obtained from the author upon request.

board can be drawn up. This document should represent the mainstream of client and staff opinion. The following are some of the specific variables that should be considered in the general proposal for the client board: (a) the number of clients composing the board; (b) the type of board members (e.g., "regular" or "rotating"); (c) the length of term for each member; (d) the authority, tasks, and responsibilities of the client board, and of each specific member (e.g., various officers); (e) procedures for electing members of the board; (f) procedures for substitutions because of sickness, discharge, etc.; (g) training of board members related to tasks and responsibilities; (h) frequency, time, and place of meetings; (i) the number and type of staff to meet with the client board; and (j) evaluation of the effectiveness of the board.

This proposal should be agreed upon, in some form, by both the staff and the elected client board as its first order of business. One should expect that the original proposal will undergo at least one revision before it is accepted by both clients and staff.

Election of Board Members

It would seem reasonable to make eligible for election to board membership only those clients who are actually willing to serve on the board. To have all the clients in a facility elect the most popular or most vocal client accomplishes nothing if that client does not want to become a board member. And if in many community settings it is almost impossible to hold a general election by all clients, one may opt for an alternative. That is, one could announce an informal get-together or party for all clients willing to serve in any capacity on such a board. During this get-together, the volunteers for the board could become better acquainted and thus vote more meaningfully for those volunteers who can most adequately represent them. At this party-election, clients can express in "campaign speeches" why the board would be important for them and what they would do for clients if elected. Volunteers for the board can be originally ascertained by soliciting the total client population by letter, telephone, or both.

Conclusion

In spite of the obstacles to creating a client advisory board, I believe that such boards can be successfully established and that their advantages far outweigh the disadvantages. It makes sense for the actual consumers of services to have more say about the quantity, quality, and delivery of those services. It also seems eminently reasonable for these consumers to have a forum in which to evaluate staff effectiveness. And with some training, the client board members will be able to devise methods of evaluating services and program. If as I have argued, the mental patient is a much more responsible and capable person than we have traditionally construed him or her to be, then psychologists and psychologist administrators in the field of mental health can no longer ethically postpone involving the consumer client in further responsibility related to his or her treatment. From the author's personal experience with a client board, there are few better methods of inducing a client toward independent responsibility, self-confidence, and a secure feeling, for once, of some control over his or her life.

Reference Notes

1. National Association of Social Workers. *Position statement on community mental health.* Washington, D.C.: Author, 1968. (Mimeo)
2. Morrison, J. K., Fasano, B. L., Becker, R. E., & Nevid, J. S. *Changing the "manipulative-dependent" role performance of psychiatric patients in the community.* Manuscript submitted for publication, 1975.

References

Arieti, S. *American handbook of psychiatry.* New York: Basic Books, 1959.

Bellak, L. *Schizophrenia: A review of the syndrome.* New York: Logos Press, 1958.

Braginsky, B., Braginsky, D., & Ring, K. *Methods of madness.* New York: Holt, Rinehart & Winston, 1969.

Daniels, D., & Rubin, R. S. The community meetings: An analytical study and a theoretical statement. *Archives of General Psychiatry,* 1968, *18,* 60–75.

Darley, P. J. Who shall hold the conch? Some thoughts on community control of mental health programs. *Community Mental Health Journal,* 1974, *10,* 185–191.

Erikson, K. T. Patient roles and social uncertainty—a dilemma of the mentally ill. *Psychiatry,* 1957, *20,* 263–272.

Fanning, V. L., Deloughery, G. L., & Gebbie, K. M. Patient involvement in planning own care: Staff and patient attitudes. *Journal of Psychiatric Nursing and Mental Health Services,* 1972, *10,* 5–8.

Goffman, E. *Asylums: Essays on the social situation of mental patients and other inmates.* Garden City, N.Y.: Doubleday, 1961.

Joint Commission on Mental Illness and Health. *Action for mental health.* New York: Basic Books, 1961.

Klein, M. M., & Grossman, S. A. Voting competence and mental illness. *Proceedings of the 76th Annual Convention of the American Psychological Association,* 1968, *3,* 701–702. (Summary)

Laing, R. D. *The politics of the family and other essays.* New York: Vintage Books, 1972.

Lemert, E. M. Paranoia and the dynamics of exclusion. *Sociometry,* 1962, *25,* 2–20.

Mardikian, B., & Glick, I. D. Patient-staff meetings: A study of some aspects of content, tone, and speakers. *Mental Hygiene,* 1969, *53,* 303–305.

Mayer, J. E., & Rosenblatt, A. Clash in perspective between mental patients and staff. *American Journal of Orthopsychiatry,* 1974, *44,* 432–441.

Morrison, J. K. Labeling: A study of an "autistic" child. *Journal of Family Counseling,* 1974, *2,* 71–80.

Parsons, T. *The social system.* Glencoe, Ill.: Free Press, 1951.

Petroni, F. A. Correlates of the psychiatric sick role. *Journal of Health and Social Behavior,* 1972, *13,* 47–54.

Robins, A. J., & Blackburn, C. Governing boards in mental health: Roles and training needs. *Administration in Mental Health,* 1974, *3,* 37–45.

Rooney, H. L. Roles and functions of the advisory board. *North Carolina Journal of Mental Health,* 1968, *3,* 33–43.

Rosenhan, D. L. On being sane in insane places. *Science,* 1973, *179,* 250–258.

Sarbin, T. The scientific status of the mental illness metaphor. In S. C. Plog & R. B. Edgerton (Eds.), *Changing perspectives in mental illness.* New York: Holt, Rinehart & Winston, 1969.

Sarbin, T., & Mancuso, J. C. The failure of a moral enterprise: Attitudes of the public toward mental illness. *Journal of Consulting and Clinical Psychology,* 1970, *35,* 159–173.

Scheff, T. J. *Being mentally ill: A sociological theory.* Chicago: Aldine, 1966.

Schooler, C., & Parkel, D. The overt behavior of chronic schizophrenics and the relationship to their internal state and personal history. *Psychiatry,* 1966, *29,* 67–77.

Searles, H. *Collected papers on schizophrenia and related subjects.* New York: International Universities Press, 1965.

Szasz, T. *The myth of mental illness.* New York: Hoeber-Harper, 1961.

Szasz, T. *Ideology and insanity.* New York: Doubleday, 1970.(a)

Szasz, T. *The manufacture of madness.* New York: Delta, 1970.(b)

Weitz, W. A. Experiencing the role of a hospitalized psychiatric patient: A professional's view from the other side. *Professional Psychology,* 1972, *3,* 151–154.

The Impact of a Client Advisory Board on a Community Mental Health Clinic

James K. Morrison and Michael S. Cometa

IN RECENT YEARS community mental health professionals have increasingly focused on the psychiatric client-consumer as evaluator of services. Thus, the staff of mental hospitals and community mental health centers have placed stronger emphasis on the importance of having clients evaluate the effectiveness of the services they receive (Denner & Halprin, 1974; Hart & Bassett, 1975; Powell, Shaw & O'Neal, 1971; Zusman & Slawson, 1972). The senior author (Morrison, 1976) has argued that such periodic evaluations are not sufficient, and that a mechanism is needed to ensure systematic feedback from the client-consumer related to the quality of services. Although citizen advisory boards (Kane, 1975; Meyers, Dorwart, Hutcheson & Decker, 1972; Robins & Blackburn, 1974; Rooney, 1968) have become increasingly accepted in the field of community mental health, such boards seldom, if ever, allow the actual consumers the opportunity for input.

A number of arguments can be put forward which demonstrate the utility and advantages of establishing client advisory boards in community mental health facilities. Such boards would ensure that the citizens most familiar with a clinic's operations have the opportunity to recommend changes in the delivery of

113

services. Furthermore, membership on such boards may enable psychiatric patients to adopt more responsible roles at the clinic. Thus, by taking part in the determination of the optimum delivery of services, such client board members assume a certain degree of responsibility for the success or failure of their own treatment.

The present report concentrates on the impact one client advisory board (CAB) has had on a community mental health clinic's programs and staff. An attempt will be made to demonstrate the effectiveness of the CAB, as well as its acceptance by the clinic staff.

The Development of a Client Advisory Board

The client advisory board is a concept which derives logically from a view of psychiatric clients as reasonably competent, responsible, and rational persons in spite of their social/psychological/medical problems. The client-consumers at our clinic are viewed as persons who have the right and the ability to evaluate the services they receive from mental health professionals. This type of reasoning led the professional staff at our community mental health center satellite clinic to encourage our clientele to organize a client advisory board. We were convinced that clients should become involved in evaluating clinic programs, because such involvement might lead both to increased client self-reliance, as well as to invaluable feedback from clients to staff about the clinic's services.

Although a more complete description of the CAB, and its establishment, can be found elsewhere (Morrison, 1976), a succinct description will be provided here.

Initially, after five preliminary meetings with staff and clients, an initial proposal was drafted, describing the functioning of a client board. (Eighteen percent of the total patient population and all of the staff participated in those meetings.) Twenty-three percent of the client population expressed interest in such a board, and a party-election was held to allow clients to become acquainted, to make campaign speeches, and to conduct an election for board membership.

The client advisory board was established to provide clients with an opportunity: (a) to assist staff in the development and/or evaluation of mental health services; (b) to evaluate and make recommendations for appropriate changes in the physical setting of the clinic; and, (c) to evaluate and make recommendations for appropriate changes in the roles of staff and students, as well as in the procedures of the clinic. The client board consists of three elected regular members, who serve three month terms, and as many rotating members (all other interested clients) as desire to participate in weekly, one hour board meetings. Since the clinic is a state facility, the power and authority of the board derive from the willingness of the staff to establish and support such a board. To ensure the "actual" power of the board, the staff recommended that at meetings twice as many clients as staff be present. The staff were also aware of the fact that a client board would be only a token affair unless they took very seriously the board's recommendations for changes.

Brief History of the Client Advisory Board

To properly understand the impact of the board on the clinic it is necessary to delineate the board's transactions in its first twelve months of its existence. In that period the board:

(a) thoroughly evaluated ten clinic programs (e.g., group psychotherapy, assertive training group)

(b) arranged two seminars presenting clients with different points of view on electroshock therapy in order to ensure informed consent

(c) inspected and made recommendations concerning the client waiting room areas

(d) evaluated the possible benefits of a nonclinic program (i.e., Recovery, Inc.) for clients

(e) appraised the effectiveness of the team's family care system

(f) evaluated the problems of telephone communication with the staff

(g) investigated the legal rights of clients related to consent to treatment

(h) evaluated and approved the role descriptions of two new employees and four students, and the firing of one parttime employee

(i) regularly reviewed clients' suggestions left in a suggestion box

(j) surveyed clients as to whether they would be interested in seeing their clinical records

(k) provided consultation to staff in the development of two new clinical programs, in the organization of a planning committee for a social-educational program, and in the reorganization of a client newsletter

(l) conducted program for clinical staff to orient them to the problems of becoming and remaining a client

(m) actively assisted staff in the development of a Social Adaptation Questionnaire

(n) recommended and assisted staff in developing a citizen advisory board

(o) approved a research project

(p) assisted two clinical staff in resolving their conflicts over the goals of a clinical program

(q) surveyed clients on their opinions of programs

(r) made presentations on the concept of a client board to other community teams

(s) assisted staff in evaluating clinicians on the level of therapy skills

(t) periodically elected new board members

Some of these transactions involved two to four board meetings. At program evaluations staff who conducted the programs were asked to justify the existence of these services by providing empirical research evidence attesting to the effectiveness of those services. A client board member usually had surveyed patients who had attended those programs, and reported their evaluations of those programs to protect client anonymity.

Demographic Profile of Board Members

Forty-two one-hour board meetings were conducted during a twelve month period. (Initially the board had decided to meet biweekly.) On the average, 4.0 clients, 2.0 staff, 0.8 students (observers), and 0.4 nonclient visitors (observers) attended each meeting. In the first twelve months of the board, a total of 27 (33 percent of the total patient population) clients attended one or more CAB meetings. Five of those clients attended from 41 percent to 93 percent of the forty-two meetings, thus providing a reliable core group of interested members.

Board members tended to be primarily unemployed ($n = 24$), females ($n = 21$) with a mean age of 36.4 years, and 11.3 years of formal education. Most ($n = 21$) members had been hospitalized for psychiatric reasons on at least one occasion. Board members had been agency clients an average of 18.2 months prior to their attendance at board meetings. The demographic profile of board members quite closely paralleled that of the total patient population, with the exception that board members tended to be slightly younger, better educated. Thus, one can with some assurance conclude that CAB members were quite representative of the total client population.

The Implementation of Board Recommendations

One way of evaluating the effectiveness of a client advisory board is to focus on the concrete changes which it has effected in the clinic. To determine the CAB recommendations for changes, the minutes of each board meeting were scrutinized and the specific recommendations by the board were categorized as follows: (a) recommendations for changes in ongoing programs (e.g., more careful screening of clients for a "women's group") and for the development of new programs (e.g., a discussion group for parents of children with severe behavior problems) ; (b) recommendations for changes in the physical environment of the clinic (e.g., carpeting on stairs, a more comfortable waiting room) ; and, (c) recommendations for procedural and personnel changes (e.g., clarification of emergency on-call system, firing an employee). Table 1 presents the number of CAB recommendations made, and the number

Table 1
Number of CAB Recommendations, and Number and Percentage
Implemented, by Recommendation Category

Recommendation Category	Total No. of Recommendations by CAB	No. & Percentage of total Recommendations Implemented
1. Changes in programs.	72	59 (82%)
2. Changes in physical environment of clinic.	28	25 (89%)
3. Changes in procedures and personnel.	9	9 (100%)
Totals	109	93 (85%)

and percentage of those recommendations implemented. These percentages ranged from 82 percent to 100 percent, indicating the very high number of board recommendations implemented by the clinic staff. If one combines all of the above mentioned recommendation categories and determines the percentage of all such recommendations implemented by staff, the overall implementation figure is

85 percent. Few boards of any type can boast of a more impressive record in getting their recommendations implemented. This implementation record also attests to the willingness of the staff to make the recommended changes, most of which were seen as reasonable, practical, and appropriate.

Staff Evaluation of the CAB

We developed a 20-item Staff Evaluation Index (SEI) to determine the attitudes of clinic staff ($n = 11$) toward the client advisory board. Items were worded both positively and negatively. Staff were asked to rate, anonymously, their degree of agreement or disagreement (on a 7 point scale) with statements describing the functioning of the CAB. The instrument is scored by assigning scores of 7, 6, and 5 for responses indicating a positive view of the CAB; 3, 2, and 1 for responses suggesting a negative impression of CAB; and a score of 4 for responses indicating lack of certainty. Thus, the maximum total score is 140; the minimum 20.

Table 2 presents the mean staff ratings (in rank order) for each of the 20 items, along with the total number of "negative" ratings (1,2,3) made by the 11 staff for each item. Since the total number of negative ratings were small, we considered it of some interest to examine which items induced such evaluations. The overall ratings indicate that staff have a very positive view of the CAB. Responses to item 20 suggest that staff are generally divided as to whether the CAB is clearly the clinic's most valuable program. It is not surprising that such an item produced responses reflecting differences of opinion, since some of the staff would naturally tend to see their own programs as more valuable than the client board. What is surprising is that seven of the eleven staff indicated that the client board was more valuable than nine other clinic programs. The only item which produced a slight tendency toward an overall negative view of the board was item 4 ("At the present time, CAB members do not reflect the opinions of our total clientele"). This item produced six negative responses (agreement with the statement). In group discussion, staff explained this response by stating that they thought the board's recommendations reflected the opinions of the more verbal, intelligent clients who had less severe problems. Although this is undoubtedly true, the total number of clients who have attended CAB meetings actually do adequately represent the total client population.

The total mean score for the staff ($n = 11$) was 113.9, again suggesting the staff's overall positive view of the CAB. (Note that

Table 2
Rank-order Mean Staff Ratings, and Number of Negative Ratings,
on SEI Items

Rank Order	Item No.	Abbreviated Item Content[a]	Mean Staff Rating	No. of Negative Ratings
1	10	My experiences with CAB have, unfortunately, made me too guarded with clients.	6.7	0
2	12	I do not approve of staff being subjected to client grievances.	6.5	0
3	19	I only pretend to follow CAB recommendations.	6.4	1
4	8	I'm afraid a manipulative CAB member could get staff members fired without real justification.	6.4	0
5	1	Staff have experienced unnecessary discomfort during CAB evaluations of their programs.	6.1	0
6	5	CAB made large number of valuable suggestions on improving services.	6.1	1
7	17	CAB is actually a mere token gesture since board members do not have an important role in the clinic.	6.0	1
8	14	CAB has been definitely successful in making many changes at the clinic.	5.9	1
9	6	CAB provides assessments and suggestions comparable to those of staff.	5.9	0
10	2	CAB has definitely provided clients with a means of expressing positive and negative feelings about services and programs.	5.8	1
11	13	CAB has improved my respect for client ability to assume responsibility.	5.7	1
12	7	I've found all CAB suggestions reasonable and acceptable.	5.7	1
13	16	In most cases, a client is better able to assess programs than staff.	5.6	0
14	9	Because of CAB, I have more respect for client awareness of problems and issues.	5.6	1

Table 2 (cont'd.)

Rank Order	Item No.	Abbreviated Item Content[a]	Mean Staff Rating	No. of Negative Ratings
15	3	CAB has allowed clients to assume more control over treatment than is often desirable.	5.6	2
16	18	Staff have received valuable feedback on programs from CAB.	5.5	2
17	15	CAB clients have improved their self-concept due to CAB membership.	5.3	0
18	11	The CAB has no real power.	5.0	4
19	20	CAB is clearly the clinic's most valuable program.	4.6	3
20	4	CAB presently does not reflect the opinions of our total clientele.	3.6	6

[a]Complete wording of items available in Appendix.

the most negative score possible is 20; the most positive score, 140.) This is perhaps surprising since certain members of the client board have at times pressured staff to produce evidence of program effectiveness, or otherwise abandon or radically change a particular program. Apparently, such pressure was not construed too negatively by clinic staff.

Staff were also asked to provide estimates of the number of CAB meetings they had attended, how many of their own programs they were asked to justify before the board, and how often they read the posted minutes of each CAB meeting. There did not appear to be a clear relationship between the number of their own programs staff justified before the board and the total number of negative responses made on the SEI. However, those staff ($n = 8$) who generally made positive ratings tended to have attended approximately two times as many CAB meetings, and to have more frequently read the minutes of board meetings, than staff ($n = 3$) who made the most number of negative ratings (3 to 8). These results suggest that the more exposure (through actual attendance at meetings, reading of minutes) staff have to a client advisory board, the more positive their evaluations become of the board.

Some Problems

The members of the board who have been most prominent in positions of leadership (e.g., chairperson) have been primarily nonpsychotic, well-educated persons. The less educated and the more "chronic" patients have attended some meetings but certainly cannot be expected to assume leadership roles in what is really a middle-class medium, a board meeting. It is not surprising that if a board is to function at a high level of effectiveness, it must greatly rely on the intellectual skills of the less chronic, more middle-class persons who have adequate verbal and social skills. The only alternative would be to develop a different forum for the less skilled, a forum which does not rely on the verbally complex and organized transactions usually characterizing board meetings. To date we have not found such an alternative.

Another problem is that, even though in the minority at board meetings, staff persons often exert too much influence on board members. We have tried to dilute this influence by rotating staff representatives, rather than having one representative over a long period.

On occasion we have witnessed a client board member unnecessarily harass a staff person over a program. On one occasion the client seemed to relish making a staff person squirm amidst a barrage of questions on the failure of a particular program. The questions were excellent, probing ones, but seemed to issue from feelings of hostility which had been unresolved in group therapy. Such excesses can be expected. After all, nonclients are also guilty of such excesses in analogous situations.

A final problem is the constant need to replenish the board with new members. Although we were fortunate in having a highly motivated and reliable core of board members, other less involved, less interested nonregular members needed to be coaxed at times to attend meetings. Attendance at board meetings seems to be a perennial problem for all boards, and only constant efforts at finding new members can resolve this problem.

Final Comments

Another study (Morrison & Yablonovitz, in press) has demonstrated that client advisory board membership can also have a positive effect on the board members themselves. In this study, board members, as opposed to non-board clients, appeared to significantly increase their attitudes of independence and in their awareness of clinic staff and programs over equivalent three-month periods. Such changes suggest that in assuming responsible roles (board member), certain clients have less of a tendency to become passive-dependent mental patients. And, since such members become better acquainted with the clinic, they are in a better position to choose for themselves, in some cases, the type of services which most interest them. Thereby, such clients assume more responsibility for their own treatment.

We feel that our client advisory board has substantially changed our clinic's delivery of services: programs are now more consonant with the actual needs of our client-consumers. Considering the positive input of this client board on our community mental health clinic, we would enthusiastically recommend such a board for those mental health professionals involved in service delivery.

References

Denner, B., & Halprin, F. Measuring consumer satisfaction in a community outpost. *American Journal of Community Psychology*, 1974, *2*, 13–22.

Hart, W. T., & Bassett, L. Measuring consumer satisfaction in a mental health center. *Hospital and Community Psychiatry*, 1975, *26*, 512–515.

Kane, T. J. Citizen participation in decision making: Myth or strategy. *Administration in Mental Health*, 1975, *4*, 29–33.

Meyers, W. R., Dorwart, R. A., Hutcheson, B. R., & Decker, D. Methods of measuring citizen board accomplishment in mental health and retardation. *Community Mental Health Journal*, 1972, *8*, 311–316.

Morrison, J. K. An argument for mental patient advisory boards. *Professional Psychology*, 1976, *7*, 127–131.

Morrison, J. K., & Yablonovitz, H. Increased clinic awareness and attitudes of independence through client advisory board membership. *American Journal of Community Psychology*, in press.

Powell, B. J., Shaw, D., & O'Neal, C. Client evaluation of a clinic's services. *Hospital and Community Psychiatry*, 1971, *22*, 45–46.

Robins, A. J., & Blackburn, C. Governing boards in mental health: Roles and training needs. *Administration in Mental Health*, 1974, *3*, 37–45.

Rooney, H. L. Roles and functions of the advisory board. *North Carolina Journal of Mental Health*, 1968, *3*, 33–43.

Zusman, J., & Slawson, M. R. Service quality profile: Development of a technique for measuring quality of mental health services. *Archives of General Psychiatry*, 1972, *27*, 692–698.

Increased Clinic Awareness and Attitudes of Independence Through Client Advisory Board Membership*

James K. Morrison and Harold Yablonovitz

RECENTLY, THE SENIOR author has argued for the establishment of client advisory boards so that the consumers of psychiatric services might be safeguarded against ineffective and ethically questionable treatment (Morrison, 1975; Morrison, 1976; Morrison, note 1). A previous report (Morrison & Cometa, note 2) indicated that a client advisory board can be an effective means of changing the delivery of mental health services. This study revealed that 85 percent of the board's recommendations were implemented by the clinic staff. The present study focuses on the effectiveness of client advisory board membership in increasing clients' attitudes of independence, as well as their awareness of clinic staff and services.

Although it has been argued that traditional psychiatric treatment can lead to increased patient dependence on psychiatric staff (Goffman, 1961; Howe, 1972; Morrison & Nevid, 1976; Straight,

---

*This article was originally published in the *American Journal of Community Psychology,* 1978, *6*, 363–369. Reprinted with the permission of Plenum Publishing Corporation.

Schaffer & Folsom, 1973), only infrequently has empirical evidence (e.g., Morrison, Fasano, Becker & Nevid, in press) been offered which demonstrates that such a dependency orientation can be decreased. If it can be reasonably assumed that one of the objectives of a community mental health clinic is to gradually increase a client's independence from psychiatric staff, then a client advisory board's effectiveness can, in part, be measured by the degree to which board membership promotes such independence. Thus, learning independent and responsible roles (e.g., evaluator of clinic services; promoter of productive program changes) through board membership may lead clients to increased attitudes of self-confidence and self-reliance. Such positive self-attributions should induce clients to feel less helpless, and less willing to turn over to mental health professionals the primary responsibility for the success or failure of treatment (Morrison & Gaviria, note 3). Specifically, clients who are accustomed to taking some responsibility for resolving clinic problems are less likely to find it necessary to rely completely on professional staff for the resolution of their own personal problems.

Clients who adopt passive, dependent roles in the community cannot really be expected to actively investigate the range of services and staff skills available to them. Instead, they often rely on their primary therapist to design a specific treatment program for them. Thus, another problem facing clients who frequent community mental health clinics is that such clients are seldom aware of the variety of treatment programs and services available to them (Morrison & Yablonovitz, note 4). Clients may thus overlook effective services, programs, and skill-training because they do not know that some of these exist. Moreover, clients are also quite unknowledgeable of staff other than their own therapist. Such lack of familiarity with staff places clients at a disadvantage since they are less likely to agree to certain types of services (e.g., group therapy, assertive-training) offered by staff who are strangers to them. Moreover, if a client knows only one staff person, the clinic can hardly become a comfortable place in which to resolve problems. Should membership in an advisory board increase client awareness of staff and services, then such a board may enable clients to assume greater responsibility for the course of their treatment.

In this study, it is hypothesized that even limited three month board membership will significantly increase: (1) client awareness of clinic staff and services, and (2) client attitudes of independence.

Method

Subjects. The 13 experimental subjects, participating in a mean number of 6.5 advisory board meetings, were primarily young (*M* = 30.6 years), non-psychotic[1] (*n* = 10), females (*n* = 9), with a mean number of 1.9 psychiatric hospitalizations. These advisory board members had attained an average of 11.9 years of formal education and, when pretest measures were administered, had been clients of the agency an average of 14.5 months. The 13 "control" subjects, none of whom attended client advisory board meetings, were balanced with the 13 experimental subjects on all of the above mentioned variables (except age and board meetings attended), as well as on pretest scores on the two measures used in this study. Both experimental and control subjects received the type of psychiatric treatment judged most appropriate by their therapists.

Test Measures. 1. *Client Independence Questionnaire* (CIQ) is a reliable[2] self-report measure of mental patients' attitudes of independence from a psychiatric clinic and its staff. The scoring of "dependent" and "independent" responses (true; false) to each item was decided upon after consulting with the staff members of a community mental health team. (When the eight staff members were asked to take the CIQ test and indicate the "independent" response, it was found that there was, overall, 93.0 percent agreement with the authors' scoring of the measure.)[3] Examples of the measure's items, as well as responses scored as "independent," are as follows: No. 1: "Whatever happens to me in the future depends mostly on the psychiatric help I receive." (false). No. 5: "The clinic staff should ask me more often about what I think should be done about my problems" (true). Independent and dependent responses were scored 3 and 1 respectively, with a score of 2 being assigned to responses which indicated indecision (e.g., checking both responses). The maximum score possible was 48, the minimum score, 16.

---

1. Determined by lack of evidence of hallucinations or delusions during the period of the study.
2. Test-retest reliability coefficient of .78 $p < .01$, $n = 15$, over 3 months.
3. As a check on the ability of the CIQ to distinguish clients on an independence-dependence dimension, primary therapists were asked to categorize 38 clients as either "dependent" or "independent". Analysis indicated that these ratings were significantly correlated ($r = .51$, $n = 38$, $p < .001$) with clients' CIQ scores.

2. The *Clinic Recognition Test* (CRT) is a reliable[4] self-report instrument measuring the degree to which a client is acquainted with clinic staff and programs. After seeing the first names of staff listed on the measure, clients are asked to supply (1) the last names, as well as (2) the professional identifications of each staff person from a list of professions (e.g., psychologist, social worker, secretary). Clients are also asked to circle the first names of all staff they would (3) recognize on sight, and to list (4) all the clinic's programs (e.g., group therapy, social club). Each correct listing is assigned a score of 1. Since there are 14 clinic staff (and thus 14 last names, 14 professional identifications, and 14 sight recognitions possible) and 13 clinic programs, the maximum and minimum scores possible are 55 and 0, respectively.

Procedure.   All 41 clients coming to a small community mental health center satellite office for services were administered the CIQ and CRT. The 13 clients,[5] who were involved in one or more client advisory board meetings during a three month period, were administered the CIQ and CRT three months after their pretest administration. Attrition (e.g., due to moving, discharge, etc.) reduced the non-board clients from 28 to 15. Those 15 clients were given the posttest three months after having taken the original measure. From these 15 clients, 13 were selected for a control group based on those demographic variables and pretest scores which allowed this group to be matched with the experimental group. (Clients were selected for the control group before posttest scores were known.)

Results

Table 1 presents the pre and posttest means and standard deviations for experimental and control groups on both the CIQ and CRT. Analysis of variance (2 conditions X 2 phases) of the data

---

4. Test-retest reliability coefficient of .89, $p < .001$, $n = 15$, over 3 months.
5. Related to the board member selection process, it should be noted that the entire client population of the clinic was invited through personal letters to become members of the client advisory board. Although most clients expressed interest in board membership, actual attendance at at least one board meeting during the three month period of the study was as used as the determinant of the total number of board members.

Table 1
Means and Standard Deviations on CIQ and CRT
over Test Phases by Condition

| Condition | Test Measure | Test Phase | | | |
| | | Pretest | | Posttest | |
		M	SD	M	SD
Exper.	CIQ	34.23	4.99	37.46	6.17
	CRT	11.38	6.83	21.46	8.25
Contr.	CIQ	32.38	6.56	32.54	5.39
	CRT	9.23	5.78	10.92	4.73

indicated the following: (1) Condition main effects reached significance in the predicted direction for both CIQ, F $(1,24) = 4.41$, $p < .05$, and CRT, F $(1,24) = 12.29$, $p < .01$. (2) The test phase main effect reached significance only for the CRT, F $(1,24) = 10.56$, $p < .01$. (3) Only on the CRT did the interaction effect attain significance, F $(1.24) = 5.36$, p $< .05$. In summary, the differences between conditions, presumably induced by the experimental manipulation, appeared to account for most of the variation of test scores on the CIQ. On the CRT, apparently due to the change in both conditions, the condition, phase and interaction effects were all significant.

Analysis employing t-tests were performed on the responses to the CIQ and CRT to determine whether the data conformed to the hypotheses. (Neither the CIQ nor the CRT yielded significant between-group differences on pretest.) Related to between group differences on posttest, analysis of the data provided by both measures indicated that on both the CIQ, t $(24) = 2.21$, $p < .025$, and on the CRT, t $(24) = 3.99$, p $< .0005$, the experimental group reported significantly greater clinic independence and awareness, respectively, than did the control group.

Analysis with t-tests of the data provided by the CIQ indicated that only the experimental subjects significantly increased their attitudes of independence, t $(12) = 2.41$, $p < .025$. Both the experimental, t $(12) = 6.43$, $p < .00005$, and control subjects, t $(12) = 2.24$, $p < .05$, increased their awareness of the clinic.

In breaking down the experimental group's changes on the CRT, we find that from pre to posttest these client board members increased their knowledge of staff last names by 137 percent, their awareness of staff professions by 69 percent, and their on-sight recognition of staff by 62 percent. Finally, this group increased their awareness of the clinic's programs by a startling 254 percent. Any increases in these categories by the non-board members (controls) were insignificant by comparison.

Even though the experimental and control groups were not matched for age, analysis indicated that, for the experimental group, correlations of age with change scores on both the CIQ and CRT did not attain significance. This finding enables us to conclude with some confidence that most of the reported change in test scores by board members was the result of client advisory board membership, rather than the result of age.

Discussion

Analysis of the data provided by both measures (CRT, CIQ) used in this study demonstrates the effect which even limited client advisory board membership has on client awareness of a clinic, and on client attitudes of independence. By comparison, clients (controls) who received treatment at the same clinic, and who were similar to the CAB members on a number of important variables, did not undergo significant change in attitudes of independence. And, even though the control clients did experience an increase in awareness over a three month period, their increased awareness was significantly less than that of CAB members. It is not difficult to understand why non-board members, who come to a mental health clinic over a three month period, would become better acquainted with clinic staff and programs. However, membership on the client board appears to greatly accelerate a client's awareness of a clinic.

Professionals in the field of community mental health have long undervalued the opinions of mental patients (Mayer & Rosenblatt, 1974). The experience of the authors with a client board attests to the benefits which a mental health facility can receive if such boards are established (Morrison & Cometa, note 2). The present study has demonstrated that a client board also brings positive benefits to the board members themselves. These latter findings are especially promising since they suggest that client boards may be one way of ensuring that psychiatric clients do not become overly dependent on clinic staff during their treatment. This is especially important for those community mental health centers which wish to avoid making their satellite clinics and residential facilities (e.g., family care homes) mini-hospitals where the clients maintain the same passive-dependent roles (Morrison & Nevid, 1976) which were adopted in the mental hospital.

If board membership not only fosters client attitudes of independence, but also greatly increases clients' awareness of clinic programs and staff (as this study indicates), then such results are again encouraging. In those clinics where staff wish clients to assume more responsibility for solving their own problems, extensive client knowledge of clinic programs and staff should enable those clients to take a more active role in selecting appropriate services. If a client is familiar with what services and programs are available, and if he feels comfortable with the staff who provide those services, it would seem reasonable that this patient would be more willing to actively pursue alternative treatment modalities. Thus, awareness may lead to freedom of choice related to treatment.

Although the present study has focused on the effect of client advisory board membership on client attitudes and level of awareness, the authors acknowledge the need of engaging in future research to determine whether board membership induces positive change in the behavior of board members. Research efforts in this regard are presently under consideration.

Reference Notes

1. Morrison, J. K. The client as consumer and evaluator of community mental health services. Manuscript submitted for publication, 1976.
2. Morrison, J. K., & Cometa, M. S. The impact of a client advisory board on a community mental health clinic. Manuscript submitted for publication, 1976.
3. Morrison, J. K., & Gaviria, B. The psychiatrist under siege: A responsible way out. Manuscript in preparation, 1976.
4. Morrison, J. K., & Yablonovitz, H. A survey of psychiatric clients' awareness of clinic staff and services. Manuscript in preparation, 1976.

References

Goffman, E. *Asylums: Essays on the social situation of mental patients and other inmates.* Garden City, N.Y.: Doubleday, 1961.

Howe, L. The concept of community. In A. Biegel, & A. I. Levenson (Eds.), *The community mental health center.* New York: Basic Books, Inc. 1972.

Mayer, J. E., & Rosenblatt, A. Clash in perspective between mental patients and staff. *American Journal of Orthopsychiatry,* 1974, *44,* 437–441.

Morrison, J. K. A client advisory board: Real consumers evaluate services. *Mental Hygiene News,* 1975, *46*(22), 2.

Morrison, J. K. An argument for mental patient advisory boards. *Professional Psychology,* 1976, *7,* 127–131.

Morrison, J. K., Fasano, B. L., Becker, R. E., & Nevid, J. S. Changing the "manipulative-dependent" role performance of psychiatric patients in the community. *Journal of Community Psychology,* in press.

Morrison, J. K., & Nevid, J. S. Demythologizing the attitudes of family caretakers about "mental illness." *Journal of Family Counseling,* 1976, *4,* 43–49.

Straight, E. M., Schaffer, R. C., & Folsom, J. C. Patient selfcare: Its impact on psychiatric hospital staff. *Psychiatric Quarterly,* 1973, *47,* 377–385.

5
Client-Consumer Involvement in the Delivery of Psychological Services

Overview

If a consumer approach is a really meaningful one, then it should encourage clinicians to involve clients more directly in service delivery. In this chapter's first article my colleagues and I describe a research study designed to determine the feasibility of involving clients in goal-definition and in goal-attainment evaluation. Such client involvement can be of immeasurable help to clinicians who rightfully want to reduce discordant expectations between themselves and their clients as to what specific problems will be the focus of clinical interventions. The results of this pilot study are promising in that both clients and staff were able to meaningfully engage in the setting of goals and the evaluation of goal-attainment.

The second article is a case study illustrating how contracting procedures can benefit both client and clinician. Instead of being satisfied that a "paranoid" client was just being "irrational" or "psychotic" in her fear of being arbitrarily hospitalized, the clinician specified in detail what behaviors could and could not lead to involuntary hospitalization. Satisfied that most of the behaviors in which she engaged would not, as she had feared, warrant hospitalization, a contract was drawn up and signed by all parties to that effect. The contract appeared to change this client's cycle of frequent hospitalization, and resulted in a smoother working relationship between client and clinician.

The third article of this chapter illustrates how contracts for group therapy clients can increase self-disclosure and group trust. Such contracts seem to provide more adequate legal remedies for clients who reveal confidential information in group therapy only to have that confidentiality breached by other group members.

All three articles highlight the importance of involving clients in various aspects of service delivery. A consumer approach necessarily implies that service-deliverers should involve their clients in every step of service delivery from the initial definition of treatment goals to the final evaluation of goal attainment. Treatment contracts and contracts which protect the client-consumer are other ways of actually involving the client in important aspects of treatment.

Problem-Oriented Goal Attainment Scaling on a Satellite Community Mental Health Team*

Jeffrey S. Nevid, James K. Morrison, and Bernardo Gaviria

WITH THE INCREASING emphasis in recent years on accountability in the delivery of mental health services, the organization of the clinical record has become of prime importance. The Weed[8] Problem-Oriented Record (POR) has been seen[9] as an attractive means of decreasing informational deficiencies in patient charting, increasing the user's skills through continued reading and writing of notes, assessments and plans, and most importantly, tailoring treatment modalities to specific problem needs. However, as McLean & Miles[5] have noted, many of the previous psychiatric adaptations of the Weed System[2, 7] have relied on a dichotomized treatment evaluation component in which the clinician-evaluator is generally restricted to two options: no report (problem not yet resolved); or date problem resolved. The descriptive criteria for problem resolution are generally unstated and the system does not allow for graduations of goal attainment. McLean & Miles recognize the need for a goal attainment scaling component in the POR system which would provide empirical indices of treatment progress.

*This manuscript is based upon a paper presented at the NIMH Region II conference on program evaluation in Monticello, New York, May, 1976.

A recently described goal modified POR system[6] also fails to provide for scaling of goals to descriptive criteria. One system which does scale treatment goals to behaviorally stated criteria is the pioneering Goal Attainment Scaling (GAS) procedure of Kiresuk and Sherman[4]. Each selected goal is partitioned in terms of a five point scale of graded likely outcomes; each outcome or attainment level is keyed to behaviorally specified criteria. Each targeted goal is initially weighted according to its judged priority. Goal attainment is measured by progress along a five point scale, ranging from -2 ("most unfavorable treatment outcome thought likely") to +2 ("best anticipated treatment success"). As discussed by Kiresuk and Sherman, the responsibility for goal selection and scaling is assigned to an overseer goal selector or goal selection committee. Following goal selection, patients are randomly assigned to treatment modes, and, following a predetermined interval, goal attainment ratings are given by a specialized follow-up unit.

The Kiresuk and Sherman paradigm allows systematic evaluation of program effectiveness. Nonetheless, this system, as originally conceived, has certain practical limitations for routine use. First, random assignment of patients to treatment modes is contrary to the clinically more appropriate tailoring of plans to specific needs. Secondly, a specialized evaluation team may be unfeasible in terms of staffing limitations. Finally, since the patient and therapist are the primary sources of information about the treatment process, it would seem profitable to involve these parties in selecting and scaling goals, and rating of goal attainment. Modifications of the GAS system along these lines have been described by Cline, Rouzen and Bransford.[1]

From the definition of problem areas to the scaling of goals and the ratings of goal attainment, the patient's involvement in the entire evaluation process may be therapeutically desirable in increasing client-therapist communication,[5] and second, in directing both parties toward mutually defined ends. Patient involvement is also consistent with the community psychiatry goal of promoting societal reintegration of ex-institutionalized patients by providing patients with access to self-responsible, decision-making roles.

This study was directed toward designing a goal attainment scaling procedure applicable to the POR charting system. In addition, this study sought to involve the primary participants in the treatment process (the patient and therapist) as fully as possible in the evaluation process. The evaluation procedure was designed to be easily comprehensible to patients from varying educational backgrounds, and to be economical in time, effort, and administration. Finally, this study sought to assess the degree of commonality between patients' and therapists' goal attainment ratings, and to determine whether this commonality varies as a function of certain patient variables.

Method

Subjects. An eight-member community mental health center satellite team was selected for implementation on a limited basis of Problem-Oriented Goal Attainment Scaling (POGAS). Team members had previously been trained in the POR recordkeeping method, and had been utilizing the POR system in patient charting for fifteen months.

Twenty randomly selected clinic patients were asked by their therapists if they would cooperate in a research study designed to help the patient and therapist work more closely together in defining the patient's present problems and rating progress toward solving these problems. Although eighteen patients in the original sample agreed to participate, attrition due to patient dropouts over the course of this study resulted in a final sample of sixteen patients. The mean age for this final study sample was 35.9 years and the mean educational level completed was 11.4 years. Diagnostic group membership was partitioned into two categories: psychotic; and nonpsychotic. Six subjects with primary psychotic diagnoses were assigned to the former category, with the remaining ten subjects (nonpsychotic) assigned to the latter. Eight of the sixteen subjects had previously been psychiatrically hospitalized.

Procedure. The team clinicians were informed that the goals of the project were: (1) to develop a goal attainment evaluative component for determining patient progress as plans developed in the POR charting; (2) to involve patients in the problem definition, goal selection and scaling, and goal attainment rating process; and (3) to evaluate whether patients' ratings of goal attainment correspond with therapists' ratings. The staff were trained by the authors in the experimental procedure during four, regularly scheduled POR hour-long training sessions. Training included didactic seminars on the technique of goal attainment scaling, as described below, and videotaped presentations by the senior author and team staff members of practice goal attainment recording sessions with patients.

Problem-Oriented Goal Attainment Scaling (POGAS)

For the purposes of our study, the construction of the POR problem list` was seen as a joint responsibility of the patient and therapist. The patient provided the data base for the construction of the problem list, while the therapist's task was to focus attention on the most salient problem needs. The patient and therapist were expected to resolve a mutually agreed upon problem list and to key scaled goal statements to each of these problem areas. Problem areas which lacked consensus, but were nonetheless considered salient by the therapist, were charted in the POR record. Thus, a patient expressing "paranoid ideation" may have resisted an attempt by the therapist to focus on this alleged problem, yet the therapist may have considered the problem important enough to continue its charting in the POR system. Although goal attainment scales for these problems could have been constructed independently by the therapist, goal attainment scaling was restricted to the subset of problems for which there was patient-therapist consensus. Assessments and treatment plans, keyed to each problem, were derived by the therapist independently, according to POR format. Each mutually defined problem was rated by the patient on a three point scale, weighted in terms of the problem's relative significance or priority within the problem list.

Following the construction of the POR problem list, patients and therapists established treatment goals for each mutually defined problem. Goals were scaled to increasing attainment levels according to the following five point attainment scale: (-2) further away from goal; (-1) no change; (0) goal slightly achieved; (+1) goal mostly achieved; (+2) goal completely achieved. Thus, the descriptors on the Kiresuk & Sherman goal attainment scale (e.g., "expected level of treatment success") were changed to descriptors considered more easily interpretable by patients and therapists. In addition, the Kiresuk & Sherman procedure of designating expected levels of treatment success prejudges the predictive accuracy of clinician judgments of therapeutic outcome. As Cline et al.[1] have reported, these judgments may be overly optimistic, and there is no internal check on their accuracy. A scale of graduated levels of goal attainment was constructed to avoid this difficulty, by obviating the need to make prior predictions of expected clinical outcome.

Goal-attainment statements, or anchors, expressed in behavioral terms, if possible, were keyed to at least three points on the five point scale. An example of Problem-Oriented Goal Attainment Scaling is presented in Table 1. The intent of constructing these goal attainment statements was to provide more objective criteria for the ratings of goal attainment than would be expected from ratings keyed simply to such descriptors as "goal mostly achieved," and so on. Goals were scaled according to possible outcomes of psychiatric intervention, rather than remission of problems. For a problem defined as "stomach ulcers," the criteria for "goal completely achieved"—from the standpoint of psychiatric care—might be: (1) adjustment of diet within medical guidelines; (2) regular medical visits; and (3) daily practice of relaxation exercises. The psychiatric treatment goal of changing certain patient behavioral patterns may be just to provide or monitor physician or medical facility contacts. Thus, a goal might be "completely achieved" in the absence of any change in the patient's underlying medical condition.

At a three month interval, goal attainment ratings for each mutually defined problem were made independently by patient and therapist. Ratings for each problem were indicated by means of a check mark along this five point goal attainment scale. Patients were instructed to make their ratings in terms of the anchoring criteria (see Table 1). Patients were also instructed to be as honest as possible, even with negative ratings ("further away from goal"), in order that the therapist might structure treatment plans more effectively in the future. It was made clear to patients and therapists that the ratings were not intended to measure the therapists' and/or the patients' competence in therapy, but rather to evaluate the therapy process. Treatment progress was determined by transforming these scale ratings into a weighted and standardized composite goal attainment score, derived by Kiresuk & Sherman[1] as a standard variable with a mean of 50 at the mid-point (0) descriptor ("goal slightly achieved" in this case) and a standard deviation of 10.

Patient Predictor Variables. Zigler-Phillips social competency scores[10] were obtained on each patient participating in the study. The purpose of obtaining Zigler-Phillips scores was to determine whether the concordance between patients' and therapists' goal attainment ratings varied as a function of the patients' social background. The Zigler-Phillips score is a composite index which takes into account the subject's age, educational level completed, job skills, employment history, I.Q. score and marital status.

A patient's primary diagnosis was used to determine his mem-

Table 1
Sample Problem-Oriented Goal Attainment Scaling

Problems:	Social Isolation	Housing	Depression	Anxiety in Groups
Goals:	Increased socialization	Move toward independent living	Overcome depression	Feel more comfortable in groups
Weights:* Attainment Levels	30	20	30	20
Further away from goal (−2)	No social contacts Reclusive to house	Return to hospital		Pronounced trembling of hands; heavy body perspiration + great muscular tension. Afraid to introduce own opinions.
No change (−1)		Continue living in family care; No interest in developing home-making skills.	Sleeping 3-4 hours. No appetite. Feels hopeless—no way out. No interests.	

138

Goal slightly achieved (0)	Attending social groups several times monthly.	Seeking independent living and support. Learning Adult Daily Living skills.	Same as above but making efforts (counseling, meds) to overcome depression.	Lessening of hand trembling, perspiration, plus muscle tension; beginning to communicate more freely in social groups.
Goal mostly achieved (+1)	Attends social group regularly. Making outside friends among group members.		Sleeping 5-7 hours. Appetite improved. Begins to feel hopeful about future.	
Goal completely achieved (+2)		Move to independent or cooperative apartment living.		Looks forward to group activities; no trembling, perspiration, or muscle tension; able to assert self plus opinions.

*Increased scores represent judged increased priority of problem/goal statements on three-point scale (10-20-30).

bership in one of two diagnostic categories: (1) psychotic and (2) non-psychotic. Diagnostic group membership was used as an additional patient variable to determine its relationship to the concordance between patient and therapist goal attainment ratings.

Results

Problem/goal definitions and subsequent goal-attainment ratings were obtained from sixteen patient-and-therapist dyads. As estimated by clinicians, the amount of time spent in goal attainment recording sessions I and II ranged from 20 to 45 minutes (mean of 30.66 minutes).

The computation of goal attainment scores was based on Kiresuk and Sherman's derivation formula. One goal-attainment score per subject, summed across problem areas and corrected for problem weight, was obtained from both patients and therapists. Goal-attainment scores obtained from patients' ratings ranged from 40.72 to 70.00. Goal-attainment scores based on therapists' ratings ranged from 30 to 70. Mean goal attainment scores were 52.47 ($SD = 11.79$) for patients' ratings and 50.52 ($SD = 11.40$) for therapists' ratings. These patient and therapist ratings suggested that treatment progress for the patient sample as a whole could be described as approximating the mid-point (50 point) descriptor ("goal slightly achieved"). Differences between patient and therapist mean goal attainment scores were not significant in a paired or correlated t-test. This finding suggests that overall, the patient and therapist samples did not differ significantly in their estimation of goal attainment.

Pearson product-moment correlation coefficients were computed on patients' and therapists' goal-attainment scores and individual scale ratings, in order to determine the degree of commonality between these ratings. Individual scale ratings, in addition to the composite goal-attainment scores, were entered into the analysis since the summated goal attainment score may have confounded correlational products. Correlation coefficients of .41 were obtained for comparisons of both patient and therapist goal-attainment scores and individual scale ratings. Probability level of this Pearson was less than .005 for the comparison based on individual scale ratings, but equal to .10 for the composite goal attainment score comparison, due to the reduced number of observations on which this summated score was based. In either case, the shared variance ($r^2 = .16$) may be a better index of the degree to which judgments by the patient are predictable from the therapist's judgment and vice versa. Finally, nonsignificant Pearson product-moment correlation coefficients were obtained relating patient-therapist goal-attainment score differences to patient Zigler-Phillips scores and psychotic versus nonpsychotic group membership.

Discussion

In our study there was a correlation of .41 between patients' and therapists' goal attainment ratings. This value represents a considerable change from the .10 correlation coefficient between client- and therapist-perceived therapeutic progress scores obtained by Horenstein, Houston, and Holmes.[3] One possible explanation of the difference between these two studies is that in this study, attainment levels were keyed to descriptively stated criteria for evaluating change. Whereas goal-attainment scaling anchors the traditional global descriptors ("problem worse than before," "problem completely solved") to these descriptively stated criteria along a graduated attainment scale, the system appears only as reliable as the degree to which patients and therapists objectify the criteria, interpret them similarly, and make use of the criteria in evaluating treatment progress. It may be of particular clinical interest to determine whether certain patients are "overinflators" or "underinflators" of treatment success. However, in developing a reliable and useful index of treatment progress, idiosyncratic judgments must be replaced by more objective accounts of therapeutic results, tied closely to descriptive criteria.

It was evident to the experimenters that the extent to which goal statements were tied to descriptive criteria varied across patient-therapist dyads. Concordance between therapists' and patients' goal-attainment scores may be increased, in future studies, as a result of greater staff proficiency in the technique of constructing behaviorally stated performance objectives. With sufficiently precise criteria, third-party evaluators might also determine, following a brief structured interview with the patient, how closely the therapist and/or patient goal-attainment ratings relate to their independent evaluation. In addition, further investigation of the relationship between goal-attainment ratings and other criteria (e.g., behavioral rating scale changes, MMPI changes) is needed. Our study did show, however, that the concordance between patient and therapist goal-attainment scores is relatively independent of certain patient variables, such as social competency scores or major diagnostic category.

The POGAS system was constructed to provide utmost flexibility to the individual patient-therapist dyad. The therapy participants define, in their own words, the problem areas, the anchoring goal statements, and each problem is weighted according to its judged priority. It is recognized, however, that patient involvement in defining problems, setting treatment goals, and rating treatment progress may be impractical in certain clinical situations. In many such situations, the POGAS system is equally adaptable to independent determination of problem/goal definitions and goal attainment ratings by staff members exclusively.

Utility of System

It is suggested that a problem oriented goal attainment scaling system can be of decided usefulness. It requires a minimal time investment by therapists and patients, and it may facilitate therapeutic progress by providing systematic feedback to the therapy participants regarding outcome. In addition, concrete goal setting in graduated levels of attainment may facilitate therapeutic change by focusing therapeutic efforts on specified treatment objectives.

Periodic review of problems and resetting of goals may be incorporated into usual clinical practice to provide longitudinal data about patient progress and to adjust treatment modalities in terms of feedback from the patients' and therapists' evaluative ratings. Patient progress can be graphically represented through the plotting of goal-attainment scores over time. By summing across patients, statistical analysis can reveal whether treatment progress, measured by goal-attainment ratings, relates significantly to patient variables (diagnosis, premorbid history), treatment variables (type of therapy, amount of therapeutic contact), or therapist variables (years of experience, age, sex).

The system described, an adaptation of the POGAS technique of Kiresuk and Sherman,[4] can be a powerful tool for case or program audit and planning, since it remains tied to clinical operations and criteria, providing, at the same time, a quantitative assessment of outcome.

Routine use of the POGAS system, with or without parents' participation, requires periodic auditing of the system itself. First, patient charts should be reviewed in terms of the appropriateness of the goal selection process. When treatment goals are relatively trivial, goal attainment scores may be overinflated estimates of treatment progress. In addition, goals should be realistically scaled to the five-point goal-attainment scale. Both unrealistically high expectations of treatment progress keyed to the scale point "goal completely achieved" and unrealistically low expectations keyed to the descriptor "further away from goal" should be avoided. Second, problem areas should be appropriately defined to allow for precision in developing intervention strategies. Periodic inservice training, preferably with videotaped presentations, is suggested to insure optimal use of the system.

References

1. Cline, D. W., Rouzen, D. L., and Bransford, D. Goal-attainment scaling as a method of evaluating mental health programs. *Am. J. Psychiatry*, 130: 105–108, 1973.
2. Hayes-Roth, F., Longabaugh, R. and Ryback R. The problem-oriented medical record and psychiatry. *Br. J. Psychiatry*, 121: 27–34, 1972.
3. Horenstein, D., Houston, B. K. and Holmes, D. S. Clients', therapists', and judges' evaluations of psychotherapy. *J. Counsel. Psychol.*, 20: 149–153, 1973.
4. Kiresuk, T. J. and Sherman, R. A. Goal attainment scaling: A general method for evaluating comprehensive community mental health programs. *Com. Ment. Health J.*, 4: 443–453, 1968.
5. McLean, P. D. and Miles, J. E. Evaluation of the problem-oriented record in psychiatry *Arch. Gen. Psychiatry*, 31: 622–625, 1974.
6. Meldman, M. S., Johnson, E. and McLeod, D. A goal list and a treatment methods index in an automated record system. *Hosp. Com. Psychiatry*, 26: 365–370, 1975.
7. Ryback, R. S. and Gardner, J. S. Problem formulation: The problem-oriented record. *Am. J. Psychiatry*, 130: 312–316, 1973.
8. Weed, L. L. *Medical records, medical education and patient care.* Cleveland: Case Western University Press, 1969.
9. Williams, T. A. and Johnson, C. Computer assisted multi-disciplinary psychiatric assessment unit. Project Overview as of June, 1973, V. A. Hospital, Salt Lake City, 1973.
10. Zigler, E. and Phillips, L. Social competence and the process-reactive distinction in psychopathology. *J. Abnorm. Soc. Psychol.*, 65: 215–222, 1962.

Preventing Involuntary Hospitalization:[*]
A Family Contracting Approach

Jeffrey S. Nevid and James K. Morrison[**]

THE SOCIAL ECOLOGY of the family often has a determining effect on the integration of the ex-state hospital patient in the community. Carstairs (1959) has found that the ex-hospitalized patient's maintenance in the community depends partly on the family's perception of the patient as non-dangerous. Hollingshead and Redlich (1958) have found that low socioeconomic families generally react to a "mentally ill" member with resentment and fear. Hollingshead and Redlich recognize that the family's fear and resentment of the patient, potentiated by each successive hospitalization, may be a critical factor in determining recidivism.

Recently, there has been increased interest in the role of the family as reactor to, rather than purely as the cause of, a mental

---

*This article was originally published in the *Journal of Family Counseling*, 1976, *14*, 27–31. Reprinted by permission.

**This manuscript is based on a paper presented by the authors at the American Psychological Association Convention, Chicago, 1975, entitled: "Involuntary hospitalization revisited: Contracting with the 'patient.'"

patient's problems (Kreisman and Joy, 1974). This attention to the family as a complex system with varied interactions allows one to avoid the naive approach of focusing only on the identified patient in a troubled family (Morrison, 1974). Not to focus on the reciprocal effects of fear (of the patient toward other family members and, conversely, the fear of the family toward the identified patient) would appear to be a serious clinical error. For example, if the family has taken a direct role in having a member involuntarily hospitalized, the patient, following hospitalization, may live in fear of the process reoccuring. Similarily, upon the patient's return from the hospital, the family may live in fear of his/her potential retaliation for their actions. Now that the patient has been officially declared as having "mental problems" by the psychiatric establishment, the family's fear of the identified patient may increase still further. This family reaction will in turn strengthen the patient's self-construction as "dangerous" and "unstable." One could go on *ad infinitum* describing the continuous and reciprocal effects of such an escalation of fear. The end result is often further hospitalizations and increased disruption of family life.

It has also been recognized that some families use a member's "mental illness" as a rationale for his or her continued infantilization, and as a means for denying his/her power and independent, adult status in the family (Laing, 1972). The power structure is maintained, and shared responsibility for family problems is disowned as the pathology in the family becomes interpreted as belonging solely to the stigmatized patient-member. Attention is thus deployed from family conflicts to one member's "sickness," and an equilibrium of sorts is attained when in times of crisis the scapegoated member is "removed" to the hospital for his/her "disruptive" behavior.

In the following discussion, a contracting approach is suggested to (1) help break this cycle of fear and resentment, and (2) prevent the family from using commitment to maintain a member's dependency or to eschew responsibility for intrafamily problems.

It is suggested that a family member's fear of hospitalization may be reduced by means of a family contract* strengthened by the cooperation of all mental health professionals concerned in working

---

*The term "contract" is not used in the legal sense of the mutuality of obligation. Rather it refers to a unilateral promissory statement by family and clinic staff.

with the family. The authors support involuntary hospitalization only in short-term, crisis situations where there is an immediate threat to the patient's life or to the lives of others through the patient's behavior. Regardless of the differences clinicians may have with respect to the issue of involuntary hospitalization, the authors suggest that clinicians advise their patients of the criteria they use in making judgments regarding psychiatric commitment. With patients who have been previously committed, and who are fearful of being recommitted, the authors recommend the use of explicit, written contracts which stipulate those behaviors (e.g., arguing with family, wanting to live independently of the family, discussing "delusional" material or hallucinations), however socially undesirable, not necessitating involuntary hospitalization. Furthermore, the operative contingencies for favoring commitment proceedings should be specified in the contract (e.g., "Involuntary hospitalization would only be considered by this clinic in clearly life threatening situations"). Such contracts, signed by family members and clinic staff, are considered to be binding by the signees.

Through contracting, it is hoped that patients will come to recognize that commitment proceedings have definitive antecedents in their own behavior, and that rehospitalization is not an arbitrary action exercised indiscriminately by the family. Thus, the patients live with less fear of arbitrary, family-initiated commitment actions, since they have tangible assurances against such practices. And, their retaliatory attitude following an involuntary rehospitalization (within the contractual guidelines) is diminished, as they recognize their own behavioral excesses which voided the contract.

The authors recognize the limited scope of this contracting procedure. Thus, the decision rules for involuntary hospitalization practiced by the team are not generally negotiable. The clinic is mandated to prevent, through hospital confinement, serious harm to the patient or others through the patient's actions. This contracting procedure does, however, represent a reform of present practices by delineating on paper those behaviors not falling within this mandate. Without such contracts, psychiatric patients may be faced with the uncertainty, and consequently the fear, that hospitalization may follow any unorthodox action.

Erikson (1957) has suggested that community psychiatry may actually impede the ex-hospitalized patient's progress toward independent community living by providing a setting in which patient or "sick" roles remain functional. When released to the community, the ex-hospitalized patient is often faced with the need to supplant the set of patient stereotypic role-enactments encouraged by the milieu of the hospital and the family (Goffman, 1961), with role-enactments more appropriate to personally responsible, independent living. The involuntary hospitalization contracting approach encourages patients to assume personal responsibility by making clear that they must hold themselves responsible for modifying their behavior within contractual guidelines to avoid future hospitalizations. Further, in helping patients change from dependent and helpless behaviors to full citizenry role-enactments, mental health professionals often must contend with family resistance. The family may resist efforts to share decision making tasks in the family through continuing to construe the patient as a helpless and sick dependent "child." The involuntary hospitalization contract negates the use of commitment by the family in resolving family crises and in resisting the patient's attempts at autonomous behavior. In promoting the independent role functioning of their patients, therapists must at times advocate their patients' interests before families which regard their patient-members as "incapable of acting on their own." In one sense, the contracting procedure concretizes the battle, which often must be played through in family counseling for the patient to achieve independent status.

It is suggested that family contracting for involuntary hospitalization be integrated within a broad treatment program designed to increase the self-reliance and independent community functioning of exhospitalized patients. This integrated program, though beyond the scope of the present paper, might additionally include individual and/or family therapy, structured transitional after-care homes, and special workshops in developing daily living and problem solving skills to increase the patients' repertoire of adaptive, self-reliant behaviors.

Case Study

Mary K. is a thirty-eight-year-old, single, white, unemployed female, labeled a "paranoid schizophrenic," who has been psychiatrically hospitalized on eleven different occasions for a total of four years and ten months during the last twenty years. Most hospitalizations occurred as a result of the family becoming terrified of Mary's behavior and having her committed to a mental hospital. On occasion her mother had signed commitment papers and actually taken her to the hospital.

Mary's life in her lower-class family was characterized by continuous conflict with her mother. Before his death, the client's father had acted as a buffer between his wife and daughter. Her mother, having done her utmost to keep Mary at home since birth, would often have her committed to a state hospital following family disagreements. Although the patient had an extensive history of psychotic symptoms, her hospitalizations were primarily related to family disturbances rather than internal psychopathology.

Mary's "career role" as a mental patient reinforced her continued infantilization by her mother, and kept secure mother's role as omniscient protective guradian. Mary's opposition to her mother, generally about the issue of seeking increased independence, was interpreted by her mother as "crazy" behavior and subject to psychiatric penalties through commitment. Upon discharge from the hospital, Mary would usually appear to be very docile, very apologetic to her mother for the "trouble she had caused," and willing to agree to any form of treatment. In short, she would appear as if she had "atoned" for her "sins" by being committed to a hospital, and now felt duly repentent. Though she was unsatisfied in her passive-dependent position in the family, Mary was more frightened of the consequences of opposing her mother, i.e., commitment. In short, Mary lived in fear of her mother's intervention with psychiatric professionals to recommit her. Secondly, her mother lived with great anxiety over potential (though never actualized) retaliatory behavior by, in her words, "a mental patient who obviously has no control over what she does." Each fear seemed to reinforce the other until an escalation of negative expectancies would lead to increased family conflicts and treatment strategies to separate mother and daughter. Mary is presently an active client of a state-supported community based satellite psychiatric team.

Mary's stated fear that information from clinical interviews with the senior author (her primary therapist) might be used to involuntarily hospitalize her resulted in largely unproductive and circumstantial therapy sessions. Because of these fears that her mother or clinic staff would recommit her for any unorthodox behavior, the authors decided to construct a contract with Mary which clearly specified behaviors which, by themselves, could not be used as grounds for commitment.

Contracting Procedure

One regularly scheduled therapy session was used for writing the contract. First, the authors expressed to Mary our belief that she appeared fearful of "stepping out of line" (for fear of recommitment) and that any disagreement with her family might eventuate rehospitalization. It was explained to Mary that this fear was obstructing the development of a trusting and open therapeutic relationship, and additionally, causing her to be secretive, guarded, and distant from family and friends. It was emphasized that we understood her quite justifiable fear, based on past experience, of being recommitted might negate her attempts to make concrete future plans. The contract was explained as a means for reducing fears of her mother and the clinic by providing tangible assurances against arbitrary commitment actions. Mary was then asked to describe the types of behavior she felt might cause others to have her committed. She was then informed of the commitment policy of the clinic; i.e., that immediate danger to self or others through the clients' actions was a necessary condition for involuntary hospitalization. To buttress our argument that Mary need not fear commitment for the variety of behaviors she had described, the contract was then written to include these behaviors. The contract stipulated the following set of behaviors which, by themselves, could not be used as grounds for commitment: (1) the expression of anger at family or staff; (2) experiencing hallucinations or expressing beliefs others held to be false; (3) disagreeing with staff or family; and (4) changing her living situation against her mother's advice. The contract was signed by the authors, the consulting psychiatrist and rotating psychiatric residents.

Since the contract merely stipulated, on paper, the clinic policy about commitment, there was no staff resistance to the procedure. In fact, Mary's mother raised the only objection to the contracting procedure. She claimed that the contract appeared to sanction behaviors which she considered undesirable (e.g., arguing with family or holding to false beliefs). A conjoint meeting with both Mary and her mother was called to discuss these concerns. The authors' position was expressed that commitment cannot be used as an implied threat to control a patient's undesirable behavior. Further, we expressed our belief that the contract was necessary if Mary was to trust us with her personal problems, her troubling and often delusional ideas, and her intermittent auditory hallucinations. We stated that we did not sanction these behaviors, but sought to change them within a contractual, rather than a coercive model. With this clarification, the patient's mother agreed to sign the contract, and provided at least tacit consent to our efforts to promote Mary's independent functioning.

Since the signing of the contract ten months ago, Mary has not been hospitalized, either voluntarily or involuntarily. She has been placed successfully, for the first time, in a transitional family care home. Six months ago, she moved successfully to independent apartment living, something her mother had always opposed. The client previously had never lived by herself. On this occasion, with active therapist advocacy, the patient's mother did give tacit support for this move (e.g., "Well, I don't think she'll make it, but I won't try to stop you"). It was explained to Mary that failure at independent living did not mean recommitment, as the contract makes clear.

To help promote her readjustment, Mary has participated in clinic workshops designed to teach self-reliant skills of daily living and problem-solving skills. Since the contract signing, Mary has become more open about discussing auditory hallucinations and personal constructions considered to be delusional. She has begun volunteer work at the clinic, and she has become a member of the clinic's client advisory board. The importance of the contract to Mary has been well established. On two occasions, when her advisor was changed due to rotating assignments, Mary insisted that her new counselor sign the contract. Mary continues presently to carry the contract on her person, wherever she goes.

In conclusion, it is suggested that elaboration, through contracting, of the operating contingencies for involuntary commitment proceedings may have definite therapeutic advantages for client and family. First, contracting provides a means for disrupting the cyclical pattern of fear within the patient's family, by bringing into the open the often covert decision rules for psychiatric commitment. Secondly, it is suggested that certain clients, due to the frequency of their past involuntary hospitalizations, may harbor negative expectancies regarding the possibility of continuing to live independently of the hospital for extended periods. To disconfirm this sense of inevitability, and consequent lack of future orientation and constructive planning, contracting, as described above, may represent one approach. Finally, there is the additional advantage of increasing the client's sense of security in discussing certain material which that person might otherwise conceal for fear of being committed.

References

Carstairs, G. M. *Other Social Limits of Eccentricity: An English Study.* In M. K. Opler (Ed.), Culture and Mental Health: Cross-Cultural Studies. New York: Macmillan, 1959, 373–389.

Erickson, K. T. "Patient Roles and Social Uncertainty—A Dilemma of the Mentally Ill." *Psychiatry* 20 (1957) : 263–272.

Goffman, E. *Asylums: Essays on the Social Situation of Mental Patients and Other Inmates.* New York: Doubleday, 1961.

Hollingshead, A., & Redlich, F. *Social Class and Mental Illness.* New York: John Wiley & Sons, 1958.

Kreisman, D. E., & Joy, V. D. "Family response to the mental illness of a relative: A review of the literature." *Schizophrenia Bulletin* 10 (1974) : 34–57.

Laing, R. D. *The Politics of the Family and Other Essays.* New York: Vintage, 1969.

Morrison, J. K. "Labeling: A study of an 'autistic' child." *Journal of Family Counseling* 2 (1974) : 71–80.

Morrison, J. K. "An argument for mental patient advisory boards." *Professional Psychology,* in press, 1976.

Contracting Confidentiality in
Group Psychotherapy*

James K. Morrison, Mary Federico, and Harold J. Rosenthal

THE ISSUE OF confidentiality has caused some perplexing problems for psychologists and other mental health professionals (Curran, 1969; McGuire, 1974; Mykel, 1971; Shaw, 1970; Slovenko, 1966). Such problems are actually compounded for the psychotherapist in group therapy where more than one client hears confidential information (Foster, 1975). Foster has underlined the vulnerable position of clients in group therapy, a setting in which group members reveal intimate information about themselves. As Foster points out, if a person makes a statement in the presence of others, there is a presumption in law that this person does not intend that information to remain confidential. Thus, at present, group clients are apparently not legally protected from other group members who may discuss problems revealed in group to others outside group. And, neither is there any clear legal remedy when the confidentiality of group discussions is violated. It is the purpose

---

*This article was originally published in the *Journal of Forensic Psychology*, 1975, *7, 1–6*. Reprinted by permission.

of this article to propose a more effective way of ensuring confidentiality in group, and a legally promising remedy for clients whose reputation may be jeopardized by breach of confidentiality.

Schwitzgebel (1975) has recommended the use of contracts with mental patients to protect them from poor treatment by mental health professionals. He suggests that such patients would then have legal recourse since they could sue for "breach of contract." It would seem likely that contracting may also be a legal remedy to protect group psychotherapy clients from having their intimate problems revealed to others outside the group. (Of course, in cases of criminal prosecution it has long been held that one cannot make a contract precluding the court from eliciting testimony concerning a criminal offense. It is likely that courts would find a public policy, encouraging citizens to report criminal activity to the police, to be of sufficient importance to supercede the importance of a contract of confidentiality.)

The Use of a Contract in Group Therapy

During the past year we decided to test the usefuless of a contract of confidentiality. We felt that if the contract were taken seriously by group therapy clients, we would thereby protect the confidential information revealed in group sessions, as well as facilitate client self-disclosure during therapy. It is a common concern among group therapists that confidentiality be taken seriously by the clients in order to ensure the kind of self-disclosure necessary for effective therapy (Mykel, 1971).

The senior author drew up a contract which he wished to test with his group therapy clients. All 12 clients who participated in group therapy signed what was considered as a preliminary version of a group confidentiality contract. This document included a promise not to reveal confidential information outside the group, or otherwise risk being legally sued by the offended member of the group. The exact wording of the document was as follows:

> We, the undersigned, in return for group therapy, agree not to reveal to anyone outside of the (name of the agency) staff the names of anyone in group psychotherapy. Neither will we speak of anyone in the group to anyone outside of the (name of the agency) staff, in such a way as to reveal the identity of a group member. We realize that should we so break confidentiality in this manner, we risk being legally sued by the offended member of the group.

To date, the above mentioned contract has been used only with clients who are clearly mentally competent to engage in contracting. It should be noted that the therapists witnessed the contract with their signatures.

A Follow-up Study

Since the primary reasons for instituting a contract of confidentiality were to (1) deter group clients from revealing confidential information to others, and (2) to thereby facilitate client self-disclosure in group, it was of great interest to the therapists to determine whether the contract indeed served these purposes. Near the termination of group therapy, a brief anonymous questionnaire composed of five questions, along with a copy of the contract, was sent to each of the eight clients who regularly attended the group during the twelve months of its existence. All eight of the questionnaires were returned and the results were analyzed.

In response to question 1, "On a four point scale,* how seriously or lightly did you take the contract at the time you signed it?" the mean group rating was 3.24; indicating that the group as a whole took the contract seriously. In answering question 2, "Do you think the contract at any time influenced you not to talk about the problems of group members to non-group members?" five clients responded affirmatively,** and three negatively. Responding to question 3, "Can you remember any occasion on which you revealed to a non-group member the name of a group member along with some confidential information about that person?" six clients replied "no," one "not sure," and one "yes."

In response to question 4 (Did you approve of engaging in a legal contract to ensure confidentiality of group information?), seven of the eight clients responded affirmatively; one was unsure. In answering question 5 (Would you have been less likely to reveal confidential information about yourself in group had there not been a contract?), five group members replied "yes," two "no," and one "not sure."

In summary, the anonymous survey of group therapy clients

---

*Very lightly (1), lightly (2), seriously (3), very seriously (4).
**The response choices for questions 2–5 were: yes, no, not sure.

revealed that for the most part the contract deterred clients from breaking confidentiality, and facilitated self-disclosure in group. The contract was generally acceptable and was taken seriously by all but two group members.

A Proposal for a New Contract

Although the results of the survey were on the whole encouraging, one could argue that the contract should be worded more strongly so as to strengthen its deterrant value in discouraging clients from breaking confidentiality. Furthermore, in order to strengthen the legal validity of confidentiality contracting, and to aid in the enforcement of such a contract, it may be useful to actually specify a minimum value to be placed on the damage for which the injured party may sue.

It is common in legal contracts to include what is known as a "liquidated damages clause" (Simpson, 1965). In most jurisdictions this amount would be equal to what the contracting parties estimate as the damages resulting from a breach of contract. This amount generally cannot include any type of punitive damages. Thus, we have chosen to concentrate on liquidated damages in the contract mentioned below, and to allow the court to set the amount of damages resulting from other proven damage (e.g., that resulting from business losses) to the client. A liquidated damages clause would strengthen the contract, and possibly serve as an additional admonition to group members to take the contract seriously.

The revised contract, presently in use with another group of clients, reads as follows:

We, the undersigned, in consideration of and return for receiving group psychotherapy and its possible benefits, and in consideration of and return for similar promises by other members of the psychotherapy group, consciously and willingly promise never to reveal the identity of any group member (listed below) to anyone who is not in group therapy, other than staff of the psychiatric agency from which we receive services. We realize that to relate specific problems of a group member to a nongroup member, even though the name of the group member may not be directly revealed, may at times lead to the eventual disclosure of the group member's identity. Therefore, we promise to avoid speaking of any group member's problems in any manner which would even remotely risk revealing the identity of that group member. We fully realize and strongly agree that in the event of a lawsuit for breach of contract, we give the offended party the right to recover for damage to his/her reputation the minimum amount of $_____. Also, such party may recover for any other damages which can be proven.

All clients are requested to sign this contract before being accepted into group therapy. The signatures of the clients are witnessed by the cotherapists. The minimum amount of monetary damages for breach of contract is a fixed negotiated sum unanimously accepted by all the clients.

The revised contract would appear to fulfill all the conditions for a legal contract according to the common definitions of a contract (Simpson, 1965; Williston, 1957). Should then a client reveal confidential information about another group client, the offended party could apparently sue that client for breach of contract. Even though the validity of such an argument has yet to be tested in court, there is a strong probability that the court would uphold the validity of the contract, and thus rule in favor of breach of contract.

The use of confidentiality contracts are useful at the present time as a remedy for clients whose reputation may be damaged by breach of confidentiality. Ultimately, however, the protection of client confidentiality would best be established through legislation.

References

Curran, W. J. Policies and practices concerning confidentiality in college mental health services in the U.S. and Canada. *American Journal of Psychiatry*, 1969, *125*, 1520–1530.

Foster, L. M. Group psychotherapy: A pool of legal witnesses? *International Journal of Group Psychotherapy*, 1975, *25*, 50–53.

McGuire, J. M. Confidentiality and the child in psychotherapy. *Professional Psychology*, 1974, *5*, 374–379.

Mykel, N. The application of ethical standards to group psychotherapy in a community. *International Journal of Group Psychotherapy*, 1971, *21*, 248–254.

Schwitzgebel, R. K. A contractual model for the protection of the rights of institutionalized mental patients. *American Psychologist*, 1975, *30*, 815–820.

Shaw, S. Privileged communications, confidentiality, and privacy: Confidentiality. *Professional Psychology*, 1970, *1*, 159–164.

Slovenko, R. *Psychotherapy, confidentiality and privileged communication.* Springfield, Ill.: Charles C. Thomas, 1966.

Simpson, L. P. *Handbook on the law of contracts.* St. Paul, Minn.: West Publishing Co., 1965.

Williston, S. *Williston on contracts.* Mt. Kisco, N.Y.: Baker, Voorhis and Co., Inc., 1957.

6
Accountability to the Client-Consumer

Overview

CHAPTER 6 CONCERNS itself with the issue of accountability to the client-consumer. The first article presents some innovative ways in which a community mental health team can actively involve the clients in the evaluation of clinical services. Such client involvement in research efforts, especially those directly concerned with program and service evaluation, adds a different and perhaps a needed corrective dimension to our efforts at being accountable to client-consumers. Thus, when clients anonymously make evaluations of clinic programs by relaying their judgments of program effectiveness to staff by means of client advisory board members, such evaluations may give clinic staff a rather good idea of how satisfied clients really are with services.

The second article delineates how a community team can systematically accomplish an important goal of client-consumerism; evaluating all of the programs and services which a clinic provides to clients. The clinical manager or team leader is a key person in establishing an atmosphere in which psychiatric staff of all disciplines can become enthusiastic about and involved in evaluative research. If the administrator is the member of the community team ultimately responsible to the community's consumers, then he must also take the responsibility of ensuring that the consumers are receiving effective services.

In the third article a discharge study illustrates how a community team can begin to evaluate the impact a clinic's services may have on client problem resolution. Too often in clinical work we deceive ourselves in believing that what we have done for clients in a period of months or years must have had some effect on the clients' behavior. This particular discharge study is of interest because of its focus on some rarely researched areas such as (1) the readiness of community clients for discharge, (2) the percentage of discharged clients who soon seek psychiatric help elsewhere, and (3) the comparative importance of nontreatment therapeutic events (e.g., falling in love, finding a job) which occur outside clinical interventions but which have an effect on client behavior change.

The fourth article in the chapter describes an attempt to measure the specific effects of two different group therapy styles on client problem resolution. This study also attempts to answer the question whether group therapy, in general, is effective and if so, whether the effect is lasting. Such evaluations are important to client-consumers because unless a particular clinic can justify that group therapy "works" (the outcome variable) and "how it works" (the process variable, e.g., which therapy style is most effective for a particular group of therapists), the client-consumers are risking much time and perhaps money "spinning their wheels" for nothing.

The fifth article demonstrates how, if we are truly accountable to clients, we must of necessity continually evaluate our perhaps most highly valued and most often used therapeutic intervention, individual psychotherapy. In this study the particular therapy studied is that of emotive-reconstructive psychotherapy. It seems to me to be important to periodically give the client some "objective" evidence that individual therapy indeed is having the intended effect. This article explains how feedback on therapy effectiveness can be solicited after every five sessions by means of self-report questionnaires which actively involve the client in accountability.

The sixth and final article in this chapter is another discharge followup study. Like the previously mentioned discharge study, the design is rather simple and straightforward and thus may give hope to the less experienced clinician-researcher who fears he may not have time to engage in evaluative research. This study is important primarily because it is one of the few studies which address the important question: Which of our multiple services clients judge as the most and the least effective?

Accountability is the "name of the game" in a consumer approach to community psychology. Without serious efforts at accountability we cannot claim that we are safeguarding the rights of consumers.

The Role of Client-Consumers in Evaluative Data Collection*

James K. Morrison

IN MENTAL HEALTH settings it has become increasingly common for staff professionals to solicit from clients evaluative feedback about treatment effectiveness (Denner & Halprin, 1974; Hart & Bassett, 1975; Powell, Shaw & O'Neal, 1971; Zusman & Slawson, 1972; Morrison, Pitchford, Dovberg & Smith, in press). It is not common, however, for mental health professionals to construe the client-consumer as a person capable of designing, coordinating, and implementing certain types of research projects. In other words, we too often think of the client only as the person to be researched, not the person who can do research.

Researchers have long been aware of the problem of asking clients for their judgments of treatment effectiveness. Even when such clients' responses are anonymous, the judgments tend, I suspect, to be biased in a positive direction. It would appear that most clients, especially those who have been conditioned in our mental hospital system, are inclined to "tell the doctor what he or she wants to hear" (Braginsky, Braginsky & Ring, 1969). It is

---

*Reprinted in expanded form, with permission of the publisher, from the original: Morrison, J. K. Involving psychiatric clients in evaluative data collection. *Evaluation*, 1977, *4*, 74.

not difficult to imagine the risks clients must anticipate when they contemplate rendering truly negative opinions of services. They may fear arbitrary discharge, an increase of medication, involuntary hospitalization, the ire of staff, and a host of other threatening responses by staff. Even if we feel confident that in our own clinical setting such negative staff responses are quite unlikely, still we must recognize that the clients' fears of negative responses are to be expected.

Because of the possible built-in bias in our traditional way of collecting data from clients, it may be useful to consider involving clients as researchers or data collectors. Such research is not meant as a substitute for the traditional way of construing clients—as subjects of research—but rather as a complement to it. Evaluative research, in which clients are actively involved, at least as data collectors, may help us to discover and document just how positively biased our traditional research evaluations are.

In our community mental health outpatient clinic, we have established a client advisory board (Morrison, 1976; Morrison, in press), whose primary function is to evaluate all of our treatment programs and services. Through board functioning clients have been encouraged by staff to become involved in research. In just one year the client-consumers on the board have succeeded in evaluating all of the clinic's services (Morrison & Cometa, in press). Such evaluation is especially feasible when one of the board members is actually a discharged client who has signed up as a clinic volunteer. Since a volunteer signs a statement of confidentiality, he can be allowed access to some confidential information. Thus, such a person may be given the first names and telephone numbers of clients, thereby allowing him to call other clients for their judgments of the therapeutic effectiveness of certain clinic services. I have found client evauations, gathered in this manner, to be less positive and, I suspect, more reflective of clients' real opinions. Such evaluative data, collected by clients (or former clients) themselves, serve a corrective function in that the data prevent professional staff from too easily concluding from more traditional research that programs and therapeutic interventions are justified and should be continued.

The client-consumers on the advisory board have also been able to survey clients on their real program needs. Too often clinical staff slip into the conceptual trap of developing programs and services for clients based more on staff needs than on actual client needs. Thus, client involvement in program planning research again serves a corrective function.

Another example illustrative of the utility of client involvement in data collection is a recent survey by our client advisory board members of their fellow clients' views on open records. Board members were able to reach 78 percent of the client population who had telephones and determined, first, that 37 percent of the client-consumers were not even sure that their clinician-advisors made progress notes in their charts. More importantly, the client-data-collectors determined that 82 percent of the clients indicated a clear interest in seeing notes made about them in clinic charts. Such client response has led to a staff research project studying the effect which a policy of open records may have on clients.

I might also cite an ingenious use of a former client in the data collection process. Recently, as staff began to do street surveys of one small community's perception of its program needs in the mental health area, one discharged client, who was serving as a member of the citizen advisory board, volunteered to assist the staff in the survey. Such help is invaluable in these days of limited resources for research. One might even imagine certain high-functioning clients engaging in more sophisticated, publishable research. The better-educated clients may also be capable of planning their own research projects.

It has been my experience that clinical and administrative staff need not fear the assumption by clients of data-collector and evaluator roles. On the contrary, when clients assume such responsible roles they begin to learn interpersonal and conceptual skills which are functional in other settings. For example, a client board member who can confront clinical professionals with negative evaluations would more likely be able to confront a parent or spouse when appropriate.

The psychiatric client need not remain only in the role of consumer. With some encouragement and training some of the more educated and better functioning clients can also assume the more responsible roles of data collector and evaluator.

References

Braginsky, B., Braginsky, D., & Ring, K. *Methods in madness.* New York: Holt, Rinehart, and Winston, 1969.

Denner, B., & Halprin, F. Measuring consumer satisfaction in a community outpost. *American Journal of Community Psychology*, 1974, *2*, 13–22.

Hart, W. T., & Bassett, L. Measuring consumer satisfaction in a mental health center. *Hospital and Community Psychiatry*, 1975, *26*, 512–515.

Morrison, J. K. An argument for mental patient advisory boards. *Professional Psychology*, 1976, *7*, 127–131.

Morrison, J. K. The client as consumer and evaluator of community mental health services. *American Journal of Psychology*, in press.

Morrison, J. K., & Cometa, M. S. The impact of the client advisory board on a community mental health clinic. In J. K. Morrison (Ed.) *A Consumer Approach to Community Psychology*. Chicago: Nelson-Hall, in press.

Morrison, J. K., Pitchford, B., Dovberg, N., & Smith, F. J. Correspondence of staff-client evaluations of discharge readiness and non-treatment therapeutic events. *Journal of Community Psychology*, in press.

Powell, B. J., Shaw, D., O'Neal, C. Client evaluation of a clinic's services. *Hospital and Community Psychiatry*, 1971, *22*, 45–46.

Zusman, J., & Slawson, M. R. Service quality profile: Development of a technique for measuring quality of mental health services. *Archives of General Psychiatry*, 1972, *27*, 692–698.

The Mental Health Administrator and Evaluation*

James K. Morrison, Barbara Pitchford, and Frederick J. Smith

IN AN ERA marked by proliferating demands for accountability to the consumer of mental health services (Chu and Trotter, 1974; Morrison, in press a; Morrison, in press b), the clinician-executive can no longer ignore the important role of evaluation.** Although Drucker (1972) has diagnosed the paramount weakness of service institutions as their failure to evaluate performance by results, mental health administrators have too often neglected to translate it into well-planned efforts at evaluation. Until quite recently, in fact, when accountability became the shibboleth of those administrators hard pressed to justify continued or expanded funding, evaluative studies were largely "ornamental," tacked on to support administrative decisions, and regarded with some suspicion (Rich, 1973).

---

*This article was originally published in *Administration in Mental Health*, 1977, *4*, 78–82. Reprinted by permission.

**This term encompasses a wide range of research from demographic studies to empirical research. See Zusman and Slawson (1972) for those to be evaluated within mental health services.

If accountability is really the shape of things to come, administrators and clinicians will be required to provide evidence that their activities are worthwhile. Neither good intentions, hard work, nor sophisticated demographic charts will be sufficient to justify continued funding. Accountability will increasingly be used as a wedge for making budgetary decisions. In this sense meaningful evaluation can no longer remain a luxury and mental health administrators can no longer neglect their responsibility for encouraging it within their agencies.

Systematic and well-planned evaluation is an important first step toward improved management through the assessment by performance. But, before management can become a reality, mental health administrators must implement those strategies that will promote the acceptance of evaluation as an integral part of the administrative process. At least in part, management by performance is not often used in mental health organizations because it will be sabotaged unless staff are involved in and support the necessary evaluation process.

Obstacles to Evaluation

Mental health administrators, whether at the executive or middle-management levels, can expect to meet resistance from clinical staff who are often quite successful in avoiding the anxiety arousing task of evaluating whether their clinical interventions are effective. Their resistance to evaluation is frequently manifested by claims that they are already overburdened and have no available time. This often reflects the minimal value that many clinicians ascribe to evaluations.

Other obstacles frequently cited as barriers to the development of evaluation as an essential component in mental health organizations include a shortage of trained evaluators, lack of computer systems, methodological problems, the isolation of specialized evaluation units from clinical programs, and the inability of evaluators to speak the language of clinicians. However, none of these obstacles are insurmountable.

The mental health administrator who wants to integrate evaluation results into program planning and management should take a hard look at three important factors: (1) the characteristics of the team, (2) selling the idea of evaluation, and (3) the logistical problems in initiating and continuing evaluation.

Characteristics of the Team

The larger the mental health programs, the greater the problems in developing systematic evaluation. Each team member is certain to have attitudes and perhaps biases about program evaluation. Discussing proposed projects with each individual can be effective in dealing with negative attitudes. In addition, the input of individual staff members into each project can be very helpful, though it becomes difficult in large programs. This type of input can increase staff interest and commitment.

Because it is more difficult to change the attitudes of a large group (Cartwright and Zander 1968), the mental health administrator of a large program will want to carefully plan a strategy before entering into evaluation studies. And since it is not likely that one single evaluation project will change the attitudes of a large group, the administrator may want to first work with those team members who are most open to evaluation. If successful, attempts can then be made to persuade the others. If the first project sells itself (Becker, Morrison and Fasano 1975), the word will get around.

Psychologists, sociologists and an increasing number of psychiatrists have been well exposed to evaluation research. If the mental health administrator or leader can sell the idea of evaluation to key staff in those professions, they can form an invaluable core for the evaluation team. (It should be kept in mind that this group sometimes has the most negative reactions to evaluation studies, citing previous encounters as tedious, irrelevant, and/or anxiety arousing). It may help to enlist a number of research-minded students especially from the field of psychology, to help change the atmosphere.

The team leader is the most likely candidate to organize and implement evaluation projects. Steger, Woodhouse, and Goocey (1975) have shed some light on the best qualifications for this position. The performance* of administrators in a clinical setting was primarily related to indices of management skills, as opposed to personal qualities or professional competence. The major skills needed are those associated with what has been previously termed "initiating structure," including such activities as defining job

---

*As indicated by a measure of the completion and scope of projects undertaken.

expectations, performance feedback, setting goals, allocating resources, and being objective. The team leader who is to initiate
innovative change through evaluation might also incorporate some
of the characteristics of May and Cohen's (1975) "Mental Health
Engineer" who translates clinical research into practice.

The following characteristics of the team leader seem to facilitate the establishment of evaluation as an ongoing part of a mental
hospital program:

1. A belief in evaluation as essential, even crucial, to the development and improvement of services.
2. An ability to "sell" that conviction to other staff.
3. Enough knowledge about evaluation to anticipate the obstacles
   and be able to help develop new evaluative instruments when no
   appropriate ones are available.
4. An ability to assign, schedule, and complete tasks, and to make
   sure that others complete theirs.
5. An ability to raise important questions that can be operationally defined and lead to meaningful and practical research.

Selling the Idea of Evaluation

Resistance among staff seems to spring from unhappy experiences or, among the uninitiated, a feeling of incompetence in the
face of the task (Romig 1973). Dealing with these issues openly in
individual conferences, team meetings, and workshops is vital before anything else can be done. When evaluation is perceived as
extra work, peripheral, and "jammed down one's throat," the effort may be sabotaged (Rich 1973). If the staff is comfortable with
their ability to participate in evaluative projects, and if they perceive them as important to the effective delivery of services,
resistance to the extra effort required tends to dissipate.

A client advisory board may also be helpful in gaining an
acceptance of evaluation as an integral part of the organization.
At the Capital District Psychiatric Center, a client advisory board
(CAB) (Morrison 1976) has been established to review ongoing
programs. Consistent with our model of the client as consumer and
evaluator of the center's services, the staff coordinator of each
program is required to regularly justify that program in terms of
its progress toward specified goals (Morrison and Cometa, in
press). CAB members have come to expect concrete proof of
progress. Otherwise, they advocate changes and revisions in appar-

ently less than successful programs. In this way, accountability to the consumer through the evaluation of results is regularly built into every program, and evaluation, far from being peripheral, is an integral part of each program. Clinicians often become motivated to participate in evaluation studies that may help them justify the existence of their programs to a client board. If client board meetings are conducted with some diplomacy, they can be used to promote among staff the need for evaluation.

The payoffs offered by an involvement in evaluation projects include opportunities to publish. This can be a strong incentive to many professionals and students. Evaluation that increases efficiency may also be rewarding to the resultantly less harried team members (Morrison, Fasano and Becker 1976). In addition, engaging in evaluation studies can be an intellectually stimulating and rewarding endeavor for many clinicians. It may also become a vehicle for improving communication between the professional staff.

The first evaluation project should be meaningful to all involved, produce some payoff such as a saving of clinician time (Morrison, Fasano and Becker 1976), and lead to increased feelings of competence on the part of those involved (Becker, Morrison and Fasano 1975). If it fails to satisfy at least some of the real needs of the staff, then this dissatisfaction will make future studies more difficult.

Logistical Problems

As Gottesfeld (1975), Romig (1973), and Morrison and Smith (1976) have pointed out, it is possible to find resource persons, program analysts, and statisticians to collaborate in evaluation projects when staff does not have this expertise. The prospect of publications is often a sufficient inducement to enlist academically based researchers. The mental health executive is the ideal person to make contacts with these professionals in outside agencies and universities.

One of the most important tasks of the administrator is to keep on top of the evaluation projects. This often involves ensuring agreement on research design, checking to make sure that instruments are administered to clients, and coordinating the analysis, discussion, and documentation of results.

Another task of the administrator is to ensure that the staff knows and understands the results of the study and how to apply the findings to clinical practice. According to May and Cohen (1974), the translation of research findings into effective clinical practice is one of the major problems in health care. And only rarely do evaluation data affect program decisions (Nelson 1975). Translating these data into action is a major responsibility of the mental health administrator.

A Bridge to Management by Performance

Although staff acceptance of evaluation may take a year or more, the administrator who concentrates first on promoting the need for evaluation is likely to find that staff will more easily accept the value of management by performance. Certainly that has been our experience. Once our staff, including the secretary, became actively involved in evaluation, they had little difficulty accepting new policies regarding the establishment of clearly defined goals and objectives, cost-effectiveness analyses, discharge followup studies, and measures of service rendered.

At our center, evaluation studies directly led to a number of management decisions: (1) Two clinical programs were cancelled due to lack of evidence of their effectiveness; (2) Six other clinical programs were substantially altered; (3) No clinical programs could be developed without built-in evaluation; (4) All new clinical programs had to be first approved by the client advisory board; (5) New clinical programs had to be developed in the community (a street survey had indicated the need for certain new programs); (6) More extensive in-service training in areas of clinical deficiency was mandated for some staff; (7) A "research forum" was initiated to assist staff in implementing continuing studies; and, (8) Goal-attainment scaling was adopted as a system to monitor clinical performance.

Conclusions

Mental health administrators who are seriously concerned about accountability should begin to develop a spirit of systematic evaluation among the clinical staff. To accomplish this, three basic factors must be considered: (1) the characteristics of the staff; (2) selling the idea of evaluation; and, (3) the logistical problems involved.

References

Becker, R. E., Morrison, J. K. and Fasano, B. L. The effect of evaluative research on clinicians' feelings of competence, attitudes toward research and acceptance of a new approach. In: Williams, J. S., Schwartzbaum, A. M. and Ganey, R. F. eds. *Sociological Research Symposium V.* Richmond, Va: Virginia Commonwealth University Press, 1975.

Binner, P. Program evaluation. In: Feldman, S. ed. *The Administration of Mental Health Services.* Springfield, Ill.: Charles C. Thomas, 1973.

Cartwright, D. and Zander, A. *Group Dynamics: Research and Theory.* New York: Harper and Row, 1968.

Chu, F. D. and Trotter, S. *The Madness Establishment.* New York: Grossman, 1974.

Drucker, P. F. *Management: Tasks, Responsibilities, Practices.* New York: Harper and Row, 1973.

Feldman, S. Educating the future mental health executive—A graduate curriculum. *Administration in Mental Health,* 3: 74–85, 1974.

Gottesfeld, H. Cooperative research in community mental health. *Professional Psychology,* 2: 145–147, 1971.

May, P. R., and Cohen, J. Development operations in mental health delivery systems. *American Journal of Public Health,* 65: 156–160, 1975.

Morrison, J. K. An argument for mental patient advisory boards. *Professional Psychology,* 7: 127–131, 1976.

Morrison, J. K. The client as consumer and evaluator of community mental health services. *American Journal of Community Psychology,* in press.

Morrison, J. K., ed. *A Consumer Approach to Community Psychology.* Chicago: Nelson–Hall, in press.

Morrison, J. K. and Libow, J. A. The effect of newspaper publicity on a mental health center's community visibility. *Community Mental Health Journal,* in press.

Morrison, J. K., Pitchford, B., Dovberg, N. and Smith, F. J. Correspondence of staff-client evaluation of discharge readiness and nontreatment therapeutic events. *Journal of Community Psychology,* in press.

Nelson, R. H. Psychologists in administrative evaluation. *American Psychologist,* 30: 707–708, 1975.

Rich, W. C. Accountability indices: The search for the philosopher's touchstone in mental health. *Administration in Mental Health,* 2: 6–11, 1973.

Romig, D. A Management of research and development in mental health. *Professional Psychology,* 4: 265–269, 1973.

Steger, J. A., Woodhouse, R. and Goocey, R. The clinical manager: Performance and management characteristics. *Administration in Mental Health*, 2: 76–81, 1973.

Zusman, J. and Slawson, M. R. Service quality profile: Development of a technique for measuring quality of mental health services. *Archives of General Psychiatry*, 27, 692–698, 1972.

Correspondence of Staff-Client Evaluations of Discharge Readiness and Non-Treatment Therapeutic Events*

James K. Morrison, Barbara Pitchford, Norman Dovberg, and Frederick J. Smith

THIS STUDY OF discharged psychiatric clients focuses on three relatively unresearched areas in community mental health: (1) the correspondence of staff-client evaluations of discharge readiness; (2) the frequency with which clients seek alternate psychiatric services subsequent to discharge; and (3) the perceived effect of non-treatment therapeutic events (e.g., falling in love, finding a job) on client problem resolution. The study emerged from the current emphasis on the psychiatric client as both consumer and evaluator of services received (Darley, 1974; Denner & Halprin, 1974; Hart & Bassett, 1975; Morrison, 1976; Morrison, in press a; Morrison, in press b).

Method

Participants. Of the forty-two clients (followed by sixteen clinic staff) discharged in a twelve month period from a small commu-

---

*This article was originally published in the *Journal of Community Psychology*, 1977, *5*, 241–245. Reprinted by permission.

nity mental health clinic, a total of twenty-two or 52.4 percent were contacted in a telephone survey. This percentage of clients contacted is surprisingly high (cf. Denner & Halprin, 1974) for such discharge studies. (Two contacted clients were excluded from the study since one did not seem to understand the questions and the other appeared to be answering dishonestly in a way which flattered the staff.)

The twenty clients contacted, tended to be primarily female ($n = 14$), relatively young ($M = 31.9$ yrs.), without a history of previous psychiatric hospitalization ($n = 15$), and to be discharged with the approval of their clinicians ($n = 15$). These clients had been discharged from the clinic on the average of 4.4 months when followup contact was made. The contacted and non-contacted groups did not significantly differ on any of the above-mentioned variables except "termination against staff advice" (see Discussion).

Of the twenty clients who could not be reached, ten apparently no longer had telephones, four had moved out of the area, two were institutionalized (one in a hospital and one in jail) at the time contacts were attempted, and four were telephoned repeatedly without success.

Telephone survey questionnaire. Three interviewers asked clients (by telephone) and staff (in face-to-face interviews) the following questions:

1. "At our clinic, the policy is to discharge clients when they are able to take care of their problems pretty well by themselves. Do you think you were ready to leave the agency when you were discharged?" (Questions asked of staff referred to client discharge, client nontherapeutic events, etc.)
2. "Sometimes what really makes a difference in solving problems is something that happens outside the clinic. (For instance, getting a job, moving to a nicer place, falling in love, or other things.) We're wondering if anything important like that happened to you *while* you were still coming to the clinic?"
3. "Would you say that this (these) event(s) made more of a difference in helping you to resolve your problems than any help you got from the clinic?"
4. "May I ask you if you have gone to any other psychiatric agency or professional for help since you left the clinic?"

Both staff and clients were asked to respond to each question with either "yes," "no," or "not sure." This response mode was favored over a rating scale since, in the experience of the staff, a large percentage of the clinic's clients had difficulty with such a response mode.

Procedure. A list was prepared of all discharges from a community mental health clinic in the course of a twelve month period. Three telephone interviewers (a school psychologist, a third year resident, and a clinical psychology intern) selected from the list those clients whom they did not know personally and proceeded to call each client during the next three months. If, after three attempts, a client was not contacted at the known telephone number, his/her name was eliminated from the active survey list. (When more than one call was necessary, the second and third calls were made at different times of the day—including at least one evening call—and on different days.)

In introducing themselves, the telephone callers identified themselves, encouraged the clients to be honest in their evaluations, and assured them of the confidentiality of their evaluations.*

If the clients agreed (and all did), they were then asked the four questions listed earlier. The responses were then coded by number and these coded responses were given to the senior author for analysis. A similar procedure was followed with each of the clinician-advisors.

Results

Before analyzing the respondents' answers to the four survey questions, one must ask whether the twenty contacted clients are a truly representative sample of the clinic's clients. Some researchers (Denner & Halprin, 1974) have indicated, for example, that clients who initiate termination on their own, without the agreement of the therapist, may be underrepresented among clients contacted in telephone surveys. Indeed, the data suggest that such self-terminating clients are underrepresented in the contacted group. There were almost twice as many self-terminating clients in the non-contacted group ($n = 9$) as in the contacted group ($n = 5$).

Related to client readiness for discharge (Question 1), the majority of both clients ($n = 18$) and advisors ($n = 15$) thought that the clients were ready for discharge. In fifteen of the twenty

---

*The complete wording of this introductory statement is available upon request from the senior author.

cases both clients and advisors concurred, and, according to analysis by means of the Sign Test, this concordance of ratings was significant ($Z = 2.02$, $p < .025$).

Related to Question 2, in a minority yet sizeable number of cases, both clients ($n = 8$) and advisors ($n = 7$) judged a non-treatment therapeutic event to have occurred. Again there was significant agreement ($Z = 2.02$, $p < .025$), according to the Sign Test, between client and advisor related to the occurrence of such events. In fifteen of twenty cases clients and advisors agreed. The eight clients who reported non-treatment therapeutic events were asked a further question (No. 3) regarding the comparative effectiveness of such events. Although the number of clients responding to this question was too small for statistical analysis, we can report that two of these clients rated such non-clinic events as more effective than clinic services in inducing problem resolution. Furthermore, there was 80 percent (four of five cases) agreement between client and advisor about the effectiveness of such events in inducing problem resolution.

Finally, the majority ($n = 16$) of discharged clients who were contacted reported that they had not contracted psychiatric services from other agencies since they left the clinic (Question 4). Of the four who had contracted such services, two had actually been referred to these other agencies by their advisors. Also related to this question, there was a high degree of agreement (sixteen of twenty cases) in ratings by client and advisor, and this concordance reached significance ($Z = 2.47$, $p < .01$), according to the Sign Test.

Discussion

Before discussing the results of this study, it is worth repeating that the twenty non-contacted discharged clients were different from the twenty contacted clients in that a greater proportion of the former had initiated discharge on their own without initial agreement by the advisor. This finding is in agreement with that of Denner & Halprin (1974). We concur with these researchers that such findings suggest that favorable ratings by contacted clients in discharge studies may be somewhat inflated in a positive direction.

It is imperative that community mental health clinics determine the degree of agreement between advisors and their clients related to the readiness of the latter for discharge. If either party disagrees, the termination may be unproductive and/or unpleasant. Most of the clients contacted in this study apparently felt they were ready for discharge. Furthermore, clients and staff were mostly in agreement about the decision to discharge. The reported readiness for discharge is further corroborated by our finding that only 10 percent of the discharged clients (the same percentage reported by Powell, Shaw, & O'Neal, 1971) sought other psychiatric services on their own. Even considering the relatively short average period of time ($M = 4.43$ mos.) between discharge and followup contact, it is still quite unexpected that staff would be 80 percent correct in estimating which clients had and had not contracted psychiatric services elsewhere. Perhaps our staff are so knowledgeable of discharged clients' psychiatric transactions because our agency is situated in a relatively small city (approximately eighteen thousand citizens) and thus agency staff tend to know the life situations of former clients relatively well.

Although Denner and Halprin (1974) indicated that 33 percent of the clients they surveyed reported non-clinic events to be more determinant of change than clinic treatment, they did not specify the percentage of discharged clients who felt non-treatment events were actually therapeutic. Our results revealed that 40 percent of the discharged clients in this study reported non-treatment events which are therapeutic. The staff of the clinic again appeared to be quite knowledgeable as to whether there have been non-treatment events which they (and the clients as well) perceived as therapeutic. Furthermore, there was agreement among clients and staff as to whether or not these events were more effective than clinic services in leading to client problem resolution. If, as these results would suggest, events that both client and advisor perceive as therapeutic occur with some frequency apart from formal clinic services, this may represent another treatment-effectiveness variable in need of further investigation.

In order to ascertain more information about the discharged clients, the staff decided to check with the only hospital in the county with a psychiatric ward to see if any of the study's discharged clients had been admitted to that ward for any length of time following termination. While none of the twenty contacted clients had been so hospitalized since discharge, two of the twenty non-contacted clients had. We also learned that two of the twenty non-contacted clients committed suicide in the two months after the survey study had been completed. This finding, discovered outside of the original limits of the survey, suggests that we may learn more about our services, and their effect (or lack of effect) on clients, by making more concerted attempts (e.g., more telephone calls, mailed questionnaires) to reach those clients who are difficult to contact. Unless we do, we may not receive a very accurate picture of how well (or poorly) such clients are integrated in the community after discharge.

In summary, this study revealed that there was a high degree of concordance between staff and discharged clients related to readiness for discharge, the occurrence and comparative effectiveness of non-treatment therapeutic events, and the frequency with which clients sought psychiatric services elsewhere after discharge. Moreover, two areas in need of further investigation emerge from the present study: (1) the effect of staff-client disagreement about discharge readiness on client problem resolution after discharge; and (2) the role of non-treatment therapeutic events on client problem resolution.

References

Darley, P. J. Who shall hold the conch? Some thoughts on community control of mental health programs. *Community Mental Health Journal*, 1974, *10*, 185–191.

Denner, B., & Halprin, F. Measuring consumer satisfaction in a community outpost. *American Journal of Community Psychology*, 1974, *2*, 13–22.

Hart, W. T., & Bassett, L. Measuring consumer satisfaction in a mental health center. *Hospital and Community Psychiatry*, 1975, *26*, 512–515.

Morrison, J. K. An argument for mental patient advisory boards. *Professional Psychology*, 1976, *7*, 127–131.

Morrison, J. K. (Ed.) *A Consumer Approach to Community Psychology.* Chicago: Nelson-Hall, in press (a).

Morrison, J. K. The client as consumer and evaluator of community mental health services. *American Journal of Community Psychology*, in press (b).

Powell, B. J., Shaw, D., & O'Neal, C. Client evaluation of a clinic's services. *Hospital and Community Psychiatry*, 1971, *22*, 45–46.

Involving the Client-Consumer in the Evaluation of Group Therapy*

James K. Morrison, Judith A. Libow, Robert E. Becker, and Frederick J. Smith

ALTHOUGH BEDNAR & Lawlis (1971) have emphasized the serious need for group psychotherapy research focusing on the relationship of process variables (e.g., therapist style) to therapeutic outcome (e.g., problem resolution), such research has not been reported. The absence of such research is at least partially explained by the fact that available outcome measures tend to be global, nonindividualized, and unsuitable to the task (Bednar & Lawlis, 1971).

The typical approach of *outcome* research is to compare the effectiveness of a therapy group with either that of a no-treatment control group (Pattison, Brissenden & Wohl, 1967; Kraus, 1959) or with that of individual treatment (Baehr, 1954; O'Brien, Hamm, Ray, Pierce, Luborsky & Mintz, 1972). As is generally true

*Reprinted in expanded form, with permission of the publisher, from the original: Morrison, J.K., Libow, J.A., Smith, F.J., and Becker, R.E. Comparative effectiveness of directive vs. nondirective group therapist style on client problem resolution. *Journal of Clinical Psychology*, 1978, *34*, 186–187.

of outcome research, however, such studies do not specify or quantify particular therapeutic factors responsible for the observed changes. While *process* research has attempted to more closely examine and compare the effects of certain variables (e.g., therapy style, Singer & Goldman, 1954; Rogerian facilitative conditions, Truax, 1961), such approaches can be challenged in that the dependent measures used are often irrelevant to the problems which the group members present. As emphasized by Paul (1969) and Bednar & Lawlis (1971), there is a serious need in group research to directly relate process variables to therapeutic outcome so that both can be better understood.

One of the persistent problems plaguing research on group as well as individual psychotherapy is that of developing truly meaningful outcome measures. Most available studies have relied on the measurement of rather general, nonindividualized and nonbehavioral changes in group participants. For example, such changes have previously been defined as: improved ratings of client or therapist satisfaction (Beutler, Jobe & Elkins, 1974; Sechrest & Barger, 1961); overall improvement (O'Brien, Hamm, Ray, Pierce, Luborsky & Mintz, 1972); pre-post changes on standardized personality tests (Jeske, 1973) and adjustment, as in perceived social competence (McLachlan, 1974), or self-reported discontent (Baehr, 1954). While some individualized measures (e.g., Q-sorts, Pattison, Brissenden & Wohl, 1967; repertory grids, Watson, 1972) have recently been developed, measures of individual problematic behaviors have traditionally been restricted to ratings or judgments of inpatient ward behaviors by hospital staff (Bednar & Lawlis, 1971).

In this study we have decided to use self-report measures of problem resolution. This investigation differs methodologically from most group therapy studies in that an Equivalent Time-Samples Design (Campbell & Stanley, 1963) was used. The same group and leaders alternately and repeatedly experienced each of the two styles over time, allowing a comparison of therapeutic results which eliminates many of the problems associated with differences between individual members and group leaders. Such research follows the recommendation of Paul (1969) that research specify the treatment, therapists, specific problems under investigation, circumstances, and process of therapy.

Although previous research (Abramowitz, Abramowitz, Roback & Jackson, 1974) has focused on the differential effect of directive versus nondirective therapist styles as a function of internal-external locus of control, no previous research has studied the effect of such different styles on client problem resolution. Thus, no hypotheses can be formulated with any confidence, and therefore this study must be considered a pilot study.

Method

Subjects. Five females and three males, with a mean age of 26.0 years, and a mean formal educational level of 13.6 years, served as subjects in this study. All eight clients reported experiencing problems commonly referred to as "neurotic." None of the clients had been previously hospitalized for psychiatric reasons and none of the clients were taking psychotropic medication during the course of group therapy. The clients attended a mean number of 24.9 sessions (range from 18 to 36).

Self-report measures. The two measures employed in this study were: (1) *Individualized Problem Resolution Checklist* (IPRC), a reliable* self-report list of those problems, formulated by the clients, for which they expect some problem resolution through group therapy. After listing such problems (e.g., anxiety when conversing with members of the opposite sex; inability to express appropriate anger) each client rated on a six point scale ("completely resolved" to "completely unresolved") the degree to which the problem was resolved (or unresolved). (2) *Interpersonal Improvement* Scale (IIS), a reliable** 17 item standardized list of common interpersonal problems (e.g., "fear of confronting someone with whom I disagree strongly"; "a sense of discomfort around people of the opposite sex") for which clients rate resolution on the same six-point scale. Both measures were developed by the senior author.

Procedure. In an attempt to study the differential effect of group process on therapeutic outcome, two therapist styles were utilized: *directive* (therapists controlled flow of discussion, and pointed out clients' problems), and *nondirective* (clients controlled flow of discussion and presented problems to be resolved). Therapist styles were alternated every eight weeks for 48 weeks.

The clients involved in group therapy over 48 weeks were administered the IPRC and IIS repeatedly at eight-week intervals

---

*Test-retest reliability coefficient of .89, $p < .01$, $n = 19$, over 8 weeks.
**Test-retest reliability coefficient of .74, $p < .01$ $n = 20$, over 8 weeks.

over 48 weeks, and then on followup eight weeks after treatment was terminated. Clients were admitted to group at different points during the 48 weeks; two clients finished group after the thirty-eighth and thirty-ninth sessions, respectively, after reaching high problem resolution; one client left group after the thirty-fifth session because her job situation precluded further attendance.

Results

In order to first determine an overall treatment effect, one-way repeated analyses of variance were performed on the data. Results indicated that, ignoring the effect of therapist style, group therapy treatment appeared to significantly improve problem resolution over time, as reflected in ratings on the IPRC, F (5,18) $= 4.15$, $p < .05$, and on the IIS, F (5.18) $= 307.60$, $p < .001$. Analyses by means of t-tests did not reveal significant differences between IPRC and IIS scores at the end of treatment (48 weeks) and those on an eight-week followup, suggesting that the treatment effect was stable.

Related to the differential effect of therapy style on outcome, one-way repeated analyses of variance revealed that the nondirective style produced significantly more positive change on the IIS than did the directive style, F (1,18) $= 22.90$, $p < .01$. The data supplied by the IPRC did not indicate significant outcome differences for the two styles.

Discussion

The data analyses support the utility of both instruments (IPRC and IIS) in their ability to measure selected effects of group therapy over time. One measure, the IIS, also seems useful in determining the comparative effectiveness of two different therapy styles on interpersonal problem resolution.

Although only tentative conclusions can be drawn from such a limited study, the results at least suggest that the IPRC and IIS may offer future researchers of group therapy more effective ways of measuring group process and outcome. Furthermore, one of these instruments, the IPRC, reflects the emerging philosophy of client consumerism (Morrison, in press) in that clients are encouraged to define their problems in their own words. Too often we have forced client-consumers to artificially define their problems in our terminology, or not at all. Such clinician-defined problems may account for our frustrating efforts at demonstrating group therapy effectiveness.

Further research, employing controls and different, larger samples, is obviously indicated to test the usefulness of the measures used in this study, as well as to determine the validity of our conclusions on group therapy effectiveness and the greater effectiveness of a nondirective approach. Such research is now being planned.

References

Abramowitz, C. V., Abramowitz, S. I., Roback, H. B., & Jackson, C. Differential effectiveness of directive and nondirective group therapies as a function of client I-E Control. *Journal of Consulting Clinical Psychology*, 1974, *42*, 849–853.

Baehr, G. The comparative effectiveness of individual psychotherapy, group psychotherapy and a combination of these methods. *Journal of Consulting Psychology*, 1954, *18*, 179–183.

Bednar, R. L., & Lawlis, G. F. Empirical research in group psychotherapy. In A. E. Berger and S. L. Garfield, *Psychotherapy and behavior change: An empirical analysis.* New York: John Wiley and Sons, 1971.

Beutler, L. E., Jobe, A. M., and Elkins, D. Outcomes in group psychotherapy: Using persuasion theory to increase treatment efficiency. *Journal of Consulting and Clinical Psychology*, 1974, *42*, 547–553.

Campbell, D. T., & Stanley, J. C. *Experimental and quasi-experimental designs for research.* Chicago: Rand McNally Publishing Co., 1963.

Jeske, J. O. Identification and therapeutic effectiveness in group therapy. *Journal of Counseling Psychology*, 1973, *20*, 528–530.

Kraus, A. R. Experimental study of the effect of group psychotherapy with chronic psychotic patients. *International Journal Group Psychotherapy*, 1959, *9*, 293–302.

McLachlan, J. F. Social competence and response to group therapy. *Journal of Community Psychology*, 1974, *2*, 248–250.

Morrison, J. K. The client as consumer and evaluator of community mental health services. *American Journal of Community Psychology*, in press.

O'Brien, C., Hamm, K., Ray, B., Pierce, J., Luborsky, L., & Mintz, J. Group versus individual psychotherapy with schizophrenics. *Archives of General Psychiatry*, 1972, *27*, 474.

Pattison, M. E., Brissenden, A., & Wohl, T. Assessing specific effects of in-patient group psychotherapy. *International Journal of Group Psychotherapy*, 1967, *17*, 283–297.

Paul, G. L. Behavior modification research: Design and tactics. In C. M.

Franks (Ed.). *Behavior therapy: Appraisal and status.* New Jersey: McGraw-Hill, 1969.

Sechrest, L. B., & Barger, B. Verbal participation and perceived benefit from group therapy. *International Journal of Group Psychotherapy,* 1961, *11,* 49–59.

Singer, J., & Goldman, G. Experimentally contrasted social atmospheres in group psychotherapy with chronic schizophrenics. *Journal of Social Psychology,* 1954, *40,* 23–37.

Truax, C. B. The process of group psychotherapy: Relationships between hypothesized therapeutic conditions and intrapersonal exploration. *Psychological Monographs,* 1961, *75,* 1–35.

Watson, J. P. Possible measures of change during group psychotherapy. *British Journal of Medical Psychiatry,* 1972, *45,* 71–77.

Emotive-Reconstructive Therapy and Client Problem Resolution: Periodic Accountability to the Consumer

James K. Morrison and Michael S. Cometa*

THIS STUDY IS an initial attempt to empirically determine the effectiveness of a newly developed therapeutic modality, i.e., emotive-reconstructive therapy.[11] Deriving from the theoretical postulates of cognitive theory[1,8,12] emotive-reconstructive therapy (ERT) emphasizes intrapersonal variations in levels of RAS arousal,[5,6,10] as well as a reconstructive model of human memory.[2,13] A client is viewed as an active organism constantly engaged in monitoring and interpreting experiences so as to predict events with sufficient accuracy to maintain an "optimal level of arousal."[6]

Through short-term, time limited (fifteen sessions) therapy, within which the therapist employs a series of techniques (extensive use of imagery; brief periods of selective hyperventilation; role-playing; confrontation) combined in a standard sequence by the senior author, clients learn to construe themselves and signifi-

*The authors would like to gratefully acknowledge the assistance of Ms. Susan Holdridge-Crane in obtaining the reliability data for the PPC.

cant others in a different and more self-consonant manner. Primarily via visual imagery, clients sensorially recreate early anxiety-arousing events (thus facilitating the memory of those events), and, at the direction of the therapist, examine a wide range of anxiety-arousing states (e.g., anger, fear, and so on) which they as children could neither define nor understand. Clients in ERT are induced to re-experience early stress events primarily so that they can use an adult's more elaborated construct system in order to more fully comprehend the meaning of their interaction with others in the developmental years (especially years four to eight). (The generation of this type of understanding appears to reduce the anxiety clients experience when they find they cannot adequately predict their own and others' behavior. Clarifying their styles of early interaction appears to greatly facilitate clients' understanding of how their current styles of interaction have led to frustration and a series of life problems.

As critics[3,4] of psychotherapy research have pointed out, rater (often the therapists themselves) bias in estimating therapy outcome may account for the high success rates reported by the proponents of certain styles of therapy. Furthermore, in most reports of therapy effectiveness, one frequently gains the impression that "client's increased insight" is at times the only reported positive change. This study attempts to overcome these problems by having the client-consumers themselves, during the course of therapy, regularly evaluate how well they have resolved their problems (among which "lack of insight" is not included). Client reports of therapy outcome are probably more reliable and less biased than therapist ratings, as one study[7] has indicated.

Through the specification and standardization of techniques which contribute to ERT, a number of advantages are made possible. First, ERT has the advantage of being more easily studied through empirical research than are many other forms of individual therapy. Consonant with Strupp and Bergin's[15] suggested research question (i.e., what specific therapeutic interventions produce specific changes in which type of clients and under which specific conditions?), ERT's specification and standardization of techniques enable a researcher to more easily sort out the differential effect of therapist variables and of techniques than do many traditional and less defined therapeutic modalities. A second advantage of ERT is its suitability in answering the present demands of the client-consumer. Following Strupp's[14] call for the right of client-consumers to be able to understand precisely what therapeutic service they are contracting, ERT is explained in detail to clients before therapy and a specific contract drawn up delineating, by means of a behavior checklist, which problems are targeted for change. The specification and standardization of ERT techniques seem to facilitate pretherapy description of ERT, as well as the contracting process itself.

The senior author, who acted as the sole therapist in this study, decided before the study that, for ERT to be a truly effective therapeutic modality, it ought to be effective with a wide range of clients. Furthermore, ERT should compare favorably with the high success rates (89 percent) reported by proponents of other therapeutic modalities.[9,16] Finally, to take a step further than proponents of therapy previously have, the senior author decided to arbitrarily establish a problem resolution rate of 50 percent as a minimum success criterion for determining the extent to which ERT constitutes an effective, alternate therapeutic modality. Thus, it was predicted that ERT would not only produce a significant reduction in client-reported problems, but would further reflect a minimum reduction of 50 percent of the problems which clients, as a group, experienced.

Method

Subjects. Fourteen clients (7 male and 7 female), with a mean age of 30.1 years and a mean education of 14.1 years, completed 15 sessions of ERT within a time limited period (approximately 4 months). In terms of standard diagnostic nomenclature, the group was composed of 7 neurotics, 5 character disorders, and 2 psychotics. The number of clients with other profile characteristics were as follows: (a) marital status (6 single, 6 married, 2 separated); (b) previous psychiatric hospitalization ($n = 7$); (c) social class differences (10 middle class, 4 lower class). In view of these factors, we feel comfortable in asserting that the clients came from varied populations and were, as a group, less than ideal in terms of traditional standards[3] for success in individual therapy. (For example, diagnostic predictions for 50 percent—2 psychotics and 5 character disorders—of the subjects suggest that individual therapy is not likely to be highly successful.)

Instrument. The *Psychotherapy Problem Checklist* (PPC) is a reliable (test-retest reliability coefficient of .81, p <.001, N = 15, over 5 weeks), self-report measure of client problem resolution developed by the senior author. The checklist consists of 21 items which are easily identified as problems (e.g., frequent headaches, excessive anxiety, insomnia, suicidal ideation, and so on). The PPC is scored by assigning a score of 1 for each problem/symptom designated by the client. Thus, the maximum score is 21; the minimum score, 0.

Procedure. Each client was administered 15 (one hour a week) sessions of ERT. The basic structure of each session was similar for all the clients due to the standard approach to early events, and to the systematic application of techniques in a specified order. The PPC was administered to clients before therapy, and, subsequently, after the fifth, tenth, and fifteenth sessions. Clients were encouraged to report problems honestly so that the responses could assist the therapist in his therapeutic efforts. The purpose of the multiple administrations was to provide sufficient data to allow a more detailed analysis of the progressive effect of ERT during the course of each client's treatment.

Results

Table 1 indicates the means, standard deviations, and test phase comparison t-scores derived from client scores on the ERPC.

Table 1
Means, Standard Deviations, and Test-phase Comparison t-scores
Derived from Client ERPC Scores
(n = 14)

Test	Phase	Mean	S.D.	Test-phase Comparisons	t-score
I	Pretest	11.29	4.05	I vs. II	3.73*
II	After 5	7.71	4.21	II vs. III	0.77
III	After 10	6.71	4.48	III vs. IV	4.06*
IV	After 15	4.00	3.33	I vs. IV	5.80**

*p<.005
**p<.0005

Of primary interest is the comparison of client problem resolution before and after therapy. Comparing therapy phases I and IV, analysis indicates that clients report a significant problem resolution during the course of therapy, as reflected in their pre-post treatment scores on the PPC. Two other comparisons of relevance (Phases I–II; III–IV) revealed further significant problem reduction after the first (sessions 1–5) and last (sessions 10–15) five-session periods of ERT. The other comparison (Phase II–III) indicated that the problem reduction between session 5 and session 10 did not attain significance.

The percentage of group problem resolution was obtained by dividing the number of pretherapy problems into the number of problems reduced during the course of therapy (Phase I to Phase IV). Results indicated that the fourteen clients had, as a group, resolved 64.6 percent of their PPC reported problems during the 15 ERT sessions. Seventy-one percent of the clients experienced a minimum reduction of 50 percent of their PPC problems. All clients reported a problem reduction of at least 30 percent, and in no instance did a client's problems increase from Phase I to Phase IV. Thus, results indicate that 93 percent of the therapy group report a minimum reduction of 30 percent of problems reported on the PPC. Considering the severity of problems listed on the PPC, these figures suggest more than superficial, positive change.

Discussion

The results of this study indicate the effectiveness of emotive-reconstructive therapy in reducing client problems, as defined by the PPC. As reflected in our predictions, ERT reduced more than 50 percent of the therapy group's problems, suggesting that this therapeutic modality offers promise as a short-term therapy.

Examination of each of the three five-session (or five week) periods revealed that significant problem reduction occurred during the first and last five-session periods. It remains to be explained why there was no significant problem reduction in the middle phase (sessions 5–10) of therapy. One can speculate that clients experience some immediate symptom relief during the first five sessions and that they are not as highly motivated, for a period of time (middle period of therapy), to engage as thoroughly in this high-anxiety-arousing therapy. Therefore, since their problems are only superficially resolved at this early stage of therapy, lack of therapy involvement may induce the client to fall back into prior, unproductive lifestyles. At some point after session 10, such clients again appear to seriously engage in the process of problem resolution as their fifteen-session contract is about to expire. The validity of this explanation will become clearer as more clients have the opportunity to engage in ERT, thus providing a larger sample for analysis.

We contend that therapists should examine the number of dropouts from any course of a particular therapy, to gain further evidence of the usefulness of a therapeutic modality. Of the 36 persons who began ERT, 22 (or 61 percent)did not finish the 15 sessions for a variety of reasons (e.g., lack of immediate symptom relief; relocation to another area; early symptom relief with consequent "flight into health"; high anxiety related to coming sessions). As a group these 22 clients completed a mean of 4.4 sessions. The rather high dropout rate is understandable considering the large percentage (62 percent) of clients in this group with a diagnosis of character disorder and psychosis.

We place considerable importance on the need to test a promising therapy on a group of clients who are less than ideal for therapy. There is an urgent need to develop effective therapeutic techniques for that vast population of individuals whose problems are not amenable to standard methods of therapy.[3] We feel that our initial findings offer some guarded optimism that ERT may be effective even with those less educated clients, with diagnoses of psychosis or character disorder, who are motivated to complete the 15 sessions of ERT.

We do not contend that our present research is sufficient to clearly demonstrate the effectiveness of ERT. A larger sample of clients, control groups, and different measures of change are all needed. Research, already in progress, employing control groups, and extensive one-year followup studies of all clients who have received ERT, may provide more substantial and clearer evidence of this therapy's effectiveness. Furthermore, we will be employing different measures of personality and behavior change in order to corroborate the findings of this study.

References

1. Bannister, D., & Fransella, F. *Inquiring Man: The Theory of Personal Constructs*. Baltimore, Md.: Penguin Books, 1971.
2. Bartlett, F. C. *Remembering*. Cambridge, England: Cambridge University Press, 1932.
3. Bergin, A. E. Some Implications of Psychotherapy Research For Therapeutic Practice. *Journal of Abnormal Psychology*, 1966, 71, 235–246.
4. Breger, L., & McGaugh, J. L. Critique and Reformulation of "Learning-Theory" Approaches To Psychotherapy and Neurosis. *Psychological Bulletin*, 1965, 63, 338–358.

5. Dember, W. N. The New Look in Motivation. *American Scientist,* 1965, 53, 409–427.
6. Fiske, D., & Maddi, S. *Functions of Varied Experience.* Homewood, Ill.: Dorsey Press, 1961.
7. Horenstein, D., Houston, B. K., & Holmes, D. S. Clients', Therapists', and Judges' Evaluations of Psychotherapy. *Journal of Counseling Psychology,* 1973, 20, 149–153.
8. Kelly, G. *The Psychology of Personal Constructs.* (2 Vols.) New York: Norton Co., 1955.
9. Lazarus, A. A. An Evaluation of Behavior Therapy. *Behavior Research and Therapy,* 1963, 1, 69–79.
10. Mancuso, J. C. Current Motivational Models in the Elaboration of Personal Construct Theory. In A. W. Landfield (Ed.), *Nebraska Symposium on Motivation: Personal Construct Psychology.* Lincoln: University of Nebraska Press, in press.
11. Morrison, J. K. & Cometa, M. S. Emotive-Reconstructive Psychotherapy: A Short Term Cognitive Approach. *American Journal of Psychotherapy,* in press.
12. Piaget, J. *Structuralism.* New York: Harper, 1970.
13. Singer, J. L. *Imagery and Daydream Methods in Psychotherapy and Behavior Modification.* New York: Academic Press, 1974.
14. Strupp, H. H. On Failing One's Patient. *Psychotherapy: Theory, Research and Practice,* 1975, 12, 39–41.
15. Strupp, H. H., & Bergin, A. E. Some Empirical and Conceptual Bases For Coordinated Research in Psychotherapy: A Critical Review of Issues, Trends, and Evidence. *International Journal of Psychiatry,* 1969, 7, 18–90.
16. Wolpe, J. Behavior Therapy in Complex Neurotic States. *British Journal of Psychiatry,* 1964, 110, 28–34.

Client and Therapist Ratings of the Differential Effectiveness of Clinic Services on Problem Resolution

James K. Morrison, Frederick J. Smith,
Barbara Pitchford, and Norman Dovberg

THE PURPOSE OF this study is to explore a new area of clinical research—the differential effectiveness of various community mental health services on client problem resolution. Although recently we have witnessed the proliferation of studies (Denner & Halprin, 1974; Hart & Bassett, 1975; Ishiyama, 1970; Kotin & Schur, 1969; Mayer & Rosenblatt, 1974; Powell, Shaw & Slawson, 1972) focusing on the client-consumer's view of mental health services, we know of no studies which purport to determine client-therapist ratings of the differential impact of the various treatments on client problem resolution. Although a number of studies suggest that community mental health services can be effective, there is at present a great need to determine which services are most and least effective. In this era of accountability to the consumer (Morrison, 1976), mental health professionals can no longer postpone the issue of whether much time and effort may be wasted on some therapeutic modalities which are only minimally effective in helping clients resolve their problems.

As pointed out elsewhere (Morrison, Pitchford, Dovberg & Smith, in press), it no longer makes sense to solicit either the clinician's or the client's opinion alone of the therapeutic effectiveness of certain services. Both judgments are of value and each may complement the other. For example, while therapists may overestimate (Horenstein, Houston & Holmes, 1973) treatment effectiveness, it is also reasonable that some clients may underestimate such effectiveness, thus suggesting that the truth may lie somewhere between both judgments.

Method

Subjects. Of the 42 clients (followed by 16 clinic staff) discharged in a twelve month period from a small community mental health clinic, a total of 22 or 52.4 percent were contacted in a telephone survey. This percentage of clients contacted is surprisingly high (cf. Denner & Halpren, 1974) for such discharge studies. (Two contacted clients were excluded since one did not seem to understand the questions and the other appeared to be answering dishonestly in a way which flattered the staff.) The demographic characteristics of the 20 clients who were included in the analysis, as well as those of the 20 who could not be contacted, can be found in an earlier report (Morrison, Pitchford, Dovberg & Smith, in press). Briefly, both groups tended to be primarily female, young ($M = 32.4$ years), without history of previous hospitalization, and to have been discharged a mean of four months before the survey.

Of the 20 clients who could not be reached, 10 apparently no longer had telephones, 4 had moved out of the area, 2 were institutionalized (in a hospital and jail) at the time contacts were attempted, and 4 were telephoned repeatedly without success.

Table 1 presents the number and percentage of contacted[1] discharged clients each receiving five categories of services. As indicated in this table most (80 percent) clients received some form of individual therapy.

Telephone survey questionnaire. Three interviewers asked clients (by telephone) and staff (in face-to-face interviews) the following questions:

1. Even if you were not completely satisfied with the help you got from our agency, did the agency help you even a little bit? (If the answer was negative, the interviewer then stated: "We'd be interested in finding out why you think things didn't work out when you came to the agency so we won't make the same mistakes again." Comments were noted.[2])

Table 1
Number and Percentage of Discharged Clients (n = 20)
Receiving Each of Five Categories of Services

Service Category	N	Percentage
1. Psychopharmocologic agents	7	35
2. Group therapy	11	55
3. Individual therapy	16	80
4. Ancillary programs	9	45
5. Advocacy assistance	7	35

2. (A list of services given to each client was read.) Which service do you think helped you the most to solve your problems?

3. Which service do you think helped the least in helping you solve your problems?

Both staff and clients were asked to respond to all three questions.[3] The wording of the questions was simplified to ensure that the less intelligent clients would comprehend the questions.

Procedure. A list was prepared of all discharges from a community mental health clinic during a 12 month period. (Clients who moved out of the clinic's catchment area and were thus subsequently transferred to another mental health facility, as well as clients who appeared only for an intake interview, were excluded from the survey.) Three telephone interviewers (a school psychologist, a third year psychiatric resident, and a clinical psychology intern), all unknown to the discharged clients, selected from the list those clients whom they did not know personally and proceeded to call each client during the next three months. If, after three attempts, a client was not contacted at the known telephone number, his/her name was eliminated from the active survey list. (When more than one call was necessary, the second and third calls were made at different times of the day—including at least one evening call—and on different days.)

In introducing himself, the telephone caller read the following to the client from an instruction sheet:

Hello. This is _____. The director (name provided) of the clinic has asked me to call all the people discharged in the last 12 months—about 50 people—to find out what they honestly feel about our clinic. If you will just take about three minutes, I'd like to ask your opinion of the clinic. This information will help the clinic to do a better job in the future. You can feel free to criticize as much as you need to. Everything you say will be held in strictest confidence. I will not tell anyone else who said what. Okay?

If the clients agreed (and all did), they were then asked the three questions listed earlier. The responses were then coded by number and these coded responses were given to the senior author for analysis. A similar procedure was followed with each of the advisors.

Results

Analysis of the data supplied by the three questions were analyzed with the Sign Test to determine the agreement between clients and therapists. The data supplied by respondents to question one indicated that clients ($n = 20$) and their therapists ($n = 20$) significantly ($Z = 3.36$, $p < .0005$) concurred in their judgments that the clinic had been at least minimally effective in inducing client problem resolution. Ninety percent of both clients and therapists attributed to the clinic some impact on client problem resolution.

Related to question two (most effective service?), analysis of the data indicated significant ($Z = 2.06$, $p < .025$) agreement between clients ($n = 15$) and their therapists ($n = 15$) related to the maximally effective service. (Note that in 5 cases only one service had been rendered, and thus the question could not be meaningfully asked.)

Finally, related to the responses to question three (least effective service?), analysis of the data indicated that the judgments of clients ($n = 14$) and therapists ($n = 14$) did not significantly concur.

Discussion

The analysis of the data indicated that clients and their therapists seem to share similar judgments that the clinic had been helpful, at least minimally, in client problem resolution. The ten percent of the sample's clients who did not feel the clinic was the least bit helpful related to problem resolution, compares well with the eleven percent in Denner and Halprin's (1974) study who expressed dissatisfaction with clinic services.

It is also of great significance that therapists and clients agreed on the service—when there was more than one—which helped the most. There appeared to be less agreement related to the minimally effective service.

It would be important at this point to focus on which services clients and therapists judged to be most and least effective. Even though our sample size is small, the data may at least raise some interesting questions.

Table 2 presents the percentages of clients and therapists who felt which of five categories of services were most and least effective. Of the clients who received more than one service and also

Table 2
Percentage of Clients and Therapists Rating each Service Category Most and Least Effective

	Most Effective		Least Effective	
	Clients	Therapists	Clients	Therapists
Service Category	(n = 15)	(n = 15)	(n = 14)	(n = 14)
1. Psychopharmocologic agents	0.0	16.7	40.0	40.0
2. Group therapy	36.4	36.4	30.0	10.0
3. Individual therapy	66.7*	60.0*	14.5	28.6
4. Ancillary programs	0.0	0.0	62.5*	75.0*
5. Advocacy assistant	14.3	14.3	33.3	16.7

*Largest percentage in most and least effective categories.

felt the clinic helped clients at least a little, 66.7 percent felt individual psychotherapy was the most effective service, 36.4 percent judged group psychotherapy most effective, and 14.3 percent deemed advocacy assistance to be most effective. As also indicated in Table 2, the percentages of therapists judging which services were most effective were quite similar to the percentages of clients. However, there was a slight tendency for therapists to overestimate the effectiveness of psychopharmocologic agents (e.g., Thorazine, Valium, and so on), but to underestimate the effectiveness of individual therapy.

Related to those services which clients felt to be the least effective, the service rated as having the least impact (by 62.5 percent of clients receiving at least one of those services) were ancillary programs (e.g., social club, adult basic education program, and so on). A similar percentage (75.0 percent) of therapists judged those (n = 9) of their clients in ancillary programs to have benefited least by those programs as compared to any of the other four service categories.

Overall, there was 80 percent agreement between therapists and their clients as to the most effective clinic service, and 57.1 percent agreement between the same groups as to the least effective service. Although the latter agreement was not statistically significant, it is still rather high.

Considering both client and therapist judgments of the most effective clinic services, it would appear that individual and group therapy warrant the most expenditure of time and energy, at least for clients similar to those in our study. Other services (medication, ancillary programs, and advocacy assistance) may be often only marginally effective and thus may not warrant the amount of time many clinicians devote to such services. However, the staff of each clinic must draw their own conclusions related to their own particular clients and types of treatment. Most importantly, clinical staff should take into consideration what clients perceive to be the most effective service. Granted, clients can be wrong and clinicians will at times want to overlook their opinions. But if clinicians never solicit such opinions, one might indeed question whether such staff are afraid to hear what the clients have to say.

Notes

1. It should be noted that the contacted discharge group is not typical of the clinic caseload in the services they received. For example, 70 percent of the client population are clients discharged from state mental hospitals and usually receive medication and advocacy services more frequently, and individual therapy less frequently, than the contacted clients in this discharge study.
2. Only two clients responded negatively and both declined to comment.
3. Staff were asked to respond whether the agency helped *clients,* and which services most and least helped clients to resolve problems.

References

Denner, B., & Halprin, F. Measuring consumer satisfaction in a community outpost. *American Journal of Community Psychology,* 1974, *2,* 13–22.

Hart, W. T., & Bassett, L. Measuring consumer satisfaction in a mental health center. *Hospital and Community Psychiatry,* 1975, *26,* 512–515.

Horenstein, D., Houston, B. K., & Holmes, D. S. Clients', therapists', and judges' evaluations of psychotherapy. *Journal of Consulting Psychology,* 1973, *20,* 149–153.

Ishiyama, T. The mental hospital patient-consumer as a determinant of services. *Mental Hygiene*, 1970, *54*, 221–229.

Kotin, J., & Schur, M. Attitudes of discharged mental patients toward their hospital experiences. *Journal of Nervous and Mental Disease*, 1969, *149*, 408–414.

Mayer, J. E., & Rosenblatt, A. Clash in perspective between mental patients and staff. *American Journal of Orthopsychiatry*, 1974, *44*, 432–441.

Morrison, J. K. The client as consumer and evaluator of community mental health services. *American Journal of Community Psychology*, in press.

Morrison, J. K., Pitchford, B., Dovberg, N., & Smith, F. J. Correspondence of staff-client evaluations of discharge readiness and nontreatment therapeutic events. *Journal of Community Psychology*, in press.

Powell, B. J., Shaw, D., & O'Neal, C. Client evaluation of a clinic's services. *Hospital and Community Psychiatry*, 1971, *22*, 45–46.

7

Consumer Independence from Service Providers

Overview

THE ISSUE OF which theoretical model may yield the most benefits to the client consumer is at the heart of this chapter. The first article of chapter three presents a study which was attempted to explore whether a certain conceptual approach (e.g., the antimedical model or radical psychosocial position) might be more effective in inducing client attitudes of independence than another (e.g., medical-model approach). The data indeed suggest that a client's attitudes, assumedly reflecting his or her implicit theoretical approach to psychiatric ideology and practice, do significantly correlate with that client's attitudes of dependence-independence. Specifically, the more a client appears to adopt an antimedical position, the more his attitudes reflect independence from psychiatric caregivers. Such results lend credence to our overall consumer approach which emphasizes the dangers of making clients too dependent on psychiatric professionals. It appears from the data of this study that the medical model approach to psychiatric ideology and practice may in some instances actually foster attitudes of dependence among certain clients.

The second article presents an empirical study designed to operationally demonstrate that inducing psychiatric outpatients to become more independent (e.g., to solve more problems without the help of mental health professionals) can actually have a positive effect on the way clients view themselves, the staff, and their own behavior. Although not mentioned, the staff decision to adopt a different approach to the telephone behavior of clients actually emerged from the clinicians' discouragement with a medical-model approach to clients.

The final article describes how clients can learn various vocational skills which enable them to move in the direction of increased competence, and thus increased independence from psychiatric caregivers. The project, that of establishing a client-staff newsletter, was quite successful in teaching clients various skills (e.g., editing, writing, organizing) useful in finding employment. The newsletter also increased communication between staff and clients so that the latter were more aware of available programs and services, and the former more aware of client needs. It is felt that the newsletter project more than likely would not have emerged so clearly or so easily from an approach to clients which emphasized that their problems were actually symptoms of an underlying "mental illness."

Clients' Dependency on Psychiatric Staff as a Function of a Medical Paradigm*

James K. Morrison, Johnel D. Bushell, Gregory D. Hanson,
Susan Holdridge-Crane, and Janet R. Fentiman

OUT OF THE controversy over whether mental disorder can be legitimately characterized as "illness" has emerged the related charges that the medical paradigm robs psychiatric clients of responsibility for their behavior and fosters in such clients nonassertive, passive-dependent attitudes (Goffman, 1961; Morrison, Fasano, Becker & Nevid, 1976; Szasz, 1961, 1970a, 1970b; Torrey, 1974). However, to date, no research has attempted to more clearly define whether such attitudes of dependence are closely related to attitudes toward "mental illness."

The present study was designed to assess the validity of this relationship by means of two instruments recently developed to measure attitudes toward mental illness and attitudes of dependence. Although this study was designed as correlational research and was thus unable to illuminate cause and effect relationships, it was expected that the data provided by this pilot study could at

---

*Reprinted in an expanded form, with permission of the publisher, from the original: Morrison, J.K., Bushell, J.D., Hanson, G.D., Fentiman, J.R., and Holdridge-Crane, S. Relationship between psychiatric patients' attitudes toward mental illness and attitudes of dependence. *Psychological Reports*, 1977, *41*, 1194.

least generate some initial evidence in support of the relationship
between medical-model-type attitudes and attitudes of dependence.

Methods

Subjects. Fifty-eight psychiatric outpatients, 38 of whom had
been hospitalized at least once for psychiatric reasons, served as
subjects. The clients were relatively young ($M = 35.2$ years),
mostly female ($n = 32$), and with limited formal education ($M = 12.6$ years). These clients were provided psychological and psychiatric services by one of three different community mental
health center outpatient clinics in a tri-city area.

Self-report measure. The *Client Attitude Questionnaire* or CAQ-B
(Morrison, Schwartz, & Holdridge-Crane, in press) is a reliable
($r = .90$), revised version of the CAQ-A (Morrison and Nevid,
1976). This 20 item instrument determines respondents' attitudes
toward mental illness which reflect either a psychosocial (anti-
medical) or a medical model. The *Client Independence Questionnaire* (CIQ) is a reliable ($r = .78$), 16 item attitude measure
determining a client's dependence on, or independence from, psychiatric staff (Morrison and Yablonovitz, in press). CIQ scores
significantly correlate ($r = .62$ $p < .01$) with therapists' ratings
of client dependence.

Procedure. Three clinicians (a clinical psychologist and two psychiatric social workers) at a community mental health center administered the CAQ-B and CIQ to their clients. Clients were also
asked to supply certain demographic information (age, sex, and so
on).

Results

Analysis of clients' CAQ-B and CIQ scores by means of a Pearson product moment correlations indicated that, as predicted, respective scores were significantly correlated ($r = .60$, $p < .01$),
suggesting a strong relationship between medical-model orientation
and attitudes of dependence on the one hand, and psychosocial
orientation and attitudes of independence on the other. Further
analyses by means of partial correlations indicated that of all the
variables studied (sex, age, years of formal education, number of
hospitalizations, and average length of each hospitalization), only
years of formal education appeared to significantly contribute to
the correlation of clients' CAQ-B and CIQ scores. Specifically,

when the effect of years of formal education was held constant, the relationship between CAQ-B and CIQ scores was almost halved ($r = .34$, $p < .05$). Furthermore, years of formal education significantly and negatively correlated with clients' CAQ-B ($r = .54$, $p < .01$) scores, indicating that with increased formal education, clients tend to adopt the more popular medical paradigm, as well as attitudes of dependence on psychiatric staff.

Discussion

The data provided by the responses of psychiatric clients to the CAQ-B and CIQ indicate that there is indeed a strong relationship between their attitudes of dependence and their medical-model-type attitudes toward mental illness. Conversely, client attitudes characterized on the CIQ as more independent strongly correlate with attitudes toward mental illness more characteristic of proponents of an antimedical model (e.g., Szasz).

The partial correlations mentioned above suggest that through our educatonal system psychiatric clients learn to apply the currently prevalent medical paradigm to their behavior. This finding points out the usefulness of establishing educational seminars (e.g., demythologizing courses) to provide clients (and others) with an opportunity to learn about nonmedical paradigms (Morrison, 1976; Morrison & Nevid, 1976). Only when such alternative educational opportunities are available can clients and others be said to have a choice in how they are able to construe themselves.

No one today can assert dogmatically which conceptual paradigm is more valid in explaining human behavior. However, if further research continues to corroborate the relationship between attitudes of dependence and medical-model attitudes, one must question the *usefulness* of the medical model at least within the field of community psychology where the independent functioning of clients is the ultimate goal.

References

Goffman, E. *Asylums: Essays on the social situation of mental patients and other inmates.* Garden City, N.Y.: Doubleday, 1965.

Morrison, J. K. Demythologizing mental patients' attitudes toward mental illness: An empirical study. *Journal of Community Psychology*, 1976, *4*, 181–185.

Morrison, J. K., Fasano, B. L., Becker, R. E., & Nevid, J. S. Changing the "manipulative-dependent" role performance of psychiatric patients in the community. *Journal of Community Psychology,* 1976, *4,* 246–252.

Morrison, J. K., and Nevid, J. S. Attitudes of mental patients and mental health professionals about mental illness. *Psychological Reports,* 1976, *38,* 565–566.

Morrison, J. K., Schwartz, M. P., & Holdridge-Crane, S. Differential attitudes of community agencies toward mental illness: A new dilemma for the psychiatric nurse. *Journal of Psychiatric Nursing and Mental Health Services,* in press.

Morrison, J. K., & Yablonovitz, H. Increased clinic awareness and attitudes of independence through client advisory board membership. *American Journal of Community Psychology,* in press.

Szasz, T. S. *The myth of mental illness.* New York: Hoeber-Harper, 1961.

Szasz, T. S. *The manufacture of madness.* New York: Delta, 1970a.

Szasz, T. S. *Ideology and insanity.* New York: Doubleday, 1970b.

Torrey, E. F. *The death of psychiatry.* Radnor, Pa., Chilton Book Co., 1974.

Changing the "Manipulative-Dependent" Role Performance of Psychiatric Patients in the Community*

James K. Morrison, Beverly L. Fasano, Roy E. Becker, and Jeffrey S. Nevid

AN EMPHASIS ON the importance of "role adoption" (e.g., "mental patient") in the psychopathology of psychiatric clients is clear in the writings of a number of theoreticians (Becker, 1963; Erikson, 1975; Goffman, 1961; Lemert, 1962; Scheff, 1966). Braginsky and his colleagues (Braginsky & Braginsky, 1967; Braginsky, Braginsky & Ring, 1969) have shown that psychiatric inpatients can shift from mental patient to conventional role-enactments, and vice-versa, depending on the demand characteristics predominant in the situation.

There is frequent reference in the literature (Barton, 1959; Goffman, 1961) that through differential reinforcement of patient role appropriate behaviors, the reward system of the mental hospital tends to encourage patients toward greater passivity and dependency. Within this environment, directly assertive behaviors are discouraged (Tobias & MacDonald, 1974), and the patient may

---

*This article was originally published in the *Journal of Community Psychology*, 1976, *4*, 246–252. Reprinted by permission.

learn to apply manipulative strategies (Braginsky, Braginsky & Ring, 1969) to achieve desired ends. Similarly, evidence from several drug withdrawal studies in mental hospitals (Diamond & Marks, 1960; Stanley & Walton, 1961) demonstrates that what is seen as "deterioration" or "clinical relapse" (when placebos are substituted for phenothiazine medication) is often increased assertive behaviors or increased responsiveness to the environment. Thus, the patient's independent role functioning is often sacrificed to the smooth functioning of a quiet and docile psychiatric ward.

When released to the community, the patient is often faced with the need to supplant the set of behaviors appropriate to the "sick" role with role-enactments more appropriate to self-reliant, independent, societal living. The growth of community psychiatry may actually impede patients' progress toward independent community living by providing a setting in which patient roles remain functional (Erikson, 1957).

The authors suggest that consistent with a patient stereotypic role, psychiatric outpatients may come to depend on therapeutic authorities (as in the hospital) for solving the most elementary problems in daily living. Secondly, the patients learn that the community clinic staff are ready, and often eager, to provide the social reinforcement and attention which is often lacking in their primary social groups and families. Thus, the community clinic may become a microcosm of the mental hospital, in which the clients can continue in the passive and helpless patient role, and the staff can continue to reinforce patient dependency by solving problems for clients, and succoring their needs for attention and nurturance. The telephone often becomes a prime instrument through which clients play out these dependent role-enactments and manipulate for attention. "Nuisance" calls from clients enacting these roles are familiar to most clinicians engaged in providing after-care services (e.g., "My welfare check didn't come today. What should I do?"). The authors would submit that the clinician who abidingly solves these daily "crises" is tacitly encouraging such dependent role-enactments, a policy which is self-defeating in the attempt to have the patient engage in more independent and self-reliant role-enactments.

It is the purpose of this present study to investigate a behavioral strategy for decreasing manipulative, dependent telephoning behavior by psychiatric outpatients. Although Brockopp (1970) adequately described the varieties of telephone strategies often used by persons who manipulate for attention, he neither provides quantitative data nor suggests means of changing such behavior. Redefining patients as "clients," and structuring social reinforcement contingencies to foster independent problem solving behavior, may facilitate the transition from dependent role appropriate behaviors to more self-reliant role-enactments.

In the present study, clinicians from a community based psychiatric team were asked to identify, according to strict criteria, clients who showed consistent patterns of dependent, manipulative behavior. These clinicians then attempted to give these clients, as well as clients not judged to be "manipulative-dependent," the clear message over the phone that psychiatric clients do not have to rely on clinicians to solve daily problems.

It was predicted that the telephoning behavior of those clients operationally defined as "manipulative-dependent" would be significantly different, in number and length per call, from the telephone behavior of those clients not judged to be "manipulative-dependent." It was also hypothesized that when appropriate reinforcement decision rules were consistently applied to client telephone calls, the number and length of such calls would be significantly reduced. It was also predicted that this reduction would be such that during the experimental period there would be no significant difference in telephoning behavior between the "manipulative-dependent" subjects and the non-"manipulative-dependent" subjects. Finally, it was hypothesized that on a self-report measure the clients would not report significantly more negative behavior change as a result of the decrease in telephone time with staff.

Method

Subjects. Twenty adult client subjects and five full-time clinicians on the staff of a community based psychiatric team (a clinical psychologist, two vocational counselors, two mental health therapy aids) served as subjects. The twenty clients included in this report were participants for whom there was comparable data for equivalent time periods. The subjects (15 females and 5 males) ranged in age from 21 to 61 years with a mean of 43.5 years. Nineteen of the twenty had a history of psychiatric hospitalization, 18 were using prescribed psychotropic medication, 10 were in weekly group psychotherapy, and 10 in individual psychotherapy. All clients received advocacy services.

Client Service Questionnaire. In order to determine the effect of the study on client behavior, a Client Service Questionnaire (CSQ)[1] was developed by the authors (Becker, Morrison, & Fasano).* This instrument consisted of 36 true-false items focusing on client attitudes toward staff (e.g., "At least one person on the staff really cares about me"), toward themselves (e.g., ""I rarely feel afraid"), and toward their own behavior (e.g., "Often I call the staff when it turns out I really didn't need to"). Responses indicating positive attitudes were positively keyed so that possible scores ranged from 0 to 36.[2]

Charting Instrument. The chart on which calls were recorded was posted in the community team's office. The amount of time, time of day, data of each call, as well as the name of the clinician receiving the call were recorded on the chart. Clinicians could consult the chart to determine which clients were calling and which clinicians they called. Thus, if clients ceased to call their primary advisors and began to scatter their calls to other clinicians, this could be quickly detected by consulting the chart.

Procedure. The clinicians, through discussion, decided that any client fulfilling three of the following five criteria was to be placed in the "manipulative-dependent" (MD) client group: (1) an observed tendency to blame others most of the time for problems; (2) one or more suicide gestures (not attempts) since becoming a patient of the psychiatric agency; (3) one or more suicide and/or homicide threats; (4) one or more attempts to persuade clinicians to psychiatrically hospitalize when the staff judged this to be unnecessary; and, (5) frequent (2 or more a week) and/or after-hour telephone calls. Three of the subjects (2 females and 1 male) were judged to meet the criteria for inclusion in this group, and were placed in the "manipulative-dependent" (MD) group. These three were comparatively young (ages 21, 29, 30) with their mean age of 26 years being exactly twenty years less than the mean age (46 years) for the seventeen "non-manipulative-dependent" (NMD) subjects.

In clinical team meetings, the team clinicians practiced techniques to elicit clear and direct messages from clients early in conversations so that calls could be quickly categorized and the appro-

---

*Becker, R. E., Morrison, J. K., & Fasano, B. L. *The effect of evaluative research on clinicians' feelings of competence, attitudes toward research and acceptance of a new approach.* Presented at the 5th Annual Alpha Delta Kappa Sociological Research Symposium, 1975.

priate decision rule applied. Each call was charted as either "informational," "medical," or "psychological."

A key decision rule was to terminate *informational* calls (e.g., "What time is group?" "The landlord is complaining!" etc.) as soon as possible without being rude or abrupt. In the experience of the team, such calls frequently merged into "conversational" (Brockopp, 1970) content with limited therapeutic or problem-solving outcome. Another decision rule specified that *medical* calls (e.g., focusing on somatic complaints, side effects of medication, etc.) should be terminated quickly with the recommendation that the client consult his personal physician or the team's psychiatrist. A decision rule for *psychological* calls (e.g., "I'm nervous and depressed," "I'm hearing voices") stipulated that if two such calls occurred in a seven day period a "counseling" session must be scheduled. The clinicians reviewed the calls with the client giving negative verbal reinforcement for calls which were judged to be primarily attention-getting in content. Positive verbal reinforcement was given for problem-solving aspects of the calls.

The experimental manipulation was applied in terms of an A-B-A self-control design. The clinicians charted all incoming telephone calls from clients for a period of four consecutive weeks (Phase I) to obtain a baseline for telephoning behavior. This data was analyzed to determine the validity of expected significant differences between "manipulative-dependent" clients and "non-manipulative-dependent" clients. During the eighteen consecutive weeks using the experimental approach (Phase II) charting was continued and specified decision rules were applied to the charted behaviors of both client groups. Following the experimental phase the clinicians continued to chart but did not apply decision rules (Phase III) in order to provide data relevant to estimating an extinction curve for behavior change.

Finally, the Client Service Questionnaire was administered before and after 8 week periods throughout the study.

Results

Table I presents the means and standard deviations for the number and minutes of client-initiated telephone calls by groups and phase.[3] A 2 x 3 (2 groups x 3 phases) analysis of variance was performed on both the mean number and minutes of monthly telephone calls. Results indicate that a group's main effect reached significance for both the mean number of calls, F $(1,54) = 129.16$,

Table 1
Means and Standard Deviations for Number and Minutes of Monthly
Telephone Calls by Condition and Phase

Condition	Behavior	Phase I		Phase II		Phase III	
		M	SD	M	SD	M	SD
MD	Number	1.58	0.78	0.76	0.55	0.92	0.63
	Minutes	7.15	3.42	0.65	0.29	3.37	2.61
NMD	Number	0.04	0.10	0.07	0.09	0.07	0.15
	Minutes	0.59	1.42	0.29	0.41	0.29	0.75

$p < .001$, and the mean minutes per call, $F (1,54) = 56.66$, $p < .0001$, for such calls. A phase main effect was also significant for both number $F (2,54) = 7.27$, $p < .005$, and minutes, $F (2,54) = 19.89$, $p < .0001$. Interaction effects were also significant for number $F (2,54) = 8.47$, $p < .001$, and minutes, $F (2,54) = 16.43$, $p < .0001$, of telephone transactions.

Between group t-test analyses indicate that, as predicted, the "manipulative-dependent" clients demonstrated significantly more telephoning transactions than the "non-manipulative-dependent" subjects during Phase I in both number of calls, $t (18) = 3.49$, $p < .05$, and minutes per calls, $t (18) = 3.27$, $p < .05$. Nonsignificant inter-group differences were found in charted number and minutes of telephone calls during Phase II. Inter-group differences did not reach statistical significance during Phase III as well.

Within group changes, as analyzed by t-tests, indicate that there was significant reduction in the number, $t (4) = 5.53$, $p < .05$, and minutes, $t (4) = 3.52$, $p < .05$, of MD initiated telephone calls from Phase I to Phase II. The MD subjects' calls were neither significantly different in number or minutes from Phases I to III, or from Phases II to III. NMD subjects telephone calls did not significantly change in either number of minutes from phase to phase.

Table 2 presents the Client Service Questionnaire scores by condition and test administration. A 2 x 4 (2 conditions x 4 administrations) analysis of variance revealed that the condition main effect reached significance, $F (1,72) = 56.46$, $p < .0001$, but that neither the administration main effect nor the interaction ef-

Table 2
Means and Standard Deviations for CSQ Scores
by Condition and Administration

| | Administration | | | | | | | |
| | I | | II | | III | | IV | |
Condition	M	SD	M	SD	M	SD	M	SD
MD	12.33	4.16	11.33	5.13	18.00	4.00	16.00	5.29
NMD	24.29	3.77	24.12	4.36	23.77	4.68	24.00	3.04

fect did. Analysis employing t-tests indicated that MD and NMD subjects significantly differed on their CSQ self-reports during administrations I, t (18) = 4.65, p <.05, and II, t (18) = 4.06, p <.05, but not during Administrations III and IV. CSQ self-report score changes were small throughout the study as indicated by the lack of significant changes within groups from one administration to any other, except where the MD subjects reported significantly more positive attitudes on the CSQ from Administration I to III, t (4) = 8.50, p <.025.

Discussion

The results of the present study indicate, as expected, that clients who were previously judged to be "manipulative-dependent" make more phone calls to confer with their counselors and spend more time on the phone per call, than clients not judged to be "manipulative-dependent" in their role-enactments. This telephoning behavior is consistent with a patient role defined in terms of a dependent relationship with therapeutic authorities. Whereas such dependent, manipulative behavior may be positively valued, and perhaps reinforced, in the hospital milieu (Barton, 1959), it is expected that such role-enactments are self-defeating in the client's attempt to function independently in the community.

The application of decision rules, i.e., the withdrawal of social reinforcement contingent on manipulative-dependent telephoning behavior, produced, as the results show, decreased telephoning (number and minutes per call) for the "manipulative-dependent" clients. The telephoning behavior of "non-manipulative-dependent" subjects did not change significantly across treatment phases, perhaps reflecting the relative infrequency of such calls.

Nonsignificant differences in telephoning behavior between

Phase II and Phase III for "manipulative-dependent" clients indicates that the behavior change following therapeutic manipulation
remained resistant to extinction effects following reinstatement of
baseline reinforcement contingencies. Further research efforts may
determine whether the permanence of this behavioral change would
exceed the eight week extinction period examined here. It may
prove necessary to provide a periodic application of decision rule
strategies to insure more permanent effects.

It is interesting to note that at the point in the study when
these decision rules seem to have been most effective (i.e., at the
end of Phase II) the "manipulative-dependent" subjects reported
on the CSQ (Administration III) their most positive attitudes toward themselves, the staff and their own perceived behavior
change. These results seem to indicate that when "manipulative-
dependent" clients become less dependent on the clinical staff (as
measured by their reduced telephone behavior), they appear to
also feel more positive about themselves and the staff with whom
they relate. "Nonmanipulative-dependent" clients did not report
such changes, presumably because few decision rules were actually
applied to them.

It should be emphasized that this was an experimental pilot
study. It is difficult in a community setting to find more than a few
clients who can be defined as "manipulative-dependent" according
to the relatively strict criteria used here. The paucity of such
clients thus makes it difficult to study the behavior of more than
a few manipulative clients at a time. But considering that such
clients may account for as much as 80 percent (a percentage based
on this study's baseline data for MD and NMD clients) of the
staff's time, it becomes essential to determine the contingencies of
their behavior change. This study has provided evidence that at
least some attention-seeking, dependent behavior (e.g., telephone
calls) of manipulative-dependent, clients can be reduced. And, this
reduction in telephone time did not appear to have any negative
effects on the clients' attitudes toward the staff or themselves as
indicated by a self-report measure administered periodically during
the study.

With the present emphasis on the reintegration of previously
hospitalized mental patients into the community, therapeutic intervention should be focused on increasing the client's participation
in self-reliant, independent roles. To effect the change from patient role-enactments to citizenry role-enactments, it is suggested

that the reward contingencies operating in the community milieu be structured to encourage more independent problem solving behavior. The present study demonstrated the effects of changing social reinforcement contingencies to alter one modality of manipulative-dependent role-enactments, telephoning behavior. It should be emphasized, however, that decreasing manipulative, dependent behaviors through the employment of behavioral strategies, in the absence of building alternative, more adaptive, behaviors, is a questionable strategy (Bandura, 1969). Thus, in addition to traditional group and individual psychotherapy, our clinic offers special workshops in problem solving skills, and training programs in daily living activities, particularly suited for ex-hospitalized clients.

Notes

1. Test-retest reliability coefficient of .97, $p < .001$, $N = 10$ over 2 months.
2. More specific information about the data supplied by the CSQ can be provided upon request.
3. Because the number of "psychological" and "medical" telephone calls were too few to meaningfully analyze, they have been combined with "informational" calls for the purposes of the present analysis.

References

Bandura, A. *Principles of behavior modification*. New York: Holt, Rinehart and Winston, 1969.

Barton, R. *Institutional neurosis*. Bristol: John Wright and Sons, 1959.

Becker, E. Socialization, command of performance and mental illness. *American Journal of Sociology*, 1962, *67*, 494–501.

Braginsky, B., & Braginsky, D. Schizophrenic patients in the psychiatric interview: An experimental study of their effectiveness at manipulation. *Journal of Consulting Psychology*, 1967, *31*, 543–547.

Braginsky, B., Braginsky, D., & Ring, K. *Methods of madness*. New York: Holt, Rinehart & Winston, 1969.

Brockopp, G. W. The telephone call: Conversation or therapy. *Crisis Intervention*, 1970, *2*, 73–75.

Diamond, L. J., & Marks, J. B. Discontinuance of tranquilizers among chronic schizophrenic patients receiving maintenance dosage. *Journal of Nervous and Mental Disease*, 1960, *131*, 247–251.

Erickson, K. T. Patient roles and social uncertainty—a dilemma of the mentally ill. *Psychiatry*, 1957, *20*, 263–272.

Goffman, E. *Asylums: Essays on the social situation of mental patients and other inmates*. Garden City, New York: Doubleday, 1961.

Lemert, E. M. Paranoia and the dynamics of exclusion. *Sociometry*, 1962, *25*, 2–20.

Scheff, T. J. The role of the mentally ill and the dynamics of mental disorder: A research framework. *Sociometry*, 1963, *26*, 436–453.

Stanley, W. J., & Walton, D. J. Tri Fluoperazine. *Journal of Mental Science*, 1961, *107*, 250–257.

Tobias, L. L., & MacDonald, M. L. Withdrawal of maintenance drugs with long term hospitalized mental patients: A critical review. *Psychological Bulletin*, 1974, *81*, 107–125.

A Client Newsletter:
The Message Becomes the Medium

Michael J. Connelly, Michael R. Harris, and James K. Morrison

IN THE PAST decade a new client consumerism has emerged within
the mental health system. Increasingly the psychiatric client is
being construed not only as the consumer, but also as the rightful
evaluator, of a variety of psychological, medical, social and rehabilitative services (Morrison, 1977). Mental patients, formerly
viewed as suffering from a variety of "mental illnesses" for which
cures were being sought through a number of medical, surgical,
and chemical interventions, are increasingly being construed as
clients who collaborate with mental health professionals to reach
resolution of their various psychological/social/vocational "problems in living." With such a changing emphasis in the field of
mental health, the vocational rehabilitation counselor has emerged
as an important change agent whose interventions can facilitate
client problem resolution through the teaching of various skills.
Thus, the psychiatric client is in need of counseling in order to
learn a variety of vocational skills which enable the client to seek
and find gainful employment. Seen as a person who is usually
seriously deficient in employable skills, the psychiatric client must
be educated and trained in such a way that his or her entrance into
the work world will lead to a certain measure of happiness and

personal satisfaction.* It is within this context of client consumer-ism that a new rehabilitative medium, that of a client newsletter, has been developed.

Although the traditional function of newsletter derives from some specific need for information sharing, in the field of community mental health a newsletter may serve another function as well. Thus, participation in the organization, writing, and production of a newsletter may become a rehabilitative tool whereby psychiatric clients learn various skills (e.g., social, literary, organizational) which may be useful in finding employment, or generally in increasing their level of interpersonal functioning in the community. In short, the message (newsletter) becomes the medium (toward rehabilitation).

The more traditional need for information sharing is also met by a client newsletter. For example, on our community mental health team there is a client advisory board (Morrison, 1976) which assists the professional staff in developing, implementing and evaluating clinical/social/education rehabilitative programs. The board members often find it necessary to communicate with other clients when evaluating a particular program, soliciting new board members, and informing clients on the functioning of the board. The client board must also frequently inform professional staff of their opinions, plans, and suggestions for program changes. A newsletter thus becomes an important medium for relaying information within the mental health system.

Newsletters have traditionally been a source of information to a wide variety of readers (e.g., parents of school children, legislators' constituents, senior citizens). Fountain House in New York City and Horizon House in Philadelphia have used newsletters to share information about inhouse events and community activities.

The newsletter created by the clients and staff of our team was developed to serve a number of purposes. First, the newsletter serves an information-sharing function (e.g., about the time and location of weekly programs of the clinic). Second, the work involved in producing a newsletter allows unemployed clients to develop needed employment skills. Third, the production setting helps clients to develop interpersonal skills, social skills still underdeveloped in those clients who may have been institutionalized for years in state mental hospitals.

---

*However, as Wilkinson (1975) points out, one can no longer expect work alone to provide personal fulfillment.

After we considered the possible benefits of a newsletter to clients, a number of clients were surveyed to determine their interest in establishing a newsletter. All of the 27 clients surveyed expressed enthusiasm for the project, and several clients volunteered to take some active role in the paper. Two community college students working on the team volunteered their time in editing and writing. The vocational rehabilitation counselor and psychiatric nurse, who conceived the basic program, helped to organize the clients and students into an effective work group. Since most of the participants were involved already in an ongoing, week-night, social-recreational program, it was decided to make the events of the social program the basis of the newsletter. In fact, the name *Whose News* was chosen from several suggested by the members of that group to avoid any negative sets which might have been created by using the name of the psychiatric agency on the front page. All clients were surveyed to find out if they wanted to receive the newsletter, and the thirty who responded made up the first mailing list.

The *Whose News* staff decided to hold weekly meetings for administrative purposes (i.e., to decide on assignments for articles and tasks, to compose and edit articles, to set timetables, and so on). The weekly meeting was also used to collate and mail the newsletter once it had been duplicated. Besides being work oriented, the production of the newsletter was also oriented toward fun and social recreation. Although timetables were established, they were not absolutely fixed, thus eliminating any pressure to meet a deadline. It was hoped that client involvement eventually would increase and that staff could assume a less responsible role while still remaining part of the program.

Weekly meetings served the important function of establishing a routine method of planning the next issue. Staff and an increasingly larger number of clients knew when the group met, and all were invited to attend and participate. Those clients involved in the newsletter who moved from the area, or who held jobs and thus could not attend meetings, were invited to mail in items of interest or articles. For some ex-clients the newsletter was the only remaining link with the agency, and an enjoyable one that provided for an easy flow of information.

Team and community events were announced in the *Whose News*, thus informing clients and other staff about activities in which they might participate. One entire newsletter was devoted to an extensive description of all of the social/educational/clinical/rehabilitative programs offered by the community mental health team. The staff of the *Whose News* decided to make the sharing of program information a regular part of the newsletter.

A regular column was devoted to the client advisory board (CAB), and three members of the CAB joined the core staff of the *Whose News*. Eventually staff decided to send the newsletter to all the clients served by the unit, as well as to any other individuals who requested it. A delivery system was established in which staff handed the newsletter out at groups and social events, inviting input and comments.

The first few publications lacked expertise and client input. Initially, two staff, two clients, and two volunteers were the only real participants. But gradually more and more clients became involved. Some were involved only marginally. Thus, some clients came once a month to help collate and staple; others contributed poems, editorials, recipes, community calendar notes, and a variety of other articles. A suggestion by one of the earliest involved clients resulted in a novel means of funding. Individuals were invited to send in one dollar for which their names were listed as a patron on a special page of the newsletter. This was so successful that for the first year *this was the only necessary source of funding*. Stencils and paper were paid for entirely by this means. Even the cost of mailing was minimal because of the relatively small number of clients who could not receive a copy in person from their clinical advisor or program coordinator. Mailing labels were provided free by a volunteer. For an entire year the newsletter operated virtually at no cost, except for staff time.

The benefits of the newsletter have been substantial. The newsletter reaches all clients served by the team and provides them with information about programs, articles on health and vocational ideas, and community happenings. Those clients involved in production have an opportunity to develop skills which are useful in finding and holding jobs, and in functioning interpersonally in the community. For the staff the newsletter has been one means of discovering the talents and undeveloped potential of their clients. For example, one especially disruptive client did all of the *Whose News* letterheads (which changed from one issue to the next). This was the only program she actually participated in at the center. For the agency, the paper has been an example of a low cost program in which client-participants can involve themselves at any level, in a nonthreatening way. Thus, clients can become part of something which has a rewarding outcome, e.g., seeing some of their poetry or art work reproduced for others.

The newsletter program has not been without its problems. As has been our experience with most programs involving psychiatric clients formerly institutionalized in state mental hospitals, there has been a problem motivating clients to become involved in, and to make a consistent commitment to, the program. The staff members of the community team thus were not as able, as they would have liked, to decrease their involvement in producing the newsletter. Staff support of the project, initially at a high level, decreased somewhat as the novelty of the program wore off. However, in spite of these problems, the staff and clients appeared to see the program as a successful and rewarding experience.

In the area of community mental health vocational rehabilitation counselors are becoming increasingly valued by their clinical coworkers. As mental health professionals gradually move in the direction of construing psychiatric clients as persons with multiple problems in living, rather than as patients with a mental illness, rehabilitation counselors are being called on to develop programs which encourage clients to develop badly needed work and work-related skills. Such programs as a client newsletter allow clients to construe themselves as having a sufficient repertoire of social and vocational skills to function in the work world with a moderate degree of success. Such programs also appear to nudge clients further in the direction of becoming reasonably self-reliant citizens. In our experience, a client newsletter is not only the message, it is also the medium.

References

Morrison, J. K. An argument for mental patient advisory boards. *Professional Psychology*, 1976, *7*, 127–131.

Morrison, J. K. The client as consumer and evaluator of mental health services. *American Journal of Community Psychology*, 1977, in press.

Wilkinson, M. W. Leisure: An alternative to the meaning of work. *Journal of Applied Rehabilitation Counseling*, 1975, *6*, 73–77.

8
A Community of Consumers

Overview

IT IS MY strong conviction that mental health professionals must avoid construing the community as an endless reservoir of psychiatric clients. It is tempting for some to think of most communities as "sick" and in need of the expertise of mental health professionals. The traps laid by such grandiose thinking are endless and are discussed in more detail in Chapters 1 and 9.

Such admonitions notwithstanding, I feel that community psychologists should avoid the other extreme: simply waiting for clients to hear of community mental health center services. Working *in* a community means just that. To confine one's work within the walls of a clinic or center precludes calling such work "community psychology."

With the above thoughts in mind I have chosen three articles for inclusion in this chapter. The first article explains how a clinic can increase its visibility in the community by using newspaper publicity. Do we not owe it to the potential consumers of our services to make sure that a healthy percentage at least know a clinic exists and what services it offers? I believe we do. This does not mean we try to propagandize people into believing they need us. As pointed out earlier in this book (see Chapter 3) a demythologizing approach to the community may correct any exaggerated zeal on our part to convince everyone they need us!

The second article in this chapter focuses on the utility of community or citizen boards. A review of the literature on such boards is offered along with a descriptive study of one such board which was established to avoid some of the problems of other previously described boards. It seems possible from our experience that citizen boards can be more than tokens. They can be functioning bodies with real power to protect the community from abuses in the mental health arena, and to develop programs and services which the community really needs. Although any community is a community of potential consumers, we must be cautious in overlabeling or overdiagnosing. Citizen boards can be most useful in helping clinical staff to avoid such errors.

The final article in this chapter is a case study, which illustrates how only the myopic community psychologist will construe one member of a family as *the* problem and then commit the double error of attempting to change the behavior of that one person without changing the thinking of that person's family and community. The case study also illustrates what is emphasized in the first article of Chapter 9, i.e., that community psychologists might well focus more on their role as "behavior explicators," or teachers, in the community. In this study progress with a child who had behavior problems seemed contingent on teaching family members and relevant teachers in the community different ways of understanding and construing the boy in question. The process of therapy with the boy consisted primarily of a reeducation of the boy's family and significant others (e.g., teachers).

The Effect of Newspaper Publicity on a Mental Health Center's Community Visibility*

James K. Morrison and Judith A. Libow

ALTHOUGH SOME RESEARCHERS (Goldman, 1970; Heinemann, Perlmutter, & Yudin, 1974; Ring & Schein, 1970; Tomlinson, 1971) have recently studied the community's awareness of available mental health services, no one has yet reported figures indicating that the community is very knowledgeable of such services. Even though it is certainly not unusual for community mental health centers to make use of the media to heighten community awareness of their services, no one has yet reported an attempt to study the effect of publicity on community awareness of psychiatric services. Unlike professionals in the advertising industry, mental health professionals have not taken the time to evaluate the effect of the media on public awareness or knowle\`ge of mental health services (Rosen & Tallman, 1965).

It was the purpose of the present study to (1) determine the level of awareness within a specific community related to a mental health center's existence, location, and services; (2) specify the

---

*This article was originally published in the *Community Mental Health Journal*, 1977, *13*, 58–62. Reprinted by permission from Human Sciences Press.

impact of limited newspaper publicity on that level of awareness; and (3) determine the stability of that impact over time.

Description of Center and Its Services

The Capital District Psychiatric Center is a comprehensive mental health facility, providing services in a four-county area through a number of satellite outreach offices. The center offers aftercare services primarily to patients living in the community who have a history of psychiatric hospitalization in state mental institutions. The center's satellite clinic in Cohoes, New York, in existence for five years, employs five full-time staff (one psychologist, one social worker, three mental health therapy aides), three part-time staff (one psychiatrist, one vocational rehabilitation counselor, one psychologist), and a number of students (psychiatric residents, psychology interns, and so on). This clinic provides a wide range of services including individual and group psychotherapy, medication, educational, and social programs, and advocacy assistance.

The Community

The Cohoes community, totaling approximately nineteen thousand people (according to a recent federal census), is situated in the midst of a large tricity area. The community is almost exclusively white, and has a high number of citizens on welfare. Once a highly industrialized community, the city presently finds itself with a large number of unemployed residents who are experiencing a wide range of social, economic, and psychiatric problems.

Method

The Survey Instrument The measure employed in this study to determine the visibility of the clinic and its services in the community is the *Visibility Survey Questionnaire* (VSQ). This instrument consists of five questions.
1. Have you ever heard of the Capital District Psychiatric Center in Cohoes?
2. Do you know the location of their offices?
3. Do you know what services this agency provides?
4. Do you know anyone in Cohoes who receives services or help from this agency?
5. Would you care to make any comments about this agency?

Only the first three questions are of concern in the present study. The sample was asked to respond to each question with one of three answers (yes, no, not sure). The questionnaire form also included space to record comments and limited demographic data (age and sex of respondent).

Procedure. Since random and stratified sampling of the community would have been too costly in terms of time and manpower, an "accidental sample" appeared to be the procedure of choice. Ten persons (five male and five female), ranging in age from sixteen to thirty-six years, conducted the visibility survey in one area of the community, that is, the one main street in the city. All of the interviewers were trained in interviewing skills and procedures by the senior author. The interviewers attempted to interview each person (sixteen years of age or older) who approached their survey area unless the interviewers were already actively engaged in the interviewing process.

After the first survey ($n = 105$) was conducted, a short article (with accompanying picture) about the Capital District Psychiatric Center's office appeared in a local newspaper. The article described the clinic, its location, and its service. The day after the article appeared, a second survey sample ($n = 100$) was taken in the same area of the community. Finally, six weeks after the newspaper article, a third survey ($n = 106$) was conducted in the same location to determine the stability of the effect of the newspaper article on the reported visibility (that is, awareness of the existence, location, and services) of the psychiatric center office. It should be mentioned that even though the sample number was limited and the sampling procedure not randomized, the three samples were comparatively similar in age and sex distribution. The age and sex distributions of the samples also compared favorably with the same distributions in the total population according to the most recent federal census.

Results

Analysis of the effect of publicity on the agency's visibility in the community was performed by using the Z test for differences between proportions. Table 1 presents the percentage of respondents in each sample who answered "yes," "no," and "not sure" to each of the three survey questions of relevance to this study.

These results indicate that the article had a significant effect on the reported visibility of the Capital District Psychiatric Center

Table 1
Percentage Response to Each Question over Sample Phases

Question	Response	Samples		
		Phase I (n = 105)	Phase II (n = 100)	Phase III (n = 106)
1	yes	28.6	53.0	49.1
	no	63.8	47.0	50.0
	not sure	7.6	0.0	0.9
2*	yes	17.1	33.0	22.6
	no	10.5	15.0	25.5
	not sure	8.6	5.0	1.9
3	yes	13.3	27.0	27.4
	no	17.2	24.0	22.6
	not sure	5.7	2.0	0.0

*The persons responding to questions 2 and 3 were those sample respondents who answered "yes" or "not sure" to Question 1.

in the community. Comparing the change in percentages over samples related to responses to question 1 (whether respondents had heard of the district center), it was evident that the agency's visibility (defined here as the percentage responding "yes") had significantly increased from sample 1 (before the article) to sample 2 (day following the article) in the predicted direction ($Z = 3.70$, $p < .01$). Similarly, the visibility increase remained relatively stable as indicated by the significant difference in visibility, evidenced in the follow-up at 6 weeks, between samples 1 and 3 ($Z = 3.15$, $p < .01$).

Related to question 2 (location of offices) the awareness of the psychiatric center office location significantly increased from sample 1 to sample 3 ($Z = 2.66$, $p < .01$). However, this effect evidently was not lasting as indicated by the comparison of sample 1 and sample 3 percentage differences ($Z = 1.00$, n.s.).

After the article, the community's awareness level of the clinic's services (question 3) appeared to increase significantly ($Z = 2.54$, $p < .05$). This effect was stable 6 weeks later as indicated by the significantly different visibility percentages from sample to sample 3 ($Z = 2.66$, $p < .01$).

None of the comparisons of sample 2 and 3 percentages differed significantly, indicating that the stability of the effect of publicity on community awareness was genuine.

In analyzing the visibility increases (questions 1, 2, and 3) related to the sex of the respondents, it was evident that the newspaper article had had its greatest initial impact on females, but that the effect was much more permanent among males. Related to the age of respondents, the newspaper publicity appeared to have the greatest impact on the forty-five to sixty-four year-old group, and the least impact on the fifteen to twenty-four year-old group. However, some caution should be taken in forming conclusions from the data related to sex and age breakdowns. The samples were actually too small to reach any firm conclusions related to the differential effect of publicity dependent on sex and age. Further study with larger samples will be necessary before any strong conclusions can be drawn.

Discussion

It was most surprising to the authors that one newspaper article could have such impact on the visibility of the Capital District Psychiatric Center satellite office. Not only was the dramatic visibility increase after the article quite unexpected, but the stability of this increase over six weeks time was equally surprising. The one exception concerned the community's awareness of the office location after six weeks. However, it is not surprising that after such a length of time people would tend to forget the location of an agency. (In the newspaper article the location of the agency had actually been mentioned only once.)

One may well question whether the change in agency visibility may have perhaps been due to other factors. Although this is, of course, always possible, the authors could recall no event from the time of sample 1 to sample 3, other than the newspaper article, that could have accounted for the dramatic change. Furthermore, the survey team was instructed on sample 2 to ask a further question ("How did you hear about the Capital District Psychiatric Center?") of those responding affirmatively to question 1. Of those responding "yes" to this question, 63 percent declared that they had heard of the psychiatric center through the newspaper article. This would suggest that the article had indeed accounted for much of the visibility change.

The results of this study, related to the percentage of respondents who had heard of the agency in question, compare favorably with the results of other studies (Goldman, 1974; Heinemann, Perlmutter, & Yudin, 1974; Tomlinson, 1971). The visibility changes of the psychiatric center seem surprisingly great in light of the visibility percentages, ranging from 4 percent to 30 percent, mentioned in the studies cited above.

Conclusions

Newspaper publicity, focusing on mental health centers and their services, can apparently have rather dramatic effects on the visibility of such facilities in the community; and the impact of such articles seems to remain quite strong even 6 weeks after the publicity event. Although such a conclusion can be only tentative at this time, preliminary results also suggest that publicity regarding community services may differentially affect persons of different sex and age. Further examination of the effectiveness of different media on reaching particular populations would allow for more effective community outreach to targeted community groups.

References

Goldman, A. Jefferson Community Mental Center, 1970. Personal communication to S. H. Heinemann, 1974.

Heinemann, S. H., Perlmutter, F., & Yudin, L. W. The community mental health center and community awareness. *Community Mental Health Journal*, 1974, *10*, 221–227.

Ring, S. I., & Schein, L. Attitudes toward mental illness and the use of caretakers in a Black community. *American Journal of Orthopsychiatry*, 1970, *40*, 710–716.

Rosen, A. C., & Tallman, F. F. A study of the use of mental health media by the lay public. *Mental Hygiene*, 1965, *49*, 36–45.

Tomlinson, F. L. A study of consumers' awareness of resources in their own community for the treatment of emotional problems. Unpublished masters thesis, School of Social Work, University of Pennsylvania, 1971.

The Citizen Advisory Board: Consumer Token or Consumer Power?

Jane E. Smith, James K. Morrison, and Margery Brown

CITIZEN OR CONSUMER advisory boards have been both severely denigrated as well as vigorously defended. In light of such divergent judgments, before attempting to establish such boards, it would seem to be essential for interested clinicians and administrators to first briefly[1] review the relevant literature in order to circumscribe the precise problems and strengths of existing boards. Secondly, much can be learned from a study of a citizen board established with the express purpose of taking advantages of the strengths, and of avoiding the weaknesses, of previously described boards. This article is thus both a review of the relevant literature as well as a study of one recently developed citizen board.

A Review of the Literature

Generally speaking, the literature concerned with citizen boards is replete with statements reflecting the importance which

---

1. A more extensive review of this literature can be found in the following: Morrison, J. K., Holdridge-Crane, S., and Smith, J. E. Citizen participation in community mental health. *Community Mental Health Review*, 1978, *3*, 1–9.

many ascribe to such boards. For example, Kane (1975) asserts that citizen boards are an essential part of a human service organization. However, the promotion of citizen boards in the literature all too often is unaccompanied by supporting evidence which attests to the viability and effectiveness of such boards. It is thus hardly surprising that Chu & Trotter (1974) found citizen boards in most community mental health centers to be ineffectual tokens.

In order to make clear decisions as to the type of citizen board which offers the most promise in terms of actual power and clear effectiveness, one must first examine the problems of previously described boards. Therefore, a brief review of the relevant literature appears to be the most logical first step toward creating a board which does not repeat the mistakes of the past.

Problems with existing boards. An apparently common problem with existing citizen boards is the lack of support these boards receive from professional clinical staff (Robins & Blackburn, 1974). Without the support of mental health professionals it is highly unlikely that any consumer board can be effective since board functioning usually depends on the active cooperation of such professionals.

A second related problem is the conflict between staff and board members which results from a failure to differentiate the specific functions of staff and board members (Robins & Blackburn, 1974; Kupst, Reidda & McGee, 1975). A lesson to be gained from such failure is that the specific tasks and objectives of a citizen board should be clearly defined and understood before a board begins to function.

Another problem arises when citizen board members relegate the responsibility for all important decisions to the professional staff. In such cases, citizen board members serve as advisors related to the raising of money, public relations, and image building, but are seldom involved to the extent that they are really committed either to the community or to the community mental health center (Holton, New & Hessler, 1973). Too frequently such token cooperation between center staff and citizen board members only creates the illusion of citizen participation (Kane, 1975). Chu & Trotter (1974) comment that few citizen advisory boards have any real fiscal control, policy-making power,[2] or program responsibility. Thus, it seems important in establishing effective

---

2. In many state-run community mental health centers fiscal control and policy-making power would not be possible without new legislation.

boards that citizen members have more than an advisory role. Real decision-making power, at least related to program development, may be a crucial ingredient in boards which aspire to be more than token boards.

A further problem with citizen boards is their weak strategic position related to board performance. When boards fail to produce, center staff can easily scapegoat the boards, even though everyone knows that the success or failure of any board depends on the performance of *both* center staff and citizen members. If board members have neglected the application of effective procedures, or the setting of realistic goals (Robins & Blackburn, 1974), such negligence is also the fault of center staff. Although it is true that board members may be unfamiliar with formal, group decision-making processes or leadership training (Briscoe, Hoffman & Bailey, 1975), as well as with the issues involved in community mental health programming (Holton, New & Hessler, 1973), board members can be familiarized with these procedures and issues if center staff take the time.

The practical problem of poor attendance plagues citizen boards just as it does all organizations, clubs, and other types of boards. Chairpersons and other officers seem to attend more regularly than other board members. The officers tend to be more commited to policy making and evaluative research, while other board members are more dedicated to ensuring that the center serves the community's needs (Kupst, Reidda & McGee, 1975). Thus, the differential attendance and commitment of officers and non-officers of the board serve to create a situation in which the attending board members (the officers) focus on what the staff of the center wants, while little heed is paid to the community's basic needs since those so interested (non-officers) are too often absent.

Another problem emerges from the composition of many boards. Boards tend to be composed mostly of community professionals and business executives who are white, married, Protestant males. The majority of these members have not asked to serve on the board and are poorly oriented toward community mental health ideology (Robins & Blackburn, 1974). The latter finding helps to explain the poor attendance which is reported at board meetings; the finding reveals another problem in that centers can easily create "elitist" boards composed of prominent citizens who are perhaps least able to represent the poor and uneducated consumers (Chu & Trotter, 1974). And because board members are not usually the type of persons who need or use a center's services, Chu and

Trotter advocate that at least some board members be actual consumers or patients of the center.

Advantages of citizen boards. In spite of the many problems with citizen boards, a number of reasons demand that consumer boards be considered as at least a potential means of improving the delivery of mental health services in the community. However, as Kane (1975) has indicated, board members may only be inclined to support board decisions when they have participated in the decision-making process. Thus, community mental health centers should seek to establish only boards which actively involve their members in all aspects of decision-making.

Citizen advisory boards may be the best available medium through which the community can voice its needs (Holton, New & Hessler, 1973; Rooney, 1968). Such boards may also be the best means of gaining community support for needed mental health programs.

Through advisory boards citizens can have some control over service and program development (Meyers, Dorwart, Hutcheson & Decker, 1947). Cohen, Reid & Berg (1975) believe that without citizen boards, continuity of care, primary prevention and community education would be extremely limited.

The advantages of creating citizen advisory boards center on the benefits to the community. Community mental centers which want to "do their own thing" should obviously not keep up the pretense of being a service center for the community. Perhaps they should drop the word "community" from their center's title. However, those centers which realize that to be effective the community must be involved should seriously consider citizen boards as an excellent means of establishing real dialog between the center and the community. From such dialog can emerge needed community programming which reflects the stamp of the client-consumer.

Dudley (1975) describes a number of guidelines developed in one geographic area for creating citizen boards. The requirement that each center must have a citizen advisory board seems reasonable to us. We also agree that board meetings should be publicized and open, that provisions be made for regular turnover of board members, and that boards should represent various age, socioeconomic, and occupational groups in the community. However, we do not feel it is practical to follow the guideline that at least 50 percent of board members be elected by the residents of the catchment area. In these days of voter apathy we find it hard to believe that an election of citizen board members would be realistic.

In our review of the literature we have circumscribed certain negative and positive aspects of citizen boards. Now we will describe one board established to avoid some of the problems, and to incorporate some of the strengths, of previous boards.

A Study of One Citizen Advisory Board

In our opinion this citizen advisory board has been effective in changing the delivery of mental health services to the community which it serves. Although the board existed for only eight months when this article was written, our evaluative efforts suggest that we have successfully resolved some of the problems of other citizen boards and have explored several new and exciting directions.

Developmental stages. The seminal stage of the citizen board began when "client advisory board" (Morrison, 1976) members met with members of a steering committee of another satellite team who were considering developing a client advisory board of their own. One member of the steering committee, upon hearing that a client board did not have much influence outside the clinic and in the community—mostly because psychiatric clients are not members of powerful and influential groups—suggested that we establish another board, a citizen board, designed to allow potential consumers (rather than actual consumers) a forum to express their veiws, as well as the opportunity to use their influence to create needed services for the community.

Following a discussion of the advantages of establishing a citizen board, the members of the client advisory board unanimously voted to further explore the possibility of creating a citizen board. The clinical staff of the satellite team also endorsed a thorough investigation of the feasibility of organizing such a board.

Both the client advisory board and the clinical team separately engaged in "brainstorming" sessions to define the tasks of a citizen board, as well as the type of membership suitable for such a board. Surprisingly the two groups terminated their separate discussions in 95 percent agreement regarding tasks and membership.

In final form both the client board and the clinical team endorsed the following tasks of the citizen board: (1) planning programs and services needed in the community; (2) planning programs to educate the community to construe the psychiatric client as a reasonably competent and responsible citizen; and (3) establishing effective communication between the citizen board and other members of the community.

The citizen board was distinguished from the client board in that the latter was designed to oversee the "direct" services delivered to actual consumers (clients), and the former was established to supervise the delivery of "indirect" services delivered to members of the community who were not clients.

The brainstorming sessions also produced agreement on the type of membership desirable for an effective citizen board. Avoiding an "elitist" model whereby a board is composed only of powerful and influential professionals, the client board and the clinical team substantially agreed to adopt a "representational" model, a board composed of citizens who represented a good cross-section of the community. Thus, the eleven board members were chosen to represent the following groups: senior citizens, businessmen, clergy, the poor, local hospital personnel, the legal establishment, school system personnel, human service agency personnel, police, city government personnel, and psychiatric clients. The latter group would be represented by a member of the client advisory board in an effort to facilitate communication, and thus cooperation, between the client and citizen boards.

The membership and tasks of the citizen board were established only after a thorough discussion of the advantages and disadvantages of the various types of boards outlined in the literature. Letters were sent out to eleven persons whom clinical staff and client board members felt were representative of the eleven interest groups mentioned above. The letters described in detail the possible tasks and procedures of the proposed board. The clinical staff called each of the eleven persons and all eleven accepted. Representing the eleven groups mentioned above were the mayor of the city, the chief of police, the superintendent of schools, the city corporation counsel, the director of the city's human service agencies, a local clergyman, the director of a local commerce and industry corporation, the director of a local senior citizens group, a social worker at the local hospital, a person representing the disadvantaged poor, and the chairperson of the client advisory board. These persons seemed to adequately represent both sexes, most major ethnic groups, different age categories, different religions, the rich and the poor, professionals and nonprofessionals, clients and nonclients. (All members of the board were Caucasian since all persons of the small community were.)

Board functioning. At its first meeting, the citizen board decided to meet once a month for an hour. Officers were elected at a subsequent meeting. Representatives of the clinical staff agreed to meet with the board and to assume the clerical duties of the board (e.g., taking minutes, sending out copies of minutes by mail, giving reminder calls, providing coffee, and so on).

In the first eight months of its existence, the board seems to have made considerable progress in carrying out the three main tasks of the board. In order to determine which mental health programs and services were needed but unavailable in the community, the board marshaled data which indicated that at least five new programs should be considered: (1) a program in local grade schools to help young children (first through sixth graders) identify, understand, and cope with problematic feelings; (2) educative seminars for the recently divorced or separated to help these persons resolve a variety of psychological, legal, and financial problems; (3) educative and experiential seminars to assist the newly married to identify and cope with the problems of early marriage; (4) instructional programs to help parents understand and resolve their problems in rearing children; and, (5) self-help groups for certain citizens (e.g., the elderly, the widowed, and so on) who feel isolated and in need of discussion groups to help them cope with life.

The board decided to take a street survey of local citizens to determine which of these programs should be given priority. Citizens were asked to check which of the programs were most needed. (The respondents were also able to suggest any other needed programs not listed on the survey checklist.) An "accidental sample" of 169 citizens was surveyed and the results indicated that the first and fourth programs listed above received the most support. Twenty-seven percent of the respondents supported both of these programs. The other three programs received less support (12–18 percent), but sufficient to warrant serious consideration. Only 3 percent of the citizens specified programs which were not listed but which they felt were needed. The respondents' program priorities did not appreciably differ according to their sex. Younger persons (e.g., 15–18 age category) most often selected program 3. Thus, self-help groups for the elderly or widowed were most often selected by persons in the 51 and older group. Otherwise, no age differences were evident in program choices.

Following the survey the citizen board successfully negotiated with another state agency specializing in services to children and their parents, to establish the programs for parents and for children (programs 1 and 4). Since the community mental health team which had helped establish the board was the appropriate team to develop the other three programs, the clinical staff consulted with the board to plan these programs. The programs for the newly married and the divorced/separated were organized and implemented. The self-help groups are still in the early planning stages.

Other agenda of the board during its first eight months included discussion of: problems of after hour clinical coverage during psychiatric crisis; the community's fear of mental patients; and problems of interagency communication. Such open discussions were invaluable since they enabled the clinical staff of the satellite team to keep in touch with the problems and feelings of the community.

On other matters, a twelfth member was added to the board in order to facilitate commu.lication between the citizen board and a similar board of another mental health agency, specializing in services to children. This member began attending meetings after the second board meeting.

An additional program was also implemented when a member of the community saw an article about the board in the local newspaper and called the chairperson to ask if a psychology course could be developed for a local adult education program. With the help of the citizen board, a course ("The Psychology of Personal Feelings") was developed which centered on the fears and myths of people about mental patients as well as on how unresolved feelings cause personal problems. The course attracted four times as many citizens as any other course in the adult education program, and served the purpose of providing community education, one of the three tasks of the citizen board.

Evaluation of the citizen board effectiveness. It had been decided before the board began to function that after eight months, attempts would be made to evaluate the board's effectiveness. One simple way of evaluating a citizen board is to determine the overall attendance rate of board members. This article's earlier review of the literature showed that attendance rates tend to be rather poor. If members attend in reasonable numbers such attendance at least suggests that the board members, despite their busy schedules, find the meetings interesting enough to justify their regular attendance. After the first eight months of its existence an overall board member attendance rate was calculated at 48 percent. Thus, on the average, about half of the twelve members attended any one meeting. However, attendance at these once-a-month, noon-hour meetings was twice as high in the first four months (64 percent) as it was in the last four months (32 percent). Although this drop in attendance may reflect what usually happens to the members of most boards as they try less and less successfully to work regular meetings into their schedule, the decrease in attendance may also reflect some problems. After much speculation the board members present at the eighth meeting decided that perhaps those members who decreased their attendance had originally construed board functioning differently than had regular attendees and the clinical staff. Following considerable discussion the board tentatively concluded that those not attending regularly were generally the same persons who had taken a very active role in early meetings before the board had begun to discuss specific programming for the community. It is possible that those members who attended irregularly preferred the discussion of issues which characterized the early meetings. At such meetings these members had been very emotionally involved as they discussed such issues as psychiatric crises, during the evening and weekends, and child abuse, and how such phenomena affected them and their interest groups.

The board members decided to return to the format of an open-forum for a period now that the new programs were being implemented. The attendance at the next meeting was expected to increase[3] since it was advertised in the minutes, sent to each member, as an open-forum to discuss how crisis intervention might be streamlined after the clinic's regular working hours.

Another way to evaluate a citizen board is to determine its success in persuading clinic staff to act on specific recommendations for the creation of new programs, services and projects. If a board is to be effective, some concrete changes should issue from board functioning. A careful reading of the minutes of the first eight citizen board meetings revealed that board members had requested 15 different and specific changes in the community's mental health delivery system. Of those 15, seven (i.e., community publicity on available mental health services; increased information on referral agencies; development of a survey questionnaire to tap community's primary mental health needs; inception of an adult education course on the myths of mental illness; encouragement of Parent Effectiveness Training [PET]) programs in

---

3. Attendance figures in the last four months of the first year of board functioning indeed indicated that board members returned to their earlier, higher attendance rates.

the community; a review of the research literature on PET; and a return of citizen board meetings to a discussion of community issues) were fully implemented in the first eight months of the board's existence. Two other recommendations (i.e., implementation of two new programs for the community: "Communication Strategies for the Newly Married" and "Problem-Solving for the Divorced-Separated") were accepted and clinical staff were in the process of establishing these programs at the end of the first eight months. Four recommendations (program for child-abusing parents; a group to assist school children in defining and resolving problematic feelings; a clinic-initiated program to instruct parents of children with behavior problems; and family counseling services for parents of school children) where considered more appropriate within the mandate of the clinic's sister agency which focuses on children under 18 and their families. Representatives of this agency were invited to attend a series of board meetings and these representatives agreed to plan for the development of these programs. Finally, two recommendations (clinical team's assistance with afterhour crisis intervention; a streamlining of the community's agency-referral system) were accepted but were not yet implemented by the end of the eight month period. Thus, of the eleven appropriate recommendations, all were accepted, and nine were implemented fully or in part by the end of the first eight months of the board's existence. That is a 77 percent implementation rate, suggesting the board had been reasonably effective in getting its recommendations implemented. Moreover, such an implementation rate indicates that the board has actual power and is not simply a token board.

Finally, the board functioning was also evaluated in terms of how successful it had been in bridging the gap between the community and the clinic. Of course a board cannot be very effective in such a role unless the community first knows about its existence. Street surveys before the board began, and after eight months, indicated that through publicity in the media, the board had been successful in increasing its visibility approximately 10 percent: no small feat indeed! There was also anecdotal evidence that certain citizens had called board members to have them raise particular issues at board meetings, thus establishing that the board was indeed a conduit for community grievances and recommendations. Furthermore, a number of citizens called to find out how they could enroll in the new mental health programs which had been publicized in the newspaper, thus suggesting that the board was serving its purpose of acting as a bridge between the community and the center.

In summary, there is evidence that the board had been successful in its first eight months in accomplishing its three primary tasks: program planning and implementation, community education, and increasing community awareness of board functioning.

Some Conclusions

Our review of the literature, although delineating a host of problems for citizen boards, also indicated that such boards offered some promise. We have described in detail the functioning of one board, delineating some of its problems and some of its successes. We doubt that a viable and effective board can emerge unless a clinic's staff is fully committed to consumer protection and involvement. The problems (e.g., decreasing attendance; members assenting to board membership for prestige rather than out of interest; and so on) will eventually token-ize a board unless clinic staff constantly evaluate the process and functioning of citizen boards. However, we remain convinced that, in spite of the problems and effort involved, citizen boards make good sense. Without them the community is liable to either get too little of what it wants and needs, or too much of what it neither wants nor needs.

References

Briscoe, R., Hoffman, D., & Bailey, J. Behavioral community psychology: Training a community board to problem solve. *Journal of Applied Behavior Analysis*, 1975, *8*, 157–168.

Chu, F., & Trotter, S. *The madness establishment.* New York: Grossman Publishers, 1974.

Cohen, S., Reid, W., & Berg, T. Measuring agency investment in community mental health. *Community Mental Health Journal*, 1975, *11*, 239–247.

Dudley, J. Citizens' boards for Philadelphia community mental health centers. *Community Mental Health Journal*, 1975, *11*, 410–417.

Holton, W., New, P., & Hessler, R. Citizen participation and conflict. *Administration in Mental Health*, 1973, *2*, 96–103.

Kane, T. Citizen participation in decision-making: Myth or strategy. *Administration in Mental Health*, 1975, *4*, 29–34.

Kupst, M. J., Reidda, P., & McGee, T. Community mental health boards: A comparison of their development, functions, and powers by board members and mental health center staff. *Community Mental Health Journal*, 1975, *11*, 249–255.

Meyers, W., Dorwart, R., Hutcheson, B., & Decker, D. Organizational and attitudinal correlates of citizen board accomplishment in mental health and retardation. *Community Mental Health Journal*, 1974, *10*, 192–197.

Morrison, J. K. An argument for mental patient advisory boards. *Professional Psychology*, 1976, *7*, 127–131.

Robins, A., & Blackburn, C. Governing boards in mental health: Roles and training needs. *Administration in Mental Health*, 1974, *3*, 37–45.

Rooney, H. Roles and functions of the advisory board. *North Carolina Journal of Mental Health*, 1968, *3*, 33–43.

Labeling:
A Study of an "Autistic" Child*

James K. Morrison

DURING THE PAST few decades, those involved in the mental health movement have conducted a "moral crusade" (cf. Sarbin and Mancuso, 1970) to induce the general public to adopt the proposition that deviant behavior is mental illness and that mental illness is similar to any other illness. Despite the immediate appeal of this crusade, the basic assumptions have evoked much criticism. Szasz (1961) has trenchantly criticized the view that mental illness is a disease similar to any other disease. Not only is the use of the disease model incorrect when applied to mental illness, but it is also dangerous in that it gives unwarranted legal power to medical practitioners who fill the role of experts on mental health (cf. Szasz, 1963, 1965). Even though mental health ideology has the aim of generating a more tolerant attitude toward norm-violating behavior, Sarbin (1967, 1969) and Sarbin and Mancuso (1970) have cogently argued that for the most part these attempts have been successful only in giving the public a new set of perjorative metaphors to replace the old ones. Indeed, despite the efforts to change

---

*This article was originally published in the *Journal of Family Counseling*, 1974, *2*, 71–80. Reprinted by permission.

the public's views toward mental illness, much of the mental health literature still views the psychotic as a strange, bizarre and extremely ineffectual person (cf. Arieti, 1959; Becker, 1964; Bellak, 1958; Downing, 1958; Fairweather, 1964; Gordon and Groth, 1961; Goffman, 1961; Joint Commission on Mental Illness and Health, 1961; Redlich and Freedman, 1966; Schooler and Parks, 1966; and Searles, 1965). As a result, others, according to Sarbin (1969) often view the psychotic as a "nonperson."

More recently, however, Braginsky and his associates (Braginsky and Braginsky, 1967; Braginsky et al., 1969; Braginsky et al., 1966; Braginsky et al., 1967; Braginsky et al., 1968) have begun to advocate a drastically different interpretation of psychotic behavior. Their research indicates that the psychotic is capable of social sensitivity in his use of manipulation as a means of reaching desired goals. Some psychotic patients engage in "crazy" behavior in order to remain in an institution, a place where they can at least find respite from the social turmoil which awaits them outside. Thus, often, persons labeled "mentally ill" engage in different behavior, not due to the inner dynamics of an "illness," but rather as a means of attaining their own desired goals. Following a similar trend, others (cf. Artiss, 1959; Levinson and Gallagher, 1964; Rakusin and Fierman, 1963; Szasz, 1961, 1965; Sarbin, 1967, 1969; Sarbin and Mancuso, 1970; and Towbin, 1966) have also portrayed psychotics in terms usually reserved for more "normal" persons.

Argument for a New Approach

It is the assumption of this study that mental illness labels are not only scientifically arid, but also very destructive in the labeled person's milieu. Once a person has been stigmatized by professionals as "mentally ill" a whole process is set in motion whereby the labeled person is sealed almost forever in his fate. The key persons in the labeled individual's milieu come to view all of his actions from a biased and distorted perspective. They begin to treat the target person differently, often becoming more permissive in the behavior which they expect and allow. This is especially true in the case of so-called autistic children. Once the professionals have attached such a label to children, their parents soon lose hope that such children can ever be "normal." They begin to tolerate deviant and embarrassing behavior in such children, whereas this would never be the case if these children were seen as "normal." When the child is taken to special schools, or introduced to anyone, the label "autistic" is propagated, thus ensuring that all will treat the child with special deference because of his "illness." Such children, so labeled and so treated, often engage in unmanageable behavior. But because few would conceive of such children as being socially sensitive in their use of manipulation to control their environment, the behavior is tolerated. After all, think the parents, if such behavior results from the child's "illness," it would be unfair to be anything but permissive! It is not the child's fault, but the fault of the "illness." The child can't help himself!

The present report pursues the following hypotheses; (1) once key persons in an "autistic'" child's milieu come to view the child within the framework they use to view any other child, and behave according to their perceptions, those persons will regain control over previously unmanageable behavior. Following this change of perspective, it is expected that (2) through education in the principles of behavior modification the parents and significant others will be able to bring about the rapid learning of new behavior on the part of the child.

The following questions guided the thinking of the behavior change specialist who worked with the boy described in this report: What will happen if the key persons in an "autistic" boy's milieu are educated to view the child from a totally different perspective? If the label "autistic" is removed, and if these persons are specially trained to act differently toward the child, will that child's behavior change? And if so, how radically? These are some of the questions which this author asked himself on his first encounter with the ten-year-old boy with whom this study is concerned. Rather than assuming the role of a "therapist," the author made a very concerted effort, within the time allowed, to treat the child within the framework of cognitive-learning theory, inducing significant others to view and treat the "autistic" boy from a new perspective. Having once changed the basic orientation toward the boy, the author was able to teach the key persons to bring about more socially desirable behavior on the part of the child by using various behavior modification techniques.

The approach of this present study issues from the basic proposition, set down so forcefully by Kuhn (1962), that one's paradigm shapes one's view. Thus, in the present study, it was expected that an alteration of the paradigms of key persons would lead to a change in behavior on the part of those persons toward the "autistic" child. One study (Shaver and Scheibe, 1967) has already demonstrated how a change in paradigm can result in an alteration of behavior. In their study of adult chronic mental patients at a summer camp, Shaver and Scheibe report that when nonmedical personnel treated the patients as "persons," the latter responded accordingly and began to act more "normally." It was the goal of this present study to induce significant individuals in the "autistic" boy's milieu to view this boy as a "person."

A Brief Behavioral History of Joey B.

Joey B., a tall handsome boy of ten years, was conceived out of wedlock, thus hastening marriage by his parents. He was delivered after extended and induced labor. From birth Joey was very energetic and restless, and his behavior became quite unmanageable. His mother felt inadequate because of her failure to maintain much control over the child's boundless activity. When he was twenty-two months old, Mike, his younger brother, was born. When Mrs. B. returned from the hospital, Joey behaved differently. He seemed withdrawn, passive and "depressed." Since Joey continued to show no real signs of verbal communication, the parents became even more concerned. Over the next eight years the parents took Joey to nine different psychiatrists and a number of other professionals (neurologists, hearing specialists, etc). The labels applied to the child varied from "emotionally disturbed" to "organic retardation." However, the most consistently applied label was that of "autistic." Although some of the staff at the various clinics and special schools attended by Joey took some time to teach him certain elementary behaviors (e.g., dressing himself, saying a few words, etc.), most seemed to do nothing more than squash further hopes of the parents that their child could be anything but hopelessly abnormal the rest of his life. And, it was no consolation for the parents to hear from so many that "autism" was a little understood illness. Following the completion and acceptance of the labeling process, the parents began to treat the boy even more specially. Hope having seemingly vanished, the parents no longer spent much time trying to teach the child any new behaviors. The parents' attitude toward the boy became passive and tolerant, with a certain degree of acceptance of their unfortunate fate.

After attending eight special schools, some producing positive and some negative behavioral changes, Joey was finally enrolled in a small school for children with "learning disabilities." Before his enrollment at this school, Joey's behavior had become intolerable.

After a psychiatrist prescribed the use of tranquilizers, Joey seemed to be in a great deal of pain, screamed constantly and became completely unmanageable in his behavior. Even the boy's father, who up to this point was able to exert some control over the child's actions, became ineffective in checking his son's enraged behavior. When first brought to this special school, Joey refused to eat and simply lay impassively on the floor away from the other eight boys. At first the staff was somewhat apprehensive about accepting Joey because of his "autistic" diagnosis. None of the other boys at the school was so labeled. However, since Joey's parents could find no other suitable arrangement, the school finally consented to accept the boy. With the patient help of the educational director at this school, Joey was gradually induced through praise and affection to explore and learn about his environment. Gradually, the boy began to eat regularly, associate with other boys and to learn rather rapidly many different sorting and matching tasks. It should be noted here that Joey was taken off tranquilizers before entering this school.

Although Joey's learning continued, after about four months in this school he began to engage in somewhat dangerous and unpredictable behavior. He would wander away from the school and at times lie down in the middle of the nearby highway, barely escaping being run over by passing vehicles. On another occasion he almost burned some of the other boys at the school when he suddenly overturned a pot of boiling water. Both because of the permissive atmosphere of the school and because Joey was treated differently because of his "autism," his disruptive behavior was not negatively reinforced in an appropriate manner. Finally, his destructive behavior reached the point where the staff at Joey's school became rather apprehensive, so they consulted with a clinical psychologist at a local state agency dealing with problem children. It was then that this author was asked to work with the child and his family for two and one-half hours a week.

The author's first encounter with Joey took place at his school. Upon entering the school, the author was soon approached by Joey. The boy stared briefly at this new visitor and then wandered off. Joey returned a few minutes later, climbed on the author's lap and began pulling the latter's hair. Joey incessantly made a variety of babbling sounds. He smiled gleefully much of the time as he was allowed to wander throughout the school at will, interrupting with little restraint the activities of the other children. While watching one of the volunteers trying to gain Joey's interest in a learning task, the author observed how often the boy was allowed to wander away from a task. None of the other boys in the school were treated in quite this manner. But then Joey was "autistic!" Needless to say, Joey was controlling his environment very nicely!

Joey engaged in various learning tasks for no more than a few seconds at a time. He flittered from task to task and from room to room. At times this author observed him engaging in socially disruptive behavior. When Joey would disturb the other boys while they were eating or playing, the other boys allowed him to do so for the most part. Even the other children in the school had learned that they must treat Joey specially!

Following this first encounter, the author saw Joey eight other times during the following nine weeks. The total time spent with the boy amounted to six and one-half hours. Approximately 18 hours were spent consulting with Joey's parents and teachers in an attempt to train them in a new approach. After nine weeks, this author took a new position with another agency and was forced to terminate his active involvement in the case. However, he did contact the boy and his mother and teachers for a two-month follow-up, during which time the author assessed the behavior of the child and the reactions of the significant persons in the child's milieu to that behavior.

Behavioral Analysis

One could theorize ad infinitum regarding the possible "causes" of Joey's original unmanageable behavior. However, emphasis on determining and maintaining the present reinforcement contingencies for Joey's behavior was considered of much more value. A behavioral analysis similar to that described by Kanfer and Saslow (1965) was conducted. With the emphasis on a "problem-solving" approach, the pitfalls of diagnostic classification or labeling were avoided. The learning theory at the base of this approach is similar to that set forth by Kanfer and Phillips (1970) and Mischel (1968).

Joey's behavior, labeled "autistic" by so many professionals, is here considered as "problem behavior," behavior which can disrupt a family in its regular everyday living. But this behavior issues not from the psychodynamics of an "illness," but rather from the environmental contingencies maintaining the behavior. Rather than calling such behavior "crazy," "abnormal," "autistic" or "mentally ill," it is more helpful to view such behavior from the perspective of learning theory. Thus the behavior can be explained like any other behavior for it is subject to the same principles which govern learning, reinforcement and extinction.

It is of crucial importance in relevant behavioral analysis to consider the effect that one's cognitive perspective can have on subsequent behavior. Certainly in the case of Joey, the frame of reference, built into key persons through the labeling process, affected the way those persons treated the child. The work of Kelly (1955) is important here in understanding how the way a person construes events determines the patterns of subsequent behaviors. Unfortunately, the importance of cognitive theory in relation to behavior has long been neglected (cf. Mancuso, 1970). In the case of "autistic" labeling it is easy to see how such a process, once having brought about a change in the perspective of key persons toward the "autistic" child, can result in the child beginning to act the way he is perceived.

In summary, Joey's behavior was viewed from the perspective of cognitive-learning theory. A problem-solving approach was used.

The Behavior Modification Program

Following the initial home visit, during which Joey was observed in his interaction with his mother and younger brother, the following two goals were considered practical in view of the short amount of time allotted to the study. First, it was important to determine the most potent and easily used negative and positive reinforcers so that a consistent behavior modification program could be set up in the tradition of Lovaas et al. (1965) and others such as Allen et al. (1964), Engeln et al. (1968), Harris et al. (1964) and Hart et al. (1964). In all of these studies contingent reinforcement was used to modify various destructive and antisocial behavior in children. It was especially important that Joey's mother be taught the most effective reinforcers, both because she spent so much time with the child, and because she felt so inadequate in the face of Joey's behavior. Once she would learn the use of the most potent reinforcers, when behavior change occurred, she would find new hope and encouragement in being able to control her son's behavior. (Joey's father seemed to have less difficulty managing the boy's behavior and thus was perhaps not motivated enough to take time off from work to attend the regular training sessions.) And once other key persons working with Joey began to use effective reinforcers they too would gain confidence in their own ability to bring about desired responses.

The second goal was that of consultation with all those concerned in order to bring about the most consistent reinforcement schedule possible for Joey, to ensure the extinction of certain behaviors and the strengthening of more acceptable behaviors, and to educate all concerned in the necessity of removing the "autistic" label and in treating Joey as one treats any other boy. Bijou (1965) in a school situation, and Hawkins et al., (1966) in a home situation, engaged in the treatment process the persons with whom the client had important daily role relations. In the Bijou study the parents were taught the principles about the conditions that affected their relations with their children and were shown concretely how to implement them. Similarly in this present study the education of the parents in cognitive-learning theory and the techniques of behavior modification were essential to the program. Other key persons (speech therapist, teachers) were also consulted so that a consistent reinforcement schedule might be established. Only through the sharing of information could a realistic evaluation of Joey's reinforcement contingencies be made.

A number of studies (cf. Engeln et al., 1968; Straughan, 1964; Wahler et al., 1965; Walder et al., 1967) have demonstrated the effectiveness of training mothers in a home situation to use behavior modification techniques. However, only the study by Engeln et al., (1968) really involved the whole family unit. No studies known to the author have involved both the family unit as well as other concerned persons (e.g., teachers).

With the cooperation of all concerned it was easier to alter the view that Joey was "autistic." It was hoped that, by viewing Joey's behavior in terms of learned maladaptive behavior, his parents and others would take a more active role in changing the boy's behavior. A change from viewing Joey as "autistic" was especially necessary for the boy's mother. Perhaps because of her psychiatric training as a nurse she tended to "psychologize" all of Joey's actions. She also seemed to have a neurotic need to have a "sick" son, a son who could, in his role as the "autistic" child, assuage her own guilt related to an unhappy marriage.

Determination of the Most Potent Reinforcers

After experimentation by this author with different types of reinforcement, dispensing affection proved to be the most effective positive reinforcement. The key persons in Joey's environment were then trained more effectively to use praise and physical affection (e.g., hug or kiss) contingent upon the execution by Joey of certain desired behaviors (e.g., changing his clothes after school, saying words, picking-up his room, etc.). At first, the consistent use of such rewards exhausted Joey's mother since she attempted, at first, to reinforce each of Joey's increasingly frequent positive behaviors. The author then showed her how she might shape Joey's behavior by dispensing rewards within a partial reinforcement schedule.

The most potent negative reinforcement proved to be a stern voice while issuing a command. This author found it necessary to have some persons, especially the mother, actually practice sounding "stern," while issuing commands to Joey. This the mother found difficult to do, perhaps because of her neurotic attachment to her son.

Consultation with and Education of Key Persons

By spending approximately two hours an afternoon each week consulting with those involved in eliciting new behavior from Joey, this author was able to accomplish much more than would have been possible had he spent all of that time working with Joey alone. Not only was the time spent with significant others effective in producing more widespread changes in behavior, it was also deemed essential in establishing lasting behavioral change. Although the author in his one-to-one relationship with Joey soon became a powerful reinforcing agent, he realized that the training of others would be more important since his contact with the child would eventually terminate.

Much of the time was spent with Mrs. B., pointing out how many of her methods of dealing with Joey were ineffectual in accomplishing positive behavior change. By discussing how she would try to "psychologize" everything her child did, she began to realize that she should act more spontaneously with Joey. Having been taught the use of reinforcements in a more efficient way, Mrs. B. found quick results, thus diminishing her despair over her failure as a mother. Once she realized what a powerful reinforcement agent she had become, she began to spend more time teaching her child new tasks. She also began to appreciate more the work of Joey's school, since this author was able to point out that many of the tasks Joey was now engaging in at home had been originally learned at school. As her control over Joey increased so did her cooperation in the treatment program. Mrs. B. quickly learned various techniques of behavior modification and felt more and more confident in using them alone and without direction. Becoming convinced that the new approach was working in changing Joey, she found new hope once again that Joey could develop more like other boys.

Mr. B. was consulted at his place of work. Through a sharing of knowledge, much insight was gained into Joey's behavior. Joey's father found new hope in the fact that his son's behavior had improved so much. Mr. B. began to talk and play with his son more than he ever had before. His negative attitude toward those in the psychiatric professions changed as a result of the successful management of his son's behavior. Mr. B. now no longer considered placing his son in an institution.

It was possible to obtain from Joey's speech therapist a list of words which the boy had been heard to say in the past. Such a list enabled the author to reward the saying of such words as "milk" and "juice" with the actual objects denoted by the words. It was felt that progress in speech development would ensue if all those in Joey's milieu made consistent efforts to give certain foods to Joey contingent upon the saying of the words. Thus Joey would learn the "magic" of words in bringing about desired objects, providing further incentive for him to say more and more words. Until the boy could *not* obtain certain desired objects without first saying the words for those objects, it was felt that he might not have the proper incentive to engage in verbal communication. To reinforce the cessation of babbling sounds would in the end be harmful, unless that silence could be filled with words. But to encourage the speaking of words Joey had to be treated differently than before, for he was already able to get most everything he wanted by other means of nonverbal communication (e.g., crying, babbling, grabbing, pulling of hair, etc.).

At conferences with the staff at Joey's school, it was decided to keep Joey at a task for longer periods of time without allowing him to escape. This was done by keeping him in a room away from the other children. Through the mutual sharing of information related to Joey's behavior both at home and at school, a better understanding of the boy's learning and behavior change was possible. Quite often all concerned would discover that they were working at cross-purposes. For example, on one occasion, a teacher was trying to induce Joey to draw loops on a blackboard, while at the same time this author had been working on extinguishing the drawing of such loops and reinforcing the drawing of horizontal and vertical lines. The author also encouraged the teachers at Joey's school to treat the boy increasingly like the other boys.

It is important to mention that Mike, Joey's younger brother, seemed to have been affected by how others treated his older brother. His parents often submitted to Joey when he acted strangely or when he persisted in disobeying his parents' commands. The lesson for Mike was clear. If you persist long enough, or if you act "crazy" as does Joey, you will get what you want! Mike had begun in the previous two years to withdraw more and more. He would seldom talk to strangers and played mostly by himself. At school he had begun to walk in a rather bizarre fashion, which aroused the concern of his teacher. He had also, according to his teacher, become so upset when his imaginary playmate had become "sick" that the teacher had to call his mother. When Mike's father heard of the incident, he decided to take some responsibilities (e.g., making the bed, doing the dishes) away from Mike, since they seemed to be too much for him! Thus Mike was escaping household chores by acting "crazy" like his brother!

It was suspected that perhaps Mike's teacher might be treating Mike as if something were "mentally" wrong with him since she knew of Mike's older brother, Joey. After conferring with this teacher and assuring her that Mike was not "mentally ill" the teacher began to treat Mike like her other students. Mike admitted that his bizarre walking and sick imaginary playmate were all part of a hoax. In order to provide Mike with a feeling of importance within the family and to establish a way he could consistently receive some positive reinforcement for "normal" behavior, Mike's cooperation was enlisted in teaching his older brother how to say words. It was arranged that Mike would receive verbal reinforcement from his parents for such behavior.

It should be noted here that Mr. and Mrs. B. were unhappy in their marriage almost from the beginning. The marriage had reached the point where neither party was actually communicating with the other anymore. When communication did take place it was more in the context of a threat or coercion to attain certain ends. Mrs. B. expressed with sadness that the only thing which kept her and her husband together were the children. One might add that it was the "sick" children which kept the parents together. Attempts to arrange marriage counseling for the parents failed because of

Mr. B.'s lack of cooperation. However, a number of individual sessions with Mrs. B. helped to alleviate her depression to the extent that she could engage in the behavioral program.

Results of the Behavior Modification Program

After proper instruction Joey's mother soon exerted extraordinary control over all of Joey's behavior. By the careful dispensation of positive and negative reinforcement she was able to bring about rapid and dramatic changes in Joey's behavior. She learned to negatively reinforce babbling sounds with a stern "no," while placing her hand over her son's mouth, and then positively reinforce silence with affection and attention. Gradually Joey's mother was able to induce her son to emit a number of words through the use of positive reinforcement (e.g., food, physical affection, etc.).

With the cooperation of all concerned, dramatic changes were brought about in Joey's behavioral repertoire. Whereas, before the behavioral modification program Joey consistently thwarted his mother's efforts to induce him to change clothes on coming home from school, now one request was often sufficient to induce Joey to go to his room and change. Formerly, Joey had very few table manners. Now he became neat and orderly at the table. Other changes included attention to a learning task for as long as two hours (rather than a few seconds), willingness to play games by himself or with his brother, quiet, gentlemanlike behavior in public (rather than crawling and babbling in stores), cessation of hair pulling, the disappearance of wandering behavior while at school and the termination of behavior which disturbed others at home or at school (e.g., breaking of objects, hitting playmates, pulling magazines out of his father's hands, etc.). Joey even submitted to having his hair cut for the first time without screaming at the top of his voice!

People who had known Joey but had not seen him since the inception of the behavioral program remarked at the dramatic change they noticed in this ten-year-old boy. The more Joey changed the easier it was for the people in Joey's environment to treat him as a "normal" boy. His behavior became positive reinforcement for his parents who now increased the time they spent with him. Enthusiasm and optimism began to replace frustration and despair. Joey seemed more content now that behavioral limits had been established.

The behavioral modification program also brought about changes in the behavior of Joey's brother, Mike. Apparently more content as a result of consistent reinforcement for more socially acceptably behavior, Mike began to spend more time on homework, was less of a distraction to his fellow students in class and was more helpful to Joey in teaching his brother new tasks. As both of their sons emitted less "crazy" behavior, Mr. and Mrs. B. felt less like failures as parents and the communication between them appeared to improve greatly.

Two-Month Follow-up

Eight weeks after this author's active involvement in the case he returned to Joey's home for a two-hour evaluation session with Joey, his parents and his teachers. In evaluating Joey's behavior both at school and at home, it was evident that the socially acceptable behavior which had been increased during the behavioral program was still a stable part of Joey's behavioral repertoire. There did not appear to be any significant decrease in this "positive" behavior, and further, Joey continued to make gains at school in his learning of concepts and tasks.

Conclusions

A number of conclusions can be drawn from this study. Although there was no attempt to empirically test a hypothesis, some of the observations made during this study are most illuminating regarding so-called autistic behavior. The short space of time spent with Joey and those in his environment would of course limit the generality of the conclusions. However, the long list of behavioral improvements which were attained in this short period of time testifies to the effectivess of the approach used.

The following conclusions seem warranted. Frequently the labeling process induces a change in the cognitive frame of reference used by key people who are working with an "autistic" child. The process of labeling may bring about a number of pernicious and pervasive effects in a child's behavior. In the case of Joey, regardless of any precipitating causes for Joey's original behavior, the labeling process seemed to benefit no one. In fact, there is evidence in this case history that Joey's parents and teachers, by viewing Joey as special, inadvertently reinforced socially unacceptable behavior. Mrs. B. certainly provided evidence of how the psychiatrists' labeling of Joey had led to her cessation of meaningful time with her son since she now believed that nothing would be of much use in changing Joey's "mysterious" behavior.

Another conclusion which can be drawn from this study is that some combination of cognitive and learning theory may be more useful in explaining behavior to laymen than are explanations couched in syncretistic medical model terminology. The former approach encourages individuals to take an active part in changing unacceptable behavior, whereas the latter approach too often encourages resignation, resentment, permissiveness and despair.

One might also conclude from this case study that those working with children might reconsider the time they spend directly with children, and spend more time coordinating and teaching others so that there will be a more unified and more effective behavioral change program. Such a program will fail eventually unless the key persons in a child's milieu are induced to cooperate fully with the program.

This study was an attempt to overcome the pernicious and pervasive effects of an "autistic" labeling process. By means of an alteration of the framework from which key persons viewed the "autistic" child and with the proper use of behavioral modification techniques, the child's socially unacceptable behavior was extinguished to a great degree and in its place more acceptable behavior was substituted. It would seem important in this day of widespread acceptance of the utility of behavior modification that the usefulness of a cognitive approach not be neglected. This study has indicated that a combined approach—behavior modification with emphasis on changing the cognitive perspective of key persons in the target person's milieu—may be the most effective. The next step is to empirically test the advantages of such a combined approach with children.

References

Allen, E. K., Hart, B. M., Buell, J. S., Harris, F. R., & Wolf, M. M. Effects of social reinforcement on isolate behavior of a nursery school child. *Child Development*, 1964, *35*, 511–518.

Arieti, S. *American handbook of psychiatry.* New York: Basic Books, 1959.

Artiss, K. L. *The symptom as communication in schizophrenia.* New York: Grune and Stratton, 1959.

Becker, E. *The revolution in psychiatry.* London: Collier-MacMillan, 1964.

Bellak, L. *Schizophrenia: A review of the syndrome.* New York: Logos Press, 1958.

Bijou, S. W. Experimental studies of child behavior, normal and deviant. In L. Krasner & L. P. Ullman (Eds.), *Research in behavior modification.* New York: Holt, Rinehart & Winston, 1965, Pp. 56–81.

Braginsky, B. & Braginsky, D. Schizophrenic patients in the psychiatric interview: An experimental study of their effectiveness at manipulation. *Journal of Consulting Psychology,* 1967, *31,* 543–547.

Braginsky, B., Braginsky, D., & King, K. *Methods of madness.* New York: Holt, Rinehart & Winston, 1969.

Braginsky, B., Grosse, M., & Ring, K. Controlling outcomes through impression management: An experimental study of the manipulative tactics of mental patients. *Journal of Consulting Psychology,* 1966, *30,* 295–300.

Braginsky, B., Holzberg, J., Finison, L., & Ring, K. Correlates of the mental patient's acquisition of hospital information. *Journal of Personality,* 1967, *35,* 323–342.

Braginsky, B., Holzberg, J., Ridley, D., & Braginsky, D. Patient styles of adaptation to a mental hospital. *Journal of Personality,* 1968, *36,* 283–298.

Downing, J. Chronic mental hospital dependency as a character defense. *Psychiatric Quarterly,* 1958, *32,* 489–499.

Engeln, R., Knutson, J., Laughy, L. & Garlington, W. Behavior modification techniques applied to a family unit—A case study. *Journal of Child Psychology and Psychiatry,* 1968, *9,* 245–252.

Fairweather, G. *Social psychology in treating mental illness: An experimental approach.* New York: Wiley, 1964.

Goffman, E. *Asylums: Essays on the social situation of mental patients and other inmates.* Garden City, New York: Doubleday, 1961.

Gordon, H. and Groth, L. Mental patients wanting to stay in the hospital. *American Medical Association Archives of General Psychiatry,* 1961, *4,* 124–130.

Harris, F. R., Johnston, M. K., Kelley, S. C., and Wolf, M. M. Effects of positive social reinforcement on regressed crawling of a nursery school child. *Journal of Educational Psychology,* 1964.

Hart, B. M., Allen, E. K., Buell, J. S., Harris, F. R., & Wolf, M. M. Effects of social reinforcement on operant crying. *Journal of Experimental Child Psychology,* 1964, *1,* 145–153.

Hawkins, R. P., Peterson, R. F., Schweid, E., & Bijou, S. W. Behavior therapy in the home: Amelioration of problem parent-child relations with the parent in a therapeutic role. *Journal of Experimental Child Psychology,* 1966, *4,* 99–107.

Joint Commission on Mental Illness and Health. *Action for mental health.* New York: Basic Books, 1961.

Kanfer, F. H. & Phillips, J. S. *Learning foundations of behavior therapy.* New York: Wiley, 1970.

Kanfer, F. H. & Saslow, G. Behavioral analysis: An alternative to diagnostic classification. *Archives of General Psychiatry*, 1965, *12*, 529–538.

Kelly, G. *The psychology of personal constructs*. Vols. 1 and 2. New York: W. W. Norton and Co., 1955.

Kuhn, T. S. *The structure of scientific revolutions*. Chicago, University of Chicago Press, 1962.

Levinson, D. & Gallagher, E. *Patienthood in the mental hospital*. Boston: Houghton and Mifflin, 1964.

Lovaas, O. I. Freitag, G., Gold, V. J., & Kassorla, I. C. Experimental studies in childhood schizophrenia: I. Analysis of self-destructive behavior. *Journal of Experimental Child Psychology*, 1965, *2*, 67–84.

Mancuso, J. C. *Readings for a cognitive theory of personality*. New York: Holt, Rinehart and Winston, 1970.

Mischel, W. *Personality and Assessment*. New York: Wiley, 1968.

Rakusin, J. & Fierman, L. Five assumptions for treating chronic psychotics. *Mental Hospitals*, 1963, *14*, 140–148.

Redlich, F. & Freedman, D. *The theory and practice of psychiatry*. New York: Basic Books, 1966.

Sarbin, T. On the futility of the proposition that some people be labeled "mentally ill." *Journal of Consulting Psychology*, 1967, *31*, 447–453.

Sarbin, T. The scientific status of the mental illness metaphor. In S. C. Plog and R. B. Edgerton (Eds.), *Changing perspectives in mental illness*. New York: Holt, Rinehart and Winston, 1969.

Sarbin, T. & Mancuso, J. The failure of a moral enterprise: Attitudes of the public toward mental illness. *Journal of Consulting and Clinical Psychology*, 1970, *35*, 159–173.

Schooler, C. & Parkel, D. The overt behavior of chronic schizophrenics and the relationship to their internal state and personal history. *Psychiatry*, 1966, *29*, 67–77.

Searles, H. *Collected papers on schizophrenia and related subjects*. New York: International Universities Press, 1965.

Shaver, P. R. & Scheibe, K. E. Transformation of social identity: A study of chronic mental patients and college volunteers in a summer camp setting. *Journal of Psychology*, 1967, *66*, 19–37.

Szasz, T. *The myth of mental illness*. New York: Hoeber-Harper, 1961.

Szasz, T. *Law, liberty, and psychiatry*. New York: Macmillan, 1963.

Szasz, T. *Psychiatric justice*. New York: Macmillan, 1965.

Towbin, A. Understanding the mentally deranged. *Journal of Existentialism*, 1966, *7*, 63–83.

Wahler, R. G., Winkel, G. H., Peterson, R. F., & Morrison, D. C. Mothers as behavior therapists for their own children. *Behavior Research and Therapy*, 1965, *3*, 113–124.

Walder, L. O., Cohen, S. I., Breiter, D. E., Daston, P. G., Hirsch, I. S., & Liebowitz, J. M. Teaching behavioral principles to parents of disturbed children. Paper read at Eastern Psychological Convention, Boston, 1967.

9
The Ethical Problems of Service Providers

Overview

CHAPTER 9, THE last chapter in this book, is appropriately devoted to some of the ethical issues which face mental health profesionals in general, and community psychologists in particular. Ethical concerns are always at the heart of a true consumer-oriented approach. The first article outlines those roles which may easily become ethical and conceptual traps for psychologists. I hope this discussion will enable those of us working in the field of community psychology to rethink our roles. Unless we do so we risk deceiving not only ourselves, but also the client-consumers who may be less able to see the subtle moral implications of our community role-enactments.

The second article is a discussion of the ethical, psychological and legal implications of offering psychological services to that special client-consumer, the child. After an extensive review of the relevant literature, a number of specific recommendations are made which may enable clinicians to deal more effectively with a relatively new issue of concern, i.e., whether children should have the right to give informed consent to treatment, before such treatment is foisted upon them. The child-consumer is a very powerless person in our society and extra precautions must be taken to ensure that his or her rights are protected within the sphere of community psychology.

Psychology in the Morals Marketplace: Role Dilemma for Community Psychologists

James C. Mancuso, Morris E. Eson, and James K. Morrison

To FOCUS MORE sharply on the psychiatric client as a consumer and evaluator of community mental health services (Morrison, in press), a psychologist must accept responsibility for scrutinizing the ethical implications of enacting a particular kind of professional role. Critics (Braginsky, & Braginsky, 1974; Sarbin, & Mancuso, 1970; Szasz, 1970) now clearly have registered the accusation that mental health professionals, including the clinical and the research psychologist, have failed to draw the needed distinctions between clinical judgments and moral judgments. This essay closely examines the issues involved in using the position of applied psychologist, particularly that of the community psychologist, to take on the role, often inadvertantly, of moralist. To conduct this examination we have identified four roles (healer, behavioral engineer, psychotechnologist, and scientist) which can be adopted by community psychologists. At the close, we identify that role which promises the best assurance that community psychologists can forestall entry into the "morals marketplace."

Moral Endeavor and Moral Entrepreneurship

The essence of the problems arising from community life has not changed over the ages. What has changed is the formulation of these problems or how they are construed and the solutions which seemed to follow from these constructions. Every society throughout history has used an ideology to regulate behavior and, thereby, to stabilize and perpetuate itself. To discover an ideology, Mannheim (1936) advises, one best looks at the sets of beliefs which become apparent only when political conflict arises. Such conflict, he argues, reveals "that ruling groups can in their thinking become so intensively interest-bound to a situation that they are no longer able to see certain facts which would undermine their sense of domination" (p. 36). Ideology of a society, then, might be considered as the core assumptive structure which guides much of the intellectual and political activity of the society. One all-pervading aspect of the ideology is the *moral* aspect which provides the "self-evident" truths in regard to judgments of "good" and "bad."

These self-evident truths of the moral ideology must be promoted, disseminated and implemented. Such activity, in a modern day society organized along national lines, requires a rather elaborate apparatus consisting of schools, churches, courts, prisons, armies and the like. The individuals who choose to work in these settings may be considered participants in a *moral endeavor*. They are assigned roles by which they help to maintain the stability of the society through inculcating and guarding the moral ideology. It is likely that they frequently fulfill this role by accepting, with little or no reservation, the basic assumptions of the ideology. They are, in this sense, true believers; and operating on these often unexamined assumptions about good and evil, virtue and sin, they do their part in setting a course and a direction to the society.

The moral ideology provides the unspoken justification for most of the systematized activities of the society, particularly, its economic institutions, or its arrangements for providing various goods and services and for the distribution of privilege and responsibility. That is to say, the justification for the maintenance of these activities is grounded within the framework of the established moral ideology. Individuals participating in these approved arrangements prove their own legitimate self-interest in that their participation earns for them an acceptable place within the community. However, they can act in such a way as to make it appear that their self-interest is secondary or non-existent by proclaiming the interests of community as primary, thus becoming participants in a moral endeavor. When such is the case we choose to call such individuals *moral entrepreneurs*. For example, moral entrepreneurship can be recognized when an organization of physicians opposes changes in the form of the delivering of medical services by appealing to percepts drawn from the social ideology (the advancement of medical knowledge, the breakdown of the valued physician-patient relationship), when in actuality the opposition is engendered by the threat to professional economic interests. When a group asserts that "what is good for X is good for the country" one reasonably suspects that a narrow interest is being camouflaged behind the broader moral ideology, and we would be jusified in considering it to be a blatant example of moral entrepreneurship.

The role of the scientist within this framework becomes somewhat ambiguous and difficult to determine. Do scientists, as scientists, play roles within the moral endeavor, promoting the ideology for the sake of the established order? In which instances may one categorize a scientist as a moral entrepreneur, exploiting the ideology for his own interest? Does he possibly stand outside the system with reference to ideology? These questions arise, we suspect, because of the short history of the professional scientist's role. They are particularly acute when addressed to the role of community psychologist, qua social scientist. When, for example, a psychologist promotes a particular model of man, is he motivated by the interests of the existing social order or by in the interest of some "new" social order? Or does such a model of man give the psychologist larger personal influence over others, under the pretense of benefiting others and the social order? Indeed, could one show that the proposed model stands altogether outside the moral ideology of one or another society?

In seeking to resolve the dilemma arising from the community psychologist's involvement with ideology we must recognize that scientists work within their own moral ideology, with a set of assumptive truths that serve to maintain the social order within the community of scientists. This ideology, of course, applies to a more restricted range of events than that subsumed by the total society's ideology—but it is not likely to be in opposition to the main suppositions of the more comprehensive ideology, simply because the scientist plays his occupational role at the same time that he plays his role as citizen-at-large. Thus, although the social scientist may assert that he is not guided by the existing norms in his analysis of a social problem, and that he offers a solution that is "best" within the framework of science, inevitably he is bound, to a greater or lesser extent, by the constraints of the existing ideologies of his profession and his society. Again we note that this problem is particularly acute in the case of the community psychologist whose subject matter is the very essence of the moral ideology, namely, man relative to the community. The recent charges (Wade, 1976) of the falsification of data collected by Sir Cyril Burt in order to make a case for the inherited basis for intelligence, is a case in point. In the sociology of knowledge it is generally accepted that the selection of a problem for investigation, the procedures adopted for elucidation and the drawing of implications from data are all intimately associated with ideological considerations. When we have clear indications of fraud, we are particularly alerted to the probability that the psychologist has crossed the line to moral entrepreneurship.

Because of his training the applied psychologist has to be painfully aware that his discipline provides few, if any self-evident truths about the value orderings of behaviors in social matrices. Is it *better* for a person to show more or less coercive behaviors? Is it *better* to be oriented toward high or low achievement motivation? Is it *better* for a person to be cautious or to be spontaneous? Is it *better* to arrange to remove "deviant" citizens to mental hospitals or to try to keep them in the community? The psychologist cannot answer these questions solely out of his discipline and we maintain that he shouldn't pretend that he can. When he promotes a "self-evident" value proposition pertaining to his subject matter, without being able to produce the same kind of validation he would offer for any other scientific principle, his stand derives from faith and not from the methodology of his science. He should expect that his proposals will be treated as would those of the clergyman. When he flaunts his scientific status to further the ideology and thereby promotes his own power and interests he becomes a moral entrepreneur.

The contrast between the clergyman in a mainstream religion and a salesman may be illuminating. The clergyman adopts the role of one participating in a moral endeavor. He generally has a vision of the "good" world and he seeks to influence others to accept his vision and to accept the behaviors that will bring about this better condition. He knows that he cannot objectively validate his position and he appeals primarily to faith, both his own and that of his followers. His followers desire to pay his salary, and the society extends special esteem and favor to him and his establishment. The salesman, on the other hand, does not have such a broad vision. He may promote his product in the name of a specific benefit, and sometimes he tries to advance his own interest in the name of the buyer's self-interest. Most salesmen, however, recognize the futility of trying to sell their products in the name of the social order—

that is, of playing the moral entrepreneur. A politician stands somewhere between the clergyman and the salesman. He is expected to support the society's moral endeavor, but he can easily disguise his self-interest within the ideology; and, in fact, most citizens assume this to be standard practice. When a psychologist claims that he can ameliorate mental illness, or childhood hyperactivity, or juvenile delinquency, is he promoting a product that stands outside of a social ideology, or does he suggest that he can improve the social order and thereby ask that he be supported by the society as is the clergyman?

Like the clergyman, or like anyone else, the psychologist may enlist his energies in the moral endeavor. His functioning becomes problematic to his professional colleagues and to the public when he ignores his moral functioning, particularly when he concurrently takes to the lectern or to the journals to describe professional roles that ring with science and value objectivity. The social system, for its own reasons, often ignores moral entrepreneurship and offers high and positive status to a variety of roles which applied psychologists may enact. Honesty demands that we direct critical analysis toward illuminating the areas where the applied psychologist uses his professional role to sell moral judgments.

Moral Entrepreneurship in the Healer Model

In the last decades of the nineteenth century when the study of human behavior emerged in the western world as an independent discipline, behavioral scientists committed themselves to the logical-empiricist* mode of explaining behavior. The disease model became the leading explanatory scheme for the understanding and treatment of unacceptable norm-violating behavior. In confronting persons who manifested behavior that could not be readily understood and whose responsibility seemed to violate the generally accepted deterministic principles of reward and punishment, society's agents resorted to the paradigm that accounted for deviant behavior as being caused by disease. Such a model of deviant behavior serves to draw attention away from the ideology of the society that undergirds its various institutions and that maintains the established patterns of social relations. Freud, who was respon-

---

*Radnitzky (1970) contrasts the logical-empiricist mode with the hermeneutic-dialectic mode. The former is exemplified in mathematics and physics, the latter in history and *Geisteswissenschaft* (The humanities).

sible more than anyone else for initiating and promoting the disease model for deviant behavior, has been criticized by Fromm (1970) for "his unquestioning belief, that his society, although by no means satisfactory, was the ultimate form of human progress and could not be improved in any essential feature" (p. 18).

The disease model in medicine had succeeded in removing value connotations from explanations of physical abnormality by extending the use of the same mechanistic principles that were being applied to explain normal physiological and anatomical processes. By an almost poetic extension of the mechanistic metaphor psychiatrists like Freud could explain behavioral deviations which disrupt "the ultimate form of human progress." A variety of mechanistic explanatory routes lay open. Behavioral deviants contain "weak" nervous systems and/or the "shock" (the energy impact) of "emotional trauma" "breaks down" the person's psychic processes. The "energy" of the libido increases to a point where it "breaks through" the "defensive system" of the ego, causing the person to "revert" to primary process behavior.

Mechanistic and reductionist metaphors, accounting for aberrant behavior, may be said to have reached a nadir in Meehl's presidential address before the American Psychological Association.

> What we are looking for [to explain schizophrenia] is a quantitative abberation in synaptic control—a deviation in amount of patterning of excitatory or inhibitory action—capable of yielding cumulative departures from normal control linkages under mixed appetive-aversive regimes; ... The defect must generate aversive drift on mixed social reinforcement regimes, and must yield a primary cognitive slippage.... (Meehl, 1962, p. 836; material in brackets ours.)

The inherited neurological defect that provides the substrate for clinical schizophrenia—schizotaxia—interferes with the appropriate exchange of those energies which are known as *reinforcement*! Cognitive slippage, Meehl's "diagnostic bell ringer," results from inappropriate control linkages within the machine.

In a world where humanitarian ideologies have demanded that persons should have unimpeded access to health care, those who assume the healer role acquire the high value status associated with the role. If outlandish behavior is regarded as a *symptom* of a *disease,* the professional who offers to alter the unusual and unacceptable behavior pattern is accorded the high value status of the healer. Within the framework of the disease model, a "behavior regulation specialist" offers services that are highly valued by the society. Such services enable the society to pretend that the problem is the problem of an individual and can be resolved without resort to overt coercion which might produce a collective reaction against the established order.

Further, the disease model easily assimilates extensions which enhance the positive status of behavior regulation and moral endeavor. A *mentally* ill person, after all, *suffers* in the maze of his *anxieties*! Schizophrenia extracts a heavy economic toll, for the disease has its greatest incidence among those persons who are at the peak of their productive years, and this disorder *debilitates* them so that they are *deprived of the benefits* of their years of educational preparation! Certainly, society owes high positive status to the behavior regulation specialists who "cure" these "sufferers" so that they can vigorously participate in the productivity and prosperity of the community!

One would need to be a cantankerous misanthrope in order to denigrate the psychologist or other community mental health professional who works within this particularly ennobling conception of the behavior regulator. Consider the seductiveness of the Rubinstein and Coelho's (1970) laudatory appraisal of the involvement of one federal agency in the moral endeavor.

> Prior to the riots of that explosive summer [of 1968] the institute (NIMH) had supported studies dealing with civil disorders ... studies relating to collective behavior, involving protest, conflict and hostility, are supported at approximately $1.5 million. Many studies focus on consequences of deviation and discrimination on self-esteem and identity as important factors in social adaptation.
>
> Insights derived from the laboratory and the clinic have been useful but are not sufficient. We know much from experimental research about the dynamics of social perception and attitude change, intergroup conflict and prejudice and the development of aggressive behavior and hostility. Important hormonal, psychological, and neurophysiological variables have been identified in laboratory work on individual reaction to stress ... (p. 52).

Rubinstein and Coelho, fortified by their disease model, romp through the following associations: Riots→ civil disorders→ collective behavior→ protest→ conflict→ hostility→ deprevation→

discrimination → self-esteem→ self identity→ laboratory→ clinic→ important hormonal, psychological and neurophysiological variables. From politics to neurophysiology in two easy paragraphs! The transition is now an integral part of our thinking about unwanted behavior within the mental disease model. Mass violence, which might best be viewed within a framework that takes into account legal, political, and economic variables, somehow connects to neurophysiology and hormones. Surely one must identify this transition as a case of mechanism triumphant over moral philosophy!

It may be small comfort to the targets of that rioter's hostility to know that should politicial activity take the form of violence, the healer can offer to cure the rioter. Rubinstein and Coelho, writing in a house organ of the American Psychological Association, assure us that behavioral scientists, in the employ of the state, have been devoting their energies to the mental health of those who would become involved in violent political activity; that is, in moral matters.

At any rate, their thesis is easily identified in the above quotation. Rubinstein and Coelho speak enthusiastically about behavioral science involvement in the moral enterprise wherein riots and aggressive problem solution are adjudged to be *bad*. They thinly disguise their involvement in this enterprise by introducing a discussion of hormones and neurophysiology. In that the most casual analysis reveals the inadequacy of their ploy, they must fail in their efforts to convert social problems into individual disorders. How could they avoid being classed as entrepreneurs?

Unfortunately, such writings have easily induced college youth to believe that their involvement in regulation of violent conflict qua psychologists or healers will be adjudged a humanitarian activity that deserves high positive evaluation. And, having become a true believer, what shall a young student do after spending five or six years pursuing a career in one of the ennobling professions that assumedly lead to the healer's role? Should he silently acquiesce to the pretense and then become a moral entrepreneur in the disguise of a healer? Or should he openly announce his intention to use his science to participate in promotion of an ideology; that is, should he join a moral endeavor? Perhaps he would become more effective as a scientist if he chose the latter course.

Anyone attempting to unmask the moral entrepreneur who hides behind the disguise of the healer should inform himself of the incisive arguments and conclusions of Thomas Szasz (1970).

For while the ethicist is supposedly concerned only with normal (moral) behavior, and the psychiatrist only with abnormal (emotionally disordered) behavior, the very distinction between the two rests on ethical grounds. In other words, the assertion that a person is mentally ill involves rendering a moral judgment about him. Moreover, because of the social consequences of such a judgment, both the "mental patient" and those who treat him as one become actors in a morality play, albeit one written in a medical-psychiatric jargon (p. 26).

A scientist might turn his scientific endeavor to explaining the social consequences of an authority pronouncing the judgment that a person is "mentally ill" In a latter section of the book containing the above quotation, Szasz speaks of psychiatric classification as a strategy of personal constraint. We turn to a quotation from this latter section.

... being placed in certain classes affects people, whereas it does not affect animals and things. You call a person "schizophrenic", and something happens to him; you call a rat "rat" and rock "granite", and nothing happens to them. In other words, in psychiatry and in human affairs generally, *the act of classification* is an exceedingly significant event. (Szasz, 1970, p. 191)

What happens to a person who is labeled? For one thing, he immediately is assigned to a degraded status. There are those who would insist that to call a person a *patient* rather than to call him a *sinner*, spares him of a value scale placement. Slogans like "Alcoholism is a disease like any other disease," assumedly encourage a "value free," medical classification, but the general public is hardly taken in by this "put on." In fact, anyone who has worked in a situation where he can listen to the coffee break conversations of clinical psychologists and psychiatrists cannot honestly contend that all members of the mental health team share the belief that "Alcoholism is a disease like any other disease." The best propaganda has not dispelled the widely held belief that persons who have been called *alcoholics* are basically *bums*. Over and over studies have shown (Sarbin and Mancuso, 1970) that the general public has not been induced to convert *sin* into *illness*. Negatively valued behavior, in the perceptions of the man on the street, has not yet become identified as the province of the psychiatrist. And it is clear that when the psychiatrist tries to induce the man in the street to believe that the unacceptable deviant shall be called a *patient,* the deviator becomes the subject of more intense rejections (Phillips, 1963, 1964).

One could hypothesize that the moral enterprise involved in the "psychiatrization" of unwanted behavior works a yet more significant, but somewhat indirect, effect. The by-standing observer of the labeling process learns something more than the fact that the deviator has been labeled. He also learns that a set of experts has invented and spelled out the particulars of a social role. He has watched the experts invent *mental illness* just as the experts, under the leadership of super-experts like Torquemada and Sprenger and Kraemer, invented the role of *witch*, which was then used as an ascription for some of the deviants who lived during the era of the Inquisition. And we can easily take a page from the studies of person perception to tell us about what happens when roles become available for attribution to one's self and to other persons (see Hastdorf, Schneider, and Polefka, 1970, pp. 61–90).

Members of our society know that there are experts who can act as critics of their role enactments, and the experts are empowered to award the role of *mentally ill person*, with all its negative status, to those who enact unacceptable, norm-violating behaviors. And the role assignment, once the society has created experts and patients, need not be direct. In a study reported by Yaffee and Mancuso (1977) observers ascribed relatively greater maladjustment, less power, and less activity to a subject toward whom an actor-interviewer had acted in a "professionally interested" manner. By contrast, where the interviewer acted in an offhand manner, or in an aggressively intrusive manner, the client was not judged to be as maladjusted or powerless.

Knowing the effects of the direct and indirect expert classification of persons who behave deviantly, does it not behoove ordinary unsophisticated members to shun the society's experts, lest they receive a "prize" for their successful enactment of the mentally ill role. What happens to a young officer in the armed forces of a powerful nation who knows that if he stands as the accused in a court martial proceeding, a healer may be called in to decide whether the defendent is *ill* rather than culpable? Which would act as a greater restraint upon his propensity to protest an inhumane military operation—his fear that his humanitarianism can be adjudged as a sign of his mental illness or his fear that he will be convicted of mutiny?

Rabkin (1972) has reviewed various studies that show how widely accepted is the mental illness model among thousands of intensively propagandized college students. In spite of the presumed air of objective neutrality with which the concept is promulgated, students are certain to be concerned lest the label "mentally ill" be assigned to them. Szasz and others have offered a convincing argument that diagnostic labeling acts as a form of personal restraint. The disease model associated with the role of the healer has been a major instrument in the exercise of social control and hence has rendered the role a moral enterprise.

Because mental health professionals have covertly meddled in the morals marketplace, critics have accused psychiatrists of being "priests" of a "new religion" (Lasch, 1976), psychologists of being "high priests of the middle class" (Braginsky & Braginsky, 1973), and psychotherapy as being a secular religion (Hall, 1974). Beit-Hallahmi (1976) has identified both religion and psychological treatment as serving social control functions. He notes that secular and religious helpers both share a value-laden ideology; in the case of the latter, however, the moral implications are patent while in the case of the former they are latent. To adopt the healer role in our society would seem to have moral/religious implications. However, few professionals writing within the field of community psychology address the matter of the healer role being extensively implicated in the moral enterprise.

The Behavioral Engineer as Moral Entrepreneur

Our age has been characterized as the age of technique. Progress is evident everywhere to a point where it seems to have become everyone's most important product. If the role of the medically oriented healer is to be rejected because of its implicit moral ideology, perhaps the role of the behavioral engineer would avoid value controversy. The engineer who designs a bigger and better rocket can allow himself the solace by limiting his responsibility to getting it up and assigning to others the value decision as to where it goes down. In his presidential address before the American Psychological Association, Albee (1970) suggests the possibility of such a course for the applied psychologist, namely that of the behavioral engineer. On the surface such an approach seems to avoid the pitfalls of the healer model. But does not the hazard appear when the rhetorical question is asked, "Who wants the psychologist to do the engineering?" Albee stood in little danger of criticism from fellow psychologists when he announced, in 1969, that racists harbor deep-seated emotional problems, and that psychologists could try to intervene meaningfully in their lives. One might wonder about the welcome that would await this same speech had it been given by the then president of a psychological association in the Union of South Africa. Would Albee have given the same speech at the APA convention had the convention been held in the State of Florida in 1889, rather than in 1969? Would he, in 1889, have been convinced that his science of psychology had clearly revealed the interconnections between racism and delusional behavior? Or would he, in 1889, have echoed the words of Sir Francis Galton, whose scientific credentials repeatedly receive commendation in the Psychology 101 textbooks that are used throughout the country?

> It strikes me that the Jews are specialized for a parasitical existence upon other nations, and that there is need of evidence that they are capable of fulfilling the varied duties of a civilized nation by themselves (cited in Hirsch, 1972, pp. 11–12).

Perhaps Albee would believe that he holds a more scientifically sound position than that which Galton held? Could such a belief, if it exists, stem from Albee's further belief that racism is overwhelmingly given negative value by his colleagues? He surely doesn't expect us to believe that any principles from modern psychology can cogently expose the folly of the racist's system of thought, and that all *good* people will accept these wonders of science, rally to his crusade, and come across with money to pay the high salaries of available behavioral engineers. And what if a group of wealthy racists have a different view of logic and wish to fund the salaries of their own behavioral engineers? One could readily find racists who would present pro-racism arguments which follow the *canons of logic* as flawelssly as do the anti-racists. Further, a racist could base his arguments on *premises* which appear to equal the soundness of any premise which can be offered by any of Albee's sympathizers and co-scientists.

It may be useful to remember that Erik Jaensch who became president of the German Association of Psychology in 1936 and whose work on Eidetic imagery is well known, sold out to the Nazis lock, stock and laboratory. In numerous articles and in an opus of more than five hundred pages, *Der Gegentypus* (the Anti-type), published in 1938, he claimed to have evidence "for the existence of a *biological* type with tissues and plasma so constructed that he is bound, even without any intention, to exercise a disintegrating (Cytic), polluting influence upon an environment that tolerates his presence" (Boder, 1942, page 25). Here is biological ecology promoted by a prominent psychologist in the service of the Nazi regime.

Albee would simply need to admit that his objectives are as subjectively derived as are those of a racist behavioral engineer; and having done this, he might be asked to justify his choice of employers. He would certainly be welcomed to declare his participation in a moral endeavor. He deserves to be chastized, however, if he declares that his objectives derive from scientifically grounded, value free operations.

To illustrate: Albee might strive for political equality. His anatagonist might blatantly advocate elitism. The ideology of elitism would certainly support a racist attitude. Can Albee offer *scientific* proof that elitism shall be negatively valued, and that behavioral engineers follow their science and avoid value controversy when they deplore racism?

Parenthetically, we need to point out the other seductive quality that is apparent in Albee's argument for behavioral engineering. One finds that some of Albee's statements invite a rejection of disease models as a framework for the explanation of unwanted behavior. But, alas, Albee's practice is to impugn the validity of the racist's moral judgments by calling him *pathological, delusional,* and *suffering* from deep unconscious troubles. Furthermore, racism is an *epidemic*! Isn't the use of these terms somewhat antithetical to the rejection of the healer's role? Or, are we once again being misled by the transformation of metaphors into substantives? The illness metaphor continues to provide the scientific aura to moral entrepreneurship! Even after verbally rejecting the healer role, Albee justifies the moral enterprise by throwing disease terminology at the target of his moralizing. And so, the *bad* racist deserves the *help* of the humane healer.

The Behavioral Engineer as a Paid Moral Arbiter. Scientific training gives no one a special power to see transcendent good. At least, the psychologist must avow his allegiance to ideology. He must be willing to state that his goal selection represents value choice, made by the same process through which all humans make value choices. Having made these declarations, he must then look at the source of his salary, and must go on to ask himself some potentially embarrassing questions. Does he advocate mental health because the federal government's National Institute of Mental Health is available to supply his salary? Would he do engineering for the local Anarchist Society if the Chief Anarchist happened to own a string of banking houses?

In short, a behavioral engineer must admit that his salary will not be paid by an agency whose interests are not served by presumed accomplishments of behavioral engineering. No honest moral arbiter would enter the employ of just any controlling agency with the implicit belief that what is good for the employer is good for all humanity. Then, the moral arbiter disguised as a behavioral engineer must know, in honesty, that he will be called upon to engineer for the benefit of an employer; else he cannot retain his position.

The behavioral engineer is privileged like everyone else to believe that the interests of his employer whom he serves represent desirable and useful goals. He stands to earn an opprobrium, however, when he allows or promotes the inference that *his science* has validated this belief. Even when he resorts to the healing metaphor, maintaining that he engineers to preserve or to restore mental health, the behavioral engineer needs to be reminded that it is his personal value system that has led to the decision about what behaviors are to be changed.

Zax and Cowen (1972), frequent and esteemed contributors to the literature of community psychology, assert that "the core methodologies of secondary prevention are early identification of dysfunction in individuals and early effective treatments" (p. 451). One may well ask how does one know a dysfunction when one sees one? The popular as well as the professional literature is replete with discussions centering on sexual dysfunction. What precisely is sexual dysfunction? Is it something like liver or cardiac dysfunction? Not likely. Is it determined according to statistical deviation from a norm? Who determined the norm? Kinsey? Masters and Johnson? or St. Paul? Could it be, as Fromm (1970) asserts, that "with the growth of a consumer society sex itself has become an article of consumption, and the trend in the direction of instant sexual gratification is part of the pattern of consumption that fits the economic needs of a cybernated society?" (p. 37). If one is unable to establish the nature of dysfunction except by the method of the weavers of emperor's clothes then how does one institute early effective treatment?

Of course, this questioning of the science-disguised value determinations that underlie the desire to stamp out putative dysfunction must be superimposed on the question of the basic value determinations. Earlier in their text Zax and Cowen indicate that mental health professionals need to be concerned with persons who present a serious community problem "because of their non-productivity and because they are generally defined as needing to be cared for by welfare and law-enforcement agencies" (p. 9). Why should behavioral engineers interfere in the lives of only those unproductive people who are brought into the care of welfare and law-enforcement agencies, while not interfering in the lives of equally unproductive people who are in the care of their highly paid brokerage firms? Would a student, trained to work as a community psychologist by people like Zax and Cowen, be able to find employment altering the "disordered behavior" of unproductive women who run up huge charges at Nieman-Marcus or Bloomingdale's? How easy to forget that all the "symptoms" of mental illness are behaviors, and that the most universal characteristic of those behaviors that are considered symptoms of mental illness is that they are deemed unacceptable by delegates of the power structure who hire the diagnostician!

It bears repeating that those who offer their services as behavioral engineers may—as may any other mortal human—undertake moral endeavors. Behavioral engineers who undertake moral endeavors must, however, disclaim any special skill in determining the value direction of the goals they pursue. A behavioral engineer, like any employee, renders service to self-interested agencies. The behavioral engineer must be castigated, however, when he becomes a moral entrepreneur and uses his scientism to cloak his mission and to mislead victims into believing that they are responsible for their own victimization (see Ryan, 1971, for a stimulating discussion of quasi-science as victimization).

More on the Scientific Mask of Behavioral Engineers. In speaking before the newly formed Division of Community Psychology Kelly (1970) proposed "a redefinition of the psychologist's job." He urged the establishment of doctoral training programs "that begin with the goal to train persons who are effective change agents and then proceed to select and train persons for that very purpose" (p. 525). Kelly argues that one can apply concepts drawn from biological ecology to the design of social intervention "if all of the stimulating ideas from biology are distilled into a single theme it is a . . . love . . . of the very community where you live and work, an involvement that engulfs your attention . . . to know . . . its political forces and its efforts to launch campaigns for social goods." Kelly decries the fact that few psychologists have been taught to be concerned about their communities and "still fewer ... have given time to see the promotion of a civic cause fulfilled" (p. 524).

One finds it difficult to resist beginning a commentary on Kelly's proposal by noting the title of his article: "Antidotes for Arrogance: Training for Community Psychology." One might well ask, "Whose arrogance shall be discussed?" Nowhere in Kelly's discussion does one find a consideration of who decides what civic causes merit the support of psychologists *qua* psychologists. Nowhere does he concern himself with the question of how a doctoral program designed to train change agents, trains these same people to determine which changes should be fostered in the community. The term "civic cause" is not a self-evident truth.

Not only does Kelly invoke "civic cause" but he justifies it by the halo of respectable science, namely, biology. It is biological ecology that teaches us a love of community. What, pray tell, in the study of biology teaches about love of community more effectively than does the study of Shakespeare, or Tolstoy, or John Fowles, or Alfred E. Newman? Is Kelly acting as a promoter in urging universities to support the training of moral entrepreneurs disguised as community psychologists?

Sentiments such as Kelly's will be presented in textbooks of psychology and sadly students will be seduced into believing that psychology is not only a noble profession but that its nobility is based on validated scientific principles. It is only when they draw nearer to the conclusion of their training that some students will come to the realization that they have been misled by an inept metaphor. We hope that our discussion will offer an alternative to these students other than proceeding in a career based on cynicism and misrepresentation.

The Psychotechnologist as Moral Entrepreneur

If the role of the healer and that of the behavioral engineer are to be rejected because of their moral entrepreneurship, then perhaps the role of the psychotechnologist may provide an acceptable alternative. The psychotechnologist is one who seeks to apply technological advances to the domain of individual and group behavior. R. L. Schwitzgebel (1970), as a leading exemplar of the psychotechnologist, notes—among other clinical considerations— that, "The greatest threat to civil liberty occurs prior to public exposure when no democratic determination has been made regarding legitimate applications of technical innovation" (p. 497). In noting this threat, Schwitzgebel has touched upon the most significant questions which confront psychotechnologists. Just as we asked in reference to the healer and the behavioral engineer: *Who decides which behaviors are to be achieved through the use of psychotechnology?* How does the psychotechnologist resolve questions about his choice of employers? The following quotation contains suggestions that Schwitzgebel, like many of the behavioral engineers, would be more comfortable with "excessive social control" than with the "sudden disorganization" of existing "complexly balanced organizations." In short, R. L. Schwitzgebel (1970) might comfortably declare his position as an ideologue.

> A more realistic and immediate threat from technological advance than excessive social control is the possibility of sudden disorganization and chaos. Complexly balanced organizations are vulnerable to manipulation by adroitly placed pressure. . . . Basic institutional stability of governments, universities, and unions appears increasingly threatened by uncompromising group action of even a relatively few individuals. Guerilla actions against public water supplies, communication networks, and transportation could temporarily paralyze, if not seriously injure, "Big Brother" (p. 497).

In this passage R. L. Schwitzgebel slides into his moralizing position by following two rather interesting techniques. First, he promotes the inference that chaos and disorganization within balanced organizations, through being classed as *threat,* shall be negatively valued. Thus, those who agree with this evaluation, following his argument, should be less concerned about the "Big Brother Effect" than by threats which emanate from a minority of uncompromising individuals. This line of thought disregards the validity of the nihilist advocacy of chaos—a validity which cannot be dismissed simply and directly through having undergone the training needed to acquire the role of a highly sophisticated psychotechnologist. In addition, Schwitzgebel adopts a ploy that has become exceedingly common among psychologists; who, having been exposed to some of the perennial questions facing students of experimental epistemology, should know better. He puts himself in a position where he poses as an arbiter of reality. He, somehow, is in a position to claim that sudden disorganization and chaos are the elements of a "realistic" threat. What part of his education as a psychotechnologist allows him the role of expert in determining the nature of reality? Were one to accept the infallibility of the psychotechnologist as the revealer of reality the psychotechnologist would then attain a rather strong position as a moral arbiter. He would then simply need to pronounce his judgment that each of his opponent's value statements represents an unclear view of the reality which he, as scientist, sees so well. But, the psychotechnologist has done little to demonstrate a special view of reality, or that he has gained a special skill in determining the value loading of an event. Again, we must assert the negative value of R. L. Schwitzgebel's moral entrepreneurship. Should he desire to join the moral endeavor associated with a particular "complexly balanced organization," he must do so as an equal with an avowed anarchist. His behavioral science has not granted him a special vision.

R. K. Schwitzgebel (1973), another psychotechnologist, writes a rather lengthy discussion of the ethical and legal aspects of behavioral instrumentation. This discussion centers around issues related to the direct effects of the machinery itself. Can the subject be injured by the machinery? (Additionally, Schwitzgebel does point up the ethical considerations surrounding informed consent and privacy.) Schwitzgebel, drawing from legal decisions and legislation regarding products such as drugs and electrical machinery, attempts to draw parallels with the legal and ethical matters connected with psychotechnology. Again, one would wonder what becomes of problems of deciding on which behaviors shall be altered and what behaviors shall be developed through applying the psychotechnology of the future.

A recent two volume compendium of psychotechnologically-oriented articles (Ulrich, Stachnik & Maybry, 1966, 1970), contains a series of essays which discuss ethical matters (Miron, 1970; Lucero, Vail & Scherber, 1970; Cahoon, 1970). These articles take up the problem of using aversive conditioning in order to regulate behaviors, and the authors of these articles find themselves struggling to weigh punishments in the balance of *good* and *bad* in order to decide if the *bad* of aversive stimulation can be balanced out by the *good* of the behaviors that are achieved through its use.

What of the patient's civil liberties? How can it be ethical to prohibit the use of devices that can result in successful placement of chronic patients in the community? The real deprivation, with which we should be concerned—the one most ethically

> suspect—is the deliberate deprivation of potential benefits to
> the patient, when the alternative clearly amounts to a life
> sentence in a mental institution. (Miron, 1970, p. 349)

As we can see in the above quotation, the psychotechnologist
can take the perennially useful approach of implying that he is
acting as the healer. Once again, one looks vainly for a discussion
of the perennially important questions of *who* has acted to judge
the inappropriateness of the behavior which commits a person to
a "life sentence in a mental institution," and who shall act as a
judge of the appropriateness of the behaviors which shall earn a
person a release from his sentence. The questions seem particularly
acute when cast in the form of a life or death issue. They are no
less difficult as value judgments when applied to the more mun-
dane settings of behavior modification, such as, the classroom or
the hospital ward.

Behavior Objectives Versus Value Choices. Few authors would
be more directly forward on this issue than Mischel (1968) has
been.

> Judgments about the consequences of an individual's be-
> havior are made both by the individual and by the members of
> the community who observe and evaluate him. Frequently a per-
> son labels himself and reacts to his own behaviors very differ-
> ently than does the bulk of society. . . .
>
> Rather than becoming embroiled in social judgment about
> the client's behaviors, or in speculative reconstructions about
> their hypothetical origins and motivational roots, behavior as-
> sessment begins with an attempt to select reasonable treatment
> objectives (p. 199).

This kind of forthright assertiveness has the ring of sharp,
technological thinking. Let's get down to business, and all that!
But, what else other than social judgments brings a client to the
psychotechnologist? Why does one feel personal pain? Somewhere
the patient confronts a conflict between his behaviors and the
value systems with which he interacts. Does one avoid a value conflict when one assumes a "brass tacks" psychotechnological approach and then directly attacks the behavior? Consider the illus-
tration of "clear objectives" with which Mischel follows his assertion.

Mischel cites Lazarus (1963). Lazarus used a desensitization
process to attack the frigidity of sixteen married women. Eventually nine of these women reported an improved sexual life. Why did

these women first present themselves for a modification of their
"frigidity?" One must conclude that someone—even, perhaps the
women themselves—disapproved of the way these women
approached their sexual activity. On what basis did the participants
decide to desensitize these women's rejection of sex? Why not join
a different moral endeavor? Why not desensitize them to social
expectations? One could then have aided them to leave their sexu-
ally demanding husbands; or to reject socially-generated approval
of sexual activity; or to accept a vow of chastity and to enter a
convent. Or, why did the participants not decide to desensitize the
husbands to their wives' rejection of sex? Lazarus might have
taught the husbands to enjoy celibacy!

These rhetorical questions reveal their easily transpar-
ent answer. Lazarus *did not* avoid "becoming embroiled in social
judgments about the client's behaviors," by avoiding the label "sexual dysfunction." Instead, he stepped right into the embroglio, and
he helped to pronounce the social judgment that intramarital sex,
practiced in certain amounts and in certain ways, is *good*.

As a last resort, the technologist might declare that he does
what the client wants to have done. As a person concerned with his
ethics, the applied psychotechnologist cannot sustain this position.
How would he approach a member of secret, politically-oriented
death squad who has developed an aversion to political execution?
Would a psychotechnologist desensitize this person to his assassina-
tion assignments?

The theme becomes repetitious. The applied psychologist who
attempts to assume the role of the psychotechnologist easily becomes a moral entrepreneur. His science gives no key insights by
which he avoids the very basic, recurrent problems of judging the
appropriateness of behaviors.

Informed Consent as a Special Issue for the Psychotechnologist.
R. K. Schwitzgebel (1973), in his article on the ethics of psychotechnology, draws upon the experiences of such agencies as the
United States Food and Drug Administration to draw guidelines
concerning psychotechnology. In this article, Schwitzgebel considers the matter of obtaining consent from a subject of psychotechnology. He refers specifically to matters of using subjects in
experimentation. In his discussion he misses major points. Whenever subjects are exposed to psychotechnology, of course, there is
an expected behavior change; whether the person participates as
an experimental subject or as a person whose behavior is deemed
changeworthy. In advocating informed consent, then, one implicitly

advocates informing a person regarding the social, political, personal, etc., consequences of having developed the behavior which is to be achieved through the psychotechnology.

This declaration again raises a series of confounding questions. Does the psychotechnologist know the current and long range consequences of adopting the behavior he is trying to instill? When is an applied psychotechnologist exempted from the informed consent clause? As one begins to think about these questions on informed consent he meets another perplexing question.

How Good Is the Product? This other perplexing question can be best raised after noting the claim made by Miron (1970) who holds psychotechnology in positive esteem. Miron contends that the rituals of behavior modification, skillfully applied, "alter behavior more effectively than do the traditional therapies" (p. 348), and that this efficacy can intensify ethical problems. One has to consider the evidence in regard to the very limited effectiveness, by whatever measure, of the "traditional therapies" (Eysenck, 1952; Cross, 1964) in weighing the claim for the greater effectiveness of behavior modification techniques. Moreover, does Miron mean that a technique that promises behavior change but doesn't produce it is less vulnerable to ethical criticism than one that presumably delivers the behavior change?

When a psychotechnologist faces a prospective subject, what shall he tell him—when working to achieve informed consent—concerning the potential outcomes of the application of psychotechnology? Shall it be sufficient to tell him that applications of the technology of operant conditioning have modified "behavior much more effectively than do the traditional therapies?" Shall he state, following the findings reported, for example, by Lazarus (1963), that approximately half of the subjects exposed to the technology show no appreciable related behavior change? Shall the subject who is to be changed, and/or the person paying for the services of the technologist, be informed of the very extended controversy surrounding the effects and nature of operant conditioning technology (Page, 1972; Levine, 1970)? Shall the person hiring the technologist be informed about the very likely possibility that the ritual of operant conditioning is no more effective in producing long term behavior change than is the simple technique of telling the subject to change his behavior?

Mabry, Stachnik, and Ulrich (1970) have discussed some of the cultural impediments to implementing behavioral technology. In their discussion, they state:

> Reservations about the nature of any contemplated program
> are often encountered in the initial stage. . . . Curiously, few ob-
> jections are raised as to the possible reaction to the effective-
> ness of a program (p. 327).

How would Mabry, Stachnik, and Ulrich respond to a person
who would raise questions about the effectiveness of their program? Would they present the results of studies which present
group statistics showing a .05 probability of significant difference
between the means of groups treated by different techniques from
which it has been concluded that technique q is more effective than
technique p? Would they present frequency distributions which
show the actual performance differences thus laying bare the concrete fact that more than half of the subjects in many basic operant
conditioning studies performed in a way that would disconfirm the
hypothesis that behavior modification is an effective technique?

In short, would the technologist offer his client an iron-clad,
five-year guarantee? If he cannot, why is he offering his high
priced services? To construct a crude analogy—Would a building
contractor take a fee for erecting a structure which would run a
fifty-fifty chance of being condemned by the building inspector?

The Failure of the Technologist's Disguise.   The applied psychologist, hiding his moral entrepreneurship behind his mask of the
technologist, also fails to remain disguised. Someone pays the psychotechnologist, and the person who pays also stands in a position
to hire or dismiss the applied psychologist's services. Pepinsky
(1966) in a searching article on the goals of the technology of help-
giving, directs attention specifically to behavior modification
therapies, and then states the following:

> In the context of Campbell's (1965) view of altruism, and
> mine of help-giving, the use of behavior modification must be
> construed as an amoral act, performed by A as an agent of B,
> his society, to reduce variability within it. To its proponents
> such action is not to be questioned; yet issues of this kind have
> contributed to an anxious soul searching among behavioral sci-
> entists (p. 214).

Old adages are hard to avoid. The piper's employer calls the
tune.

When the technologist tries to avoid the employee's dilemma
by asserting that he serves the best interest of the client, he needs
to analyse the client's reason for contracting with the technologist.

Is the subject responding to the society's pressure to "reduce variability?" If so, does the technologist have a first obligation to use his vaunted technology to teach the subject not to respond to the pressures against variability?

As a final issue; in addition to matters of the propriety of serving a paying master, at the point where the technologist seeks a subject's informed consent, does the technologist have an obligation to advise the subject on the distinct possibility that his technology will work no meaningful change? Does the science of psychology allow one easy answer to these moral matters?

The Scientist as the Model for the Applied Psychologist

In our introductory remarks we touched on the possible role of the community psychologist as a scientist. Let us examine this possibility more carefully from the standpoint of its moral implications.

In the opening address to the 1965 Conference on the Professional Preparation of Clinical Psychologists, N. Hobbs (1966) made the following statement:

> The commitment is to a method of problem-solving that differentiates the psychologist from the social worker, the physician, the clergyman, the school counselor, and others who work to help people with their problems. It should be the common bond of all psychologists whether in the laboratory, the private office, the clinic, or the community. It is basically the tradition of scientific inquiry (p. 5).

The ultimate function of the psychologist (including the community psychologist), then, is his pursuit of scientific inquiry. This statement easily evokes agreement. One might say that the systematic or scientific study of behavior *is* the "is" of a psychologist; for have we not all been taught from the beginning of our indoctrination into our discipline that it rests on four fundamental processes, description, explanation, prediction and control? Hobbs, however, allows for an easy skidding into moral entrepreneurship when he claims that:

> ... The psychologist works truly as a psychologist, **regardless** of the enterprise or setting, when he:
> (a) bases his actions on explicitly indentifiable assumptions

drawn from psychological theory; (b) defines with greatest possible precision the process of intervention he makes or recommends; (c) insists to himself and others that outcomes be constantly tested against comparable interventions or no interventions at all, using the most precise and powerful measures available; and (d) makes public the results of his work to further the development of knowledge and to maintain for psychology the benefits of a self-correcting system (pp. 6–7).

In an earlier part of his talk Hobbs had declared, "The problems with which the clinician deals are preponderantly moral and ethical in character" (p. 5). He might have offered sage advice to those who would teach future clinical psychologists had he pointed out, amoung his four salient descriptors of psychologists, that moral endeavor is interposed between point *a* and point *b*. When the psychologist exercises choices about the goals that are to be attained by his actions and recommendations (point a) and then defines a process of intervention (point b), he joins a moral endeavor and his science of intervention! At least, a psychologist must ask "Who shall decide the goals of the intervention, and for what purposes?"

In his talk Hobbs had already laid the groundwork for drawing his conclusions about the *good* which *he* would seek.

The direction of development of the social and behavioral sciences in America today will be profoundly influenced by a national decision of comparable scope: to make it possible for every citizen to develop his potential to the fullest. This decision, this momentous commitment to human development, will be the major determinant of the character of psychology in the next decade or so, provided that we are a responsive and responsible profession prepared to pick up socially significant options (pp. 1–2).

... These manifestations of a new national purpose will determine the character of the clinical psychology of the future—provided, of course, that we are ready to respond to their challenge, that we are wise enough and flexible enough to pick up the right options (p. 2).

Apparently, Hobbs would have considered psychologists to have been responsible when they pursue the national purpose of helping citizens to develop their potential to the fullest. There is some lack of clarity in Hobbs' moral endeavor, particularly as one tries to fathom the meaning of the term *potential* as related to the term *national purpose*. One could imagine that Hobbs means *potential* as a B-52 pilot! Or he might mean *potential* as a leader of organized gambling! Then, too, he could mean *potential* toward managing Ford Motor Company, especially for those persons born into the Ford family! At any rate, Hobbs advises the interventionist scientists to use wisdom and flexibility in picking up the *right* options. Applied psychologists, however, could profitably entertain the disquieting possibility that the *right* options about which *potentials* a person might seek to fulfill are more likely to be determined in the lobbies of national capitals such as Washington, D.C. than in the psychological laboratory or the clinic or the journal. One must recognize the possibility of a huge discrepancy between a personal commitment to the scientific enterprise and a personal commitment to national purposes. The national government, too, is an employer!

Conceptualization, Science, and Applied Psychology

Perhaps there is no way entirely to avoid being involved in moral issues while working as applied psychologists. However, we proceed on the assumption that within a particular metaphysic, within a particular epistemology, within a particular view of science, those who choose to present themselves as applied psychologists and to work in the clinic or the community can avoid inadvertent transformation into poorly disguised moral entrepreneurs. In our view the best framework of these particulars, one that keeps the moral issues most prominently in view, is that which encourages the psychologist to assume that each of his clients functions as a scientific psychologist and, in a sense, is involved in testing experimental hypotheses about living. (See G. Kelly [1969] for a discussion of persons as scientists.) In this student-to-teacher relationship the psychologist continually reiterates that the interpretations he offers are based on his systematic formulations about behavior. The student-client is obligated to make explicit his own values and to formulate his own goals, as he seeks to understand whether these values and goals will bring him into a harmonious or conflictful relationship with others. Which outcome he chooses is his responsibility and not the psychologist's. The major difference between the position being espoused here and those previously discussed is the role of intervention. In our view the discipline of psychology does not provide a scientific basis for intervention in the lives of others. When a client appears seeking help or when the psychologist offers his services to an agency, he does not present himself as someone who can effectively intervene in the lives of others but as someone who seeks to elaborate the ways in which people formulate problems and the consequent conceptualization of solutions.

At this point we shall not undertake the large-scaled task of defining the limits of the metaphysical, epistemological, and scientific framework within which the psychologist in the social system can cast his role as a teacher. It can be briefly stated that we would take the metaphysical position of contextualism, as defined by Pepper (1942), the epistemological position defined by Piaget (see, for example, Piaget, 1971, and Elkind, 1967), the view of science offered by Kuhn (1971) and the theory of persons propounded by Kelly (1955). In brief, our position encourages us to see a learning human as an information processor who derives most of his stimulus input and information-processing strategies from the context of the social environment in which he operates. Within this system each human is conceived as constantly striving after meaning. When the person experiences a failure to understand, that is, when he experiences a contextually produced discrepancy between his interpretation of a stimulus input and his available integrations, the striving after meaning serves to seek a reduction of the discrepancy. A reinterpretation of the stimulus input or a reorganization of the available integrations will reduce the disequilibrium and is thus functionally reinforcing. In other words psychological processes are activated and channelized by the coordination of one's current interpretations and one's anticipations. (See Mancuso [1977] for an extended elaboration of this view of motivation.)

Within the proposed view of the applied psychologist there is one aspect in which the role of scientist is enacted, namely, by engaging in what Kuhn (1971) calls the normal science of a discipline or the building of a cognitive system relating to the events subsumed by the discipline. We next assume that prior to enacting the role of teacher an applied psychologist, such as the community psychologist, should have developed his understanding of the processes involved in aiding others in the task of developing *their* cognitive systems. The applied psychologist, within this role model, serves as teacher to those who wish to understand the development of behaviors—their own behavior as well as the behavior of others. Above all, the psychologist in the society avoids the pre-determination of outcomes in order that he avoid assuming the role of moral entrepreneur.

We repeat: the applied psychologist works his psychological

science only when he works as a clarifier of behavior and behavior change processes. When he works toward specific goals, other than the goal of developing understandings about the processes of behavior, he works within a moral endeavor. (Of course, while working as a clarifier and as a definer of options he proceeds on the basic assumption that clarifying is good and that it is better to have options than to be constrained. As a scientist he should be prepared to recognize moral endeavor and its effects on behavior. And, he has an obligation to introduce this knowledge into his behavior explanation function.)

Some examples may help define the role of community psychologist as "behavior explicator." As described elsewhere (Morrison, 1976), psychologists can assume the role of teacher in "demythologizing" seminars which offer citizens the opportunity to consider and discuss the relative merits of alternative paradigms of "aberrant" behavior. People should have available the data on stigma and loss of control associated with psychiatric classification and labeling (Rabkin, 1974; Rosenhan, 1973). Furthermore, psychologists in the role of teachers can avoid the error of arbitrarily establishing for the client the goals to be attained, by actively involving the client in problem definition and in goal setting (Nevid, Morrison, Gaviria & Rathus, 1976).

The services of the applied psychologist are available to everyone, in so far as the efforts to clarify behavior change and developmental processes are available to everyone. There remains a problem regarding the remuneration of the applied psychologist. In a case where a psychologist openly declares espousal of an ideology, and then offers his services to those who support the same ideology, his remuneration problems can be easily solved. In cases where his moral commitments remain ambiguous, he faces a series of problems.

The Applied Psychologist as a Wage Earner. In a market economy, the person who would spend his days functioning as a behavior conceptualizer would need to be able to justify receiving some kind of transferrable currency. Since he seeks to stand outside of the established ideology he is likely to encounter demands that he contribute something to the economy in order to obtain that currency. Of course, there is something grand in thinking, and in then asserting, that his communication of his systems of understanding should be regarded as a sufficient *something* to earn a comfortable amount of the standard currency of the society. Several problems confront this latter assertion.

Power sources within a society can easily withhold positive

endorsement of the enterprise of understanding behavior. Indeed, in many, many instances power sources can be highly threatened by allowing for particular understandings of behavior that could undermine the ideology that maintains the existing order. For example, a market economy depends very heavily upon the belief that the prime motivation of persons is the motivation to maintain physical well-being. If people would begin to believe that spiritual peace, rather than physical well-being, is the major aspect of their motivation, then they might tend to be less willing to cooperate in a market economy. Thus, a behavioral conceptualizer-teacher who would explicate an option in regard to motivation which would de-emphasize the motivational force of physical well-being, might help to undermine the power positions of those who control large segments of market economies. Therefore, the power sources of a market economy might be more willing to offer positive endorsement to persons who would promote a conceptualization of motivation based on acquisition of "comfort." In effect, power sources would be reluctant to affirm the sufficiency of the *something* that is being contributed by a behavior-explainer who might undermine the current power base by propounding alternate views of behavior, and such power sources might advocate withholding transferrable currency from those who provided "unacceptable" behavior-explaining concepts.

It will be recalled that we showed that the Freudian explanation of behavior was one in which the established order was accepted as the "ultimate form of human progress." Fromm (1970), in writing about the crisis of psychoanalysis, indicates that access to this form of explanation can itself be considered an item in the marketplace. He notes that the fact that the therapist was paid for his listening was only a minor drawback or no drawback at all, since the payment only served to prove that the therapy was serious and respectable. "Besides," he concludes, "its prestige was high because it was, economically, a luxury item" (p. 13).

The next problem concerns the matter of what shall be judged to be a comfortable level of support for a behavior explainer. Again, a market economy attaches positive value to the acquisition of goods, and even behavior explainers seem to seek the social confirmation of their personal value which attends to their having accumulated goods. These conditions—the desire of the psychologist to earn the emoluments of a successful participant in market economies, in conjunction with the possible reluctance to offer whole-hearted support to behavior conceptualizers—place the applied psychologist in a compromising position. The blandishments of power centers encourage moral entrepreneurship or enlistment in the moral endeavor.

Some Resolutions for Those Who Would Remain Aloof. A society could treat its behavior explicators as amateurs—in the strict sense of this term. Under these circumstances a behavior explicator would make his living as a shoemaker, a lens grinder, a baker, or a longshoreman; while he devotes a part of each of his days to the careful study of behavior. In this idyllic situation he would choose his apprentices not only for their promise in becoming masters in his trade, but also for their promise as students of behavior. Imagine the joys of continuous symposia over rising hard rolls and sweet coffee cakes! And then the rush to close the shop in order to teach clients and write up symposia transcripts! There is little risk of "selling out" in this fantasy world!

Meanwhile! Can we convince those who direct market economies that they should support the academy, whose scholarly behavior explicators are available to any person in the community. Perhaps the *idea* of academy remains as the only viable social institution which can support the behavior explicator without requiring him to enter moral activity.

Perhaps as another approach, our society might eliminate the current mental health operations and replace them with a system of small autonomous behavioral explication units. Such units might be built on a model which would allow comfortable functioning under a title such as *Neighborhood Institute for Social Living*. In such institutes, the teacher-student roles would guide the interactions of the participants, and participants would work under the clear recognition that these units espouse no particular value orientations. There are in the U.S. some oases of this sort, hardly structured sufficiently even to be identified and not necessarily staffed by mental health professionals.

We have pledged ourselves, within the narrow limits of our influence, to set forth before students who wish to be clinical or community psychologists, an alternative to the traditional roles of healer, engineer, technologist or interventionist scientist. It is not likely that we shall witness the ideal conditions for the emergence of a large group of behavior explicators who derive their livelihood from a society that requires commitment to an ideology from its religious functionaries as well as its arbiters of approved and disapproved behavior explanations. However, attention to the moral implications of the usual practice of clinical psychology may serve to moderate the confidence-game quality that characterizes some of its practices. Discussions such as we have presented here may serve to encourage critical questioning on the part of clients and students being trained in clinical and community psychology.

Reprise

This essay starts with the assumption that societies function within ideologies, and that scientists are continually lured into supporting these ideologies. The problems of this situation are particularly acute for the psychologist who makes social applications from the body of his discipline. The temptation to undertake moral entrepreneurship, with scientism as a disguise for value judgment undertakings, has been a special trap for applied psychologists. Considering the cogent exposés of such entrepreneurship, psychologists must be prepared to analyse and justify their involvement in the moral implications of the professional roles which they might adopt.

As one searches through the role identities available to applied psychologists of the past decade, one notes that four role-types can be described—(1) the healer, (2) the behavioral engineer, (3) the psychotechnologist, (4) the interventionist scientist. Close inspection of the statements which have attempted to define these roles for applied psychologists reveals that the enactors of these roles often allow moral entrepreneurship to enter into the proposed role functioning.

We recommend that applied psychologists work toward fully exposing their moral endeavors. By choosing to follow one or two broad strategies the applied psychologist can avoid functioning as a disguised moral entrepreneur. He may choose to join, unequivocally and directly, into a fully apparent moral endeavor. Alternatively, he may attempt to circumscribe his activity in such a way as to reduce the possibilities that he will slip into a position where he functions as a masked moralizer.

Our analysis allows us to find repeated instances in which applied psychologists enter into the role of the moral entrepreneur. Though such entry can, unwittingly or otherwise, happen to those who would fill any of the four roles which we have identified, we regard the role of the scientifically inclined behavior explicator to be that role which least induces moral entrepreneurship. Even this role, however, is not free of insidious invitations to playing moral entrepreneur while wearing the cloak of another vocation. Thus, the scientific behavior explicator must also continuously engage in personal scrutiny, searching for ways to maintain a separation between his role as explicator, from which he also explicates social manifestations of moral endeavor, and his personal role as a purveyor of moral values. This admonition, of course, does not intend to exclude the possibility that applied psychologists will make an open declaration that they have positively espoused a particular value system and thereupon wish to apply their professional skills to the production of behaviors that are acceptable within the system which they openly promote. In all cases, we see no means by which community psychologists can evade a perpetual responsibility to work toward a satisfactory solution to the problems of isolating their moral endeavor from their behavior-explaining endeavor.

References

Albee, G. W. The uncertain future of clinical psychology. *American Psychologist*, 1970, *25*, 1071–1080.

Azrin, N. H., & Lindsley, O. R. The reinforcement of cooperation between children. *Journal of Abnormal and Social Psychology*, 1956, *52*, 100–102.

Beit-Hallahmi, B. On the "religious" functions of the helping professions. *Archiv für Religionpsychologie*, 1976, *12*, 48–52.

Boder, D. P. Nazi science. *Chicago Jewish Forum*, 1942, *1*, 23–29.

Braginsky, B. M., & Braginsky, D. D. *Mainstream psychology: A critique.* New York: Holt, Rinehart, & Winston, 1974.

Braginsky, D. D., & Braginsky, B. M. Psychologists: High priests of the middle class. *Psychology Today*, December 1973, pp. 15–20; 138–142.

Cahoon, D. D. Issues and implications of operant conditioning: Balancing procedures against outcomes. In R. Ulrich, T. Stachnik, & J. Mabry (Eds.), *Control of human behavior.* Vol. II. *From cure to prevention*, Glenview, Ill.: 1970.

Cross, H. J. The outcomes of psychotherapy: A selected analysis of research findings. *Journal of Consulting Psychology*, 1964, *28*, 413–417.

Elkind, D. (Ed.) *Six psychological studies.* New York: Vintage Books, 1967.

Eysenck, H. J. The effects of psychotherapy: An evaluation. *Journal of Consulting Psychology*, 1952, *16*, 319–324.

Eysenck, H. J. The effects of psychotherapy. In H. J. Eysenck (Ed.), *Handbook of abnormal psychology.* New York: Basic Books, 1961.

Feierabend, I., & Feierabend, R. Aggressive behaviors within politics,

1948–1962: A cross-national study. *Journal of Conflict Resolution,* 1966, *10,* 249–271.

Fromm, E. *The crisis of psychoanalysis.* Greenwich, Conn.: Fawcett Publications, 1970.

Hall, C. M. Psychotherapy as a secular religion: A middle-class urban phenomenon in post World-War II U.S. Paper presented to the 1974 meeting of the Society for the Scientific Study of Religion, Washington, D.C.

Hastdorf, A. H., Schneider, D. J., & Polefka, J. *Person perception.* Reading, Mass.: Addison-Wesley, 1970.

Hirsch, J. Genetics and competence: Do heriditability indices predict educatability? In J. McV. Hunt (Ed.), *Human Intelligence.* New Brunswick, N. J.: Transaction books, 1972.

Hobbs, N. Opening Address. In E. L. Hoch, A. O. Ross, & C. L. Winder (Eds.), *Professional Preparation of Clinical Psychologists.* Washington, D.C.: American Psychological Association, 1966.

Kelly, G. A. *The psychology of personal constructs.* New York: Norton, 1955.

Kelly, G. A. A mathematical approach to psychology. In B. Maher (Ed.), *Clinical psychology and personality.* New York: Wiley, 1969.

Kelly, J. G. Ecological constraints on mutual health services. *American Psychologist,* 1966, *21,* 535–539.

Kelly, J. G. Towards a theory of preventative intervention. In J. W. Carter, Jr. (Ed.), *Research contributions from psychology to community mental health.* New York: Behavioral Publications, 1968.

Kelly, J. G. Antidotes for arrogance: Training for community psychology. *American Psychologist,* 1970, *25,* 524–531.

Kuhn, T. S. *The structure of scientific revolutions.* Chicago: Chicago University Press, 1971.

Lasch, C. Sacrificing Freud. *New York Times Magazine,* February 22, 1976, pp. 11–12; 70–72.

Lazarus, A. A. The treatment of chronic frigidity by systematic desensitization. *Journal of Nervous and Mental Diseases,* 1963, *136,* 272–278.

Levine, M. Human discrimination learning: The subset-sampling assumption. *Psychological Bulletin,* 1970, *74,* 397–404.

Lucero, R. J. Vail, D. J., & Scherber, J. Regulating operant-conditioning programs. In R. Ulrich, T. Stachnik & J. Mabry (Eds.), *Control of human behavior.* Vol. II. *From cure to prevention.* Glenview, Ill.: Scott, Foresman, 1970.

Mabry, J., Stachnik, T., & Ulrich, R. Cultural impediments to the implementation of behavioral technology. In R. Ulrich, T. Stachnik, and J. Mabry (Eds.), *Control of human behavior.* Vol. II. *From cure to prevention.* Glenview, Ill.: Scott, Foresman, 1970.

Mancuso, J. C. Current motivational models in the elaboration of personal construct theory. In A. W. Landfield (Ed.), *Nebraska sym-*

posium on motivation: Personal construct psychology. Lincoln: University of Nebraska Press, 1977.

Mannheim, K. *Ideology and utopia.* New York: Harcourt, 1936.

Meehl, P. Schizotaxia, schizotypy, schizophrenia. *American Psychologist,* 1962, *17,* 827–831.

Mills, R. C., & Kelly, J. G. Ecology and cultural adaptation: A case study and critique. In S. Golann and C. Eisdorfer (Eds.), *Handbook of community psychology and mental health.* New York: Appleton-Century Crofts, 1973.

Miron, N. B. Issues and implications of operant conditioning: The primary ethical considerations. In R. Ulrich, T. Stachnik, & J. Mabry (Eds.), *Control of human behavior.* Vol. II. *From cure to prevention.* Glenview, Ill.: Scott, Foresman, 1970.

Mischel, W. *Personality and Assessment.* New York: Wiley, 1968.

Morrison, J. K. Demythologizing mental patients' attitudes toward mental illness: An empirical study. *Journal of Community Psychology,* 1976, *4,* 181–185.

Morrison, J. K. The client as consumer and evaluator of community mental health services. *American Journal of Community Psychology,* in press.

Nevid, J. S., Morrison, J. K., Gaviria, B., & Rathus, S. The problem-oriented goal attainment scaling system: A method of case centered evaluation. In R. Hammer, G. Landsberg, and W. Neigher, *Program evaluation in community mental health centers: A manual.* New York: D and O Press, 1976.

Page, M. M. Demand characteristics and the verbal operant conditioning experiment. *Journal of Personality and Social Psychology,* 1972, *23,* 372–378.

Pepinsky, H. B. Help-giving in search of a criterion. In E. Landy & A. M. Kroll, (Eds.), *Guidance in American Education.* Vol. 3. Cambridge, Mass.: Harvard University Press, 1966.

Pepper, S. *World hypotheses.* Berkley: University of California Press, 1942.

Phillips, D. L. Rejection: A possible consequence of seeking help for mental disorders. *American Sociological Review,* 1963, *28,* 963–972.

Phillips, D. L. Rejection of the mentally ill: The influence of behavior and sex. *American Sociological Review,* 1964, *29,* 679–686.

Piaget, J. *Biology and knowledge.* Chicago: University of Chicago Press, 1971.

Rabkin, J. G. Opinions about mental illness: A review of the literature. *Psychological Bulletin,* 1972, *77,* 153–171.

Rabkin, J. G. Public attitudes toward mental illness: A review of the literature. *Schizophrenia Bulletin,* 1974, *10,* 9–33.

Radnitsky, G. *Contemporary Schools of Metascience.* Göteborg: Akademi-förlaget, 1970.

Rosenhan, D. L. On being sane in insane places. *Science,* 1973, *179,* 250–257.

Rubinstein, E. A., & Coelho, G. V. Mental health and behavioral science: One federal agency's role in the behavioral sciences. *American Psychologist,* 1970, *25,* 517–723.

Ryan, W. *Blaming the victim.* New York: Vintage Books, 1971.

Sarbin, T. R., & Mancuso, J. C. Failure of a moral enterprise: Attitudes of the public towards mental illness. *Journal of Consulting and Clinical Psychology,* 1970, *35,* 157–173.

Schwitzgebel, R. K. Ethical and legal aspects of behavioral instrumentation. In R. L. Schwitzgebel & R. K. Schwitzgebel (Eds.), *Psychotechnology: Electronic control of mind and behavior.* New York: Holt, Rinehart & Winston, 1973.

Schwitzgebel, R. L. Behavior instrumentation and social technology. *American Psychologist,* 1970, *25,* 491–499.

Schwitzgebel, R. L. Emotions and machines: A commentary on the context and strategy of psychotechnology. In R. L. Schwitzgebel and R. K. Schwitzgebel (Eds.), *Psychotechnology: Electronic control of mind and behavior.* New York: Holt, Rinehart and Winston, 1973.

Szasz, T. *Ideology and insanity.* Garden City, New York: Anchor Books, 1970.

Tanter, R. Dimensions of conflict behavior within and between nations. *Journal of Conflict Resolution,* 1966, *10,* 41–61.

Trickett, E. J., Kelly, J. G., & Todd, D. M. The social environment of the high school: Guidelines for individual change and organizational redevelopment. In S. Golann & C. Eisdorfer (Eds.), *Handbook of community psychology and mental health.* New York: Appleton-Century-Crofts, 1973.

Ulrich, R., Stachnik, T., & Mabry, J. *Control of human behavior.* Vol. I., Glenview, Ill.: Scott, Foresman, 1966.

Ulrich, R., Stachnik, T., & Mabry, J. *Control of human behavior.* Vol. II. *From cure to prevention.* Glenview, Ill.: Scott, Foresman, 1970.

Wade, N. IQ and heredity: Suspicion of fraud beclouds classic experiment. *Science,* 1976, *194,* 916–19.

Yaffee, P. E., & Mancuso, J. C. The effects of therapist behavior on people's mental illness judgments. *Journal of Consulting and Clinical Psychology,* 1977, *45,* 84–91.

Zax, M., & Cowen, E. L. *Abnormal psychology: Changing conceptions.* New York: Holt, Rinehart & Winston, 1972.

The Child-Consumer's Informed Consent to Treatment: Ethical, Psychological and Legal Implications

Susan Holdridge-Crane, Kathleen Liston Morrison, and James K. Morrison

UNTIL QUITE RECENTLY, interest of mental health professionals in the ethical issues surrounding clinical interventions (Beit-Hellahmi, 1974; Brodsky, 1972; Daniels, 1969; Ethical Standards, 1975; Morrison, in press; Morrison, Federico, & Rosenthal, 1975; Shore, & Golann, 1964; Szasz, 1961, 1965, 1970a, 1970b) has been confined almost entirely to the adult consumers of mental health services. However, within the past five years, a new and evergrowing realization has emerged that children deserve special consideration as consumers of these same services. Quite recently the problems of child-consumers—some of which they share with their adult counterparts and some of which are unique to children—have begun to be seriously considered by both mental health professionals (LoCicero, 1976; McGuire, 1974; Koocher, 1976) and members of the legal profession (Ennis, 1976; Rada, 1976; Rodham, 1973; Worsfeld, 1974). Representatives of the first group are currently debating such issues as: Is it ethical for the parents or legal guardians of children to be able to coerce these children into psychiatric treatment and/or hospitalization without their volun-

tary and informed consent (Beyer & Wilson, 1976)? Is it ethical
for a therapist to inform legally responsible parties of information
obtained from the child during treatment, even though such information would be deemed privileged and confidential if obtained
from an adult (McGuire, 1974)?

On the legal front, similar issues are currently being argued
within the court system to the extent that the *New York Times*
(Campbell, 1976) could recently state that "... the struggle for
human rights has found a new frontier—America's children.... A
spot check of 24 states by the *New York Times* disclosed that everyone of their major cities had some legal group fighting for children's rights" (p. 26). As the *New York Times* further points out,
this trend represents a major revision in thinking about the rights
of children, one which was absent even as recently as the early
1970s. While it has traditionally been the case that "... children's
best interests were (assumed to be) synonymous with those of
their parents—except under the few circumstances where the state
is authorized to intervene in family life under the doctrine of *pares
patriae*..." (Rodham, 1973, p. 487)—a current movement
challenges these assumptions by favoring the "... extending of
more adult rights to children and by recognizing certain unique
needs and interests of children as legally enforceable rights" (Rodham, 1973, p. 487). In a few words, the Bill of Rights is not meant
only for adults, but for children as well (Sussman, 1977).

The cause of the child as consumer has been a late arrival to the
arena of debate, due partly to a tendency to view the child legally
as the responsibility of his parents. In all fairness, the late arrival
of this issue must also be, in part, laid at the feet of mental health
practitioners. As Koocher (1976) has pointed out "often ... the
standards of professional associations do not specifically address
children as a unique subset of the population" (p. 1).

For some time adults, including, unfortunately, many within
the mental health professions, have tended to look upon children
as "miniature versions of ourselves" (Koocher, 1976, p. 2). Such
a view, according to Koocher, represents an erroneous way of looking at the child.

> The subtle fallacy inherent in this reasoning is that children
> are not simply small grownups. Children are unique in at least
> two important ways. First, a child's basic equipment for adapt-
> ing and functioning in the world is quite different from that of
> an adult. Second, at the very least, children are constantly sub-

jected to benign oppression and to all the other violations that any under-represented minority experiences (p. 2).

In this treatise we intend to establish first that children as client-consumers of mental health services are a special interest group which has been traditionally deprived of various legal and psychological privileges; and, secondly, that on the basis of current knowledge of the intellectual and psychological functioning of children we should seriously consider the possibility of giving some of these consumers the right of informed consent to treatment. In order to demonstrate that children as clients are a special-interest group, three factors shall be examined: (1) the statistical frequency of children as clients; (2) the existence of intrinsic, demonstrable, and relevant differences between children and adults; and (3) the actual incidence of consumer abuse within the mental health arena.

Child Clients: A Special-Interest Group

Statistical Frequency of Child-Clients. Statistical evidence indicates that children (persons under 18 years of age) are a rather sizeable proportion of the population receiving mental health services. For example, there is some indication that while the number of institutionalized adults in the United States has decreased considerably in recent years, the number of children in mental hospitals has continued to increase (Ginsberg, 1973; NIMH, 1974a, 1974b). According to Ferleger (1976), from 1967 to 1973 the drop in total population in state and county mental institutions was 42 percent for all ages; for patients under age 18, the drop was only 12 percent. In 1967, 3 percent of all persons in those hospitals were under 18; in 1973 the under-18 age groups accounted for 4 percent of the total. Of the nearly 200,000 persons in residential institutions for the retarded, more than 40 percent are minors. In this same vein, the number of psychiatrists in the United States who specialize in treating children has also increased in recent years. From 1963 to 1973, for example, the number of child psychiatrists in the United States has grown at a rate of 200 percent, while the corresponding rate of growth for general psychiatrists within the same decade was only 46 percent (Brown, 1976). As revealed by one study (Rosen, Bahn & Kramer, 1964) which used clinic termination rates in the United States for the year ending June 30, 1961 as an index of frequency of treatment, 212 children of every

100,000 received such treatment. This rate is 16 percent higher than that for adults. The study further indicated that, considering all the various age segments of the population, children 10–14 years of age have the maximum clinic usage rate in the country, with peaks at ages 9–10 and 14–15. Children also make up a sizeable proportion of the persons receiving chemotherapy. The number of children currently receiving psychotropic drugs ranges from between 300,000 to 2 million (Brown & Bing, 1976).

Moving from national to more regional statistics, in New York City alone there are an estimated 20,000–40,000 mentally retarded children and between 160,000–200,000 children with serious emotional problems (Office of Children's Services, 1973). Thus, there seems to be little question that children are well represented among the recipients of mental health services in the United States. In terms of numbers, then, there seems to be justification for considering children as a special group within the clientele of mental health professionals. This, however, is not the only reason for treating children as a discrete interest group. As a second reason, the following factor should be considered.

Intrinsic Differences Between Children and Adults.   Children, as Koocher (1976) so aptly points out, are not merely miniature adults, i.e., persons who are much smaller, weaker or less knowledgeable than adults. Rather, they are persons who differ from their elders in some very qualitative ways. In the physical realm, of course, they tend to be smaller and lighter and to have less physical strength than adults (Tanner, 1970). But, in addition to these obvious quantitative physical differences, children also differ physically from adults in less obvious qualitative ways. For example, while many adults might not be readily aware of it, children's bodies are proportioned quite differently than the bodies of mature adults (Tanner, 1970).

Intellectually, too, children display both obvious quantitative differences from adults (e.g., they lack the amount of experience and knowledge that adults possess), and some more subtle but extremely important qualitative differences also (e.g., they lack many of the specific skills and abilities of adults for adapting and dealing with the world on a physical, emotional and social level). As several child psychologists (Inhelder & Piaget, 1969; Nelson & Kosslyn, 1975; Piaget, 1968) have demonstrated, the child's intellectual development from infancy to adulthood may be seen as a process involving a progressive increase in cognitive flexibility, spontaneity, and sophistication. Not only does the developing child acquire more and more *amounts* of knowledge, but he also develops newer and more useful methods of applying this knowledge to various problem solving situations and thus deals with his world in an increasingly more adultlike manner. Certainly, developmental evidence suggests that the child moves gradually from the point at which he is very limited in his cognitive abilities to the point at which he finally joins the adult-world as a person possessing not only a large body of knowledge but also a rather sizeable repertoire of skills and techniques for coping with life's varied problems and situations. That children lack a vast number of such adult-like skills has been amply demonstrated by many researchers working in a variety of areas as judgment and reasoning (Inhelder & Piaget, 1969; Piaget, 1969) ; language (Sinclair, 1969) ; interpersonal relations (Piaget, 1968) ; person perception (Mancuso, Morrison & Aldrich, in press; Morrison, 1973) ; and moral judgment (Kohlberg, 1963; Mancuso, Morrison & Aldrich, in press; Piaget, 1932).

Thus, as the developmental data points out, while the average adult is capable of applying intellectual abilities based upon propositional logic and abstract reasoning, in their day to day transactions—be they scholastic, social or physical—many children have not, as yet, reached the point in their own development that such skills are present and accessible. Rather, the child, generally speaking, must deal with his world armed, at best, with some very limited and, at times, even primitive means of coping and adapting. Thus, in the intellectual realm, as in the physical, the child, is, indeed, not a miniature adult. Rather, the child must be looked upon as a person who, in many ways, differs not just quantitatively (i.e., in physical size, weight, and strength and in absolute amount of knowledge and experience) but also qualitatively (especially in his cognitive abilities and skills) from his adult counterpart. Thus, children should be considered as distinct and separate from adults, since many of their particular characteristics may actually make them—because of their fewer and less sophisticated abilities—even more vulnerable to the effects of abuses by clinical professionals than are most adults. With this consideration in mind, we now will examine some actual instances of such abuses.

Evidence of Abuse Within Mental Health Profession. Rather disturbingly, an ever-increasing body of evidence suggests that children, as consumers of mental health services, may be the victims of a great deal of abuse. One such area is the use of psychotropic drugs in treating the behavioral problems of children—

giving children antidepressants to cure bed wetting, major tranquilizers to curb aggression, and amphetamines to cure hyperactivity. Within the past three decades, for example, the number of
school children receiving Ritalin and Mellaril to combat the symptoms of a condition called minimal brain dysfunction (MBD) has
skyrocketed. According to one researcher, in some school districts,
as many as 10–15 percent of the children are given potentially
dangerous drugs (Walker, 1974). In others, teachers and specialists estimate that 30 percent of the students are suitable candi-
dates for drugs. In California, one private physician admits to
treating more than 4,000 children with Ritalin (Brown & Bing,
1976). Despite the widespread use of such amphetamines to calm
the supposedly hyperactive child, one fact seems to receive little
consideration from those who are responsible for their use—that
there is a great deal of doubt as to whether the condition of MBD
actually exists. As pointed out by Schrag & Divoky (1975) in *The
Myth of the Hyperactive Child*, MBD is not a medical entity at all,
but rather a "disease by default," an ailment which puts the weight
of a spurious science against those children who have no other
problems but who don't learn to talk or read as their elders think
they should. Similarly, according to D. A. Pond (1967), professor
of child psychiatry at the University of London, and a specialist in
problems of brain damage and behavioral disturbances, "There are
. . . no absolutely unequivocal clinical signs, physiological tests or
psychological tests, that prove a relationship between brain damage
and any particular aspect of disturbed behavior" (p. 127). Two
child psychologists, Robert Y. Moore and Mitchell Blickstein, have
suggested that, in view of the current lack of evidence for the
existence of a relationship between minimal brain damage and
hyperactivity, "The concept, and hence the diagnosis, of minimal
brain damage or dysfunction should probably be discarded. It
serves no medical or educational purpose" (Moore & Glickstein,
1970, p. 640). Thus, thousands of children are being drugged in
order to combat the symptoms of a "disease" that "cannot be disclosed by a routine examination or by a specialized test such as
encephalogram" (Brown & Bing, 1976, p. 221). To make the picture even more bleak, there is evidence that, in some cases, the recipients of the drugs may actually have their health placed in
jeopardy. Walker (1974) has cited the examples of two "hyperactive" children, one with poor oxygenation and resultant behavioral problems due to a cardiac condition and another with a
prediabetic condition resulting in similar symptoms. In addition to

such short-term dangers, it must also be realized that there is virtually no evidence to assure us that such drugs are not harmful over a prolonged period (Grinspoon & Singer, 1974).

In addition to chemotherapy children have also been subjected to treatment involving psychosurgery. Older (1974) states that "children as young as four years old have been subjected to irreversible destruction of parts of their brains" (p. 669). In fact, such surgery has been performed on children diagnosed as hyperkinetic. Thus, according to Older (1974), not only are our children being drugged for a nonspecifiable and possibly nonexistent "disease," but they have also had parts of their brains destroyed for displaying such "symptoms" as "wandering tendencies" and "destructiveness."

Departing from the more medically based areas of treatment, we find evidence for other forms of abuse. The great emphasis on and credence in the administration of psychological tests and similar diagnostic and screening tools may be creating what Schrag & Divoky (1976) refer to as the "first dossierized generation," composed of children who will, upon reaching the age of adulthood, discover that they have acquired a rather extensive file filled with evidence that they are suffering from a whole variety of stigmatizing and restrictive psychological labels—"overaggressiveness," "hyperactivity," and so on. Mercer (1974) has recently cited evidence to support this possibility; "compared with preschool children and adults, school aged children are overlabeled with stigmatizing classifications such as 'retarded.' " Also, she found that "the public school system is the primary labeler in the community" (p. 127), labeling "more persons as retarded than any other organization" (p. 126) and showing a marked tendency to place potentially stigmatizing labels on members of various minority groups such as Chicanos and Blacks. Thus, she argues, our current use of psychological assessment techniques is labeling many children in a manner which fails to consider them "within a culturally appropriate normative framework" and as "multidimensional beings" (p. 125).

In the same vein, Simmonds (1976) has cited additional evidence of the tendency of mental health professionals to freely label children as suffering from various psychological disturbances. Commenting on a recent trend within family therapy, she notes that it has become increasingly common for therapists to designate a child member rather than an adult member of a family unit as the "disturbed one" when the designation of one client becomes necessary for insurance payment purposes. Simmonds believes that the child's relatively powerless state often results in his being scape-goated to avoid applying a stigmatizing label to an adult family member. Thus, many children are acquiring detrimental psychiatric labels for no other reason than that adult professionals are reluctant to apply such labels to adult clients! Considering the long-realized deleterious effects of categorizing people with various psychological terms and labels (Rosenhan, 1973; Rosenthal, & Jacobsen, 1968) as well as criticisms leveled from within the mental health profession at many of its long-revered assessment techniques (Mischel, 1968) and therapeutic procedures (Eysenck, 1952), such labeling practices seem especially unfortunate.

Another area in which children as clients seem to receive a great amount of unfair treatment involves psychiatric institutionalization of the child without his consent. In most states, a child's parent or guardian can apply to a mental hospital to have him admitted. If the hospital responds affirmatively, the child is then "voluntarily" admitted, regardless of the child's feelings (Beyer & Wilson, 1976). Additionally, in the majority of states, the child has absolutely no recourse, no legal means of appealing to any outside authority for a review of his or her admission. Unlike a voluntary adult patient, who can demand to be released at any time, or an involuntarily committed patient, who has the benefit of periodic review, the time and manner of the release of a "voluntary" child patient is entirely at the discretion of others (Beyer & Wilson, 1976). Such a situation would not be so disturbing if the parents or guardians of children always had the child's best interest at heart. However, as a recent article dealing with this subject revealed, children are often institutionalized for far different reasons. Beyer & Wilson (1976, pp. 133–134) offer the following facts:

> A review of hospital records in one state shows that children are sometimes confined to institutions for the mentally ill or mentally retarded not for their own good, but for the benefit of their parents or other family members. One child's "hyperactivity interfered with the routines of household and disturbed family members" (Ferleger, 1973, p. 4).
>
> Another child posed "no serious behavior problem; admitted due to parents' inability to provide a satisfactory home environment." Yet another child was admitted because of "emotional instability of the mother" (Ferleger, 1973, p. 6). This last case appears to fall within the ambit of a Philadelphia prehospitalization study indicating that in 25 percent of complaints of al-

leged mental illness, it was complainant, rather than the prospective patient, who evidenced signs of mental illness (Ellis,
1974, p. 860; citing Scheff, 1966, p. 171).

Adults involuntarily committed to institutions are guaranteed
due process of law: they receive procedural and substantive protections so that they will not be arbitrarily deprived of their
liberty. Children who are committed against their will to institutions by their parents are classified as having been voluntarily
committed and therefore are not guaranteed due process of law.
Whereas an adult patient's objection to such commitment is overruled in certain circumstances, the child's objection is not only
overruled but ignored.

The other side of the coin offers an equally inequitable picture.
In most states a minor, even a mature one such as a college student
living away from home, may not voluntarily elect to admit himself
to a mental hospital without parental consent (Ennis, 1976). In
addition, such a minor cannot even legally "contract or undergo
psychiatric treatment without specific permission from his parent
or guardian.... Whether living at home or away from home, a
minor must be able to furnish a physician with parental consent before the latter can lawfully initiate treatment" (Rosenberg & Katz,
1972, p. 54). Thus, children, even those living independently and
responsibly far from home, may not elect to receive psychiatric
treatment as either an inpatient or an outpatient without their
parents' express consent. Yet a parent may incarcerate them in a
mental hospital or subject them to psychiatric care as an outpatient
without the child's consent.

One further factor which is related to these issues involves the
question of confidentiality. While few mental health professionals
would challenge the importance of confidentiality in a client-
therapist relationship, in the case of the minor most laws fail to
establish whether the right of privileged communication belongs
to the parent or to the child-client (McGuire, 1974; Rosenberg &
Katz, 1972). Even the American psychological Association's Ethical Standards of Psychologists (1975) may be seen as ambiguous.
Within the Ethical Guidelines, we find the following statements:
"All materials in this official record shall be shared with the client
who shall have the right to decide what information may be shared
with anyone beyond the immediate provider of services and to be
informed of the implications of the materials to be shared." Furthermore, "Where a child or adolescent is the primary client, the

interests of the minor shall be paramount." The ambiguity lies in
the following statement which ends the APA's discussion of confidentiality: "The provider of services also has the responsibility
to discuss the contents of the record with the parents and/or child,
as appropriate, and to keep separate those parts which should remain the property of each family member." We are still faced with
the question: to whom does the privileged communication belong,
the child or his parent? To further add to the confused picture,
McGuire (1974), examined the confidentiality issue in child psychotherapy and concluded:

1. There does not seem to exist any clear, consistent, and uni-
    fied set of guidelines or principles for mental health pro-
    fessionals with regard to issues involving confidentiality and
    the child in psychotherapy.
2. There is a general lack of awareness, at least among psychol-
    ogists, of the content and applicability of the existing APA
    Code of Ethics to the child in psychotherapy.
3. There is a growing trend among mental health workers to
    operate in actual clinical situations according to an unwritten
    principle (one which seems to this author to be basically
    inconsistent with the statements of the APA Code of Ethics)
    that children or minors should be treated the same in therapy
    as their adult counterparts (p. 378).

Before considering the last example of consumer abuse in
children—that of informed consent—let us pause to summarize
our review of these abuses. On the basis of the examples already
discussed, we might well conclude that there is ample evidence of
consumer abuse of children as recipients of mental health services.
Children are continually subjected to forms of treatment and assessment that may well reflect a rather distorted interpretation of
their "best interests." Representing a very large group of persons,
children are distinguishable in many important ways from adults,
and are consumers who, in addition, are subject to many special
and frightening examples of consumer abuse. Thus, it seems that
on the basis of these examples, coupled with the large numbers of
child-clients and the great differences between children and their
adult counterparts, children should be given special consideration
as a discrete interest group of mental health consumers. With this
conclusion in mind, we now will consider one final example of con-

sumer abuse in children: informed consent. This issue has been saved for special consideration both because of its great ethical significance and because it has received less attention in the literature than many of the other issues.

The Child-Consumer and Informed Consent

Informed consent signifies a willful contracting of services following full information about treatment, its procedures, purposes, dangers, and overall implications for the client. This type of consent is of primary importance in a consideration of ethical issues in the treatment of children since informed consent may be viewed as closely related to, and even encompassing, each of the issues discussed above, i.e., the questionable effects of drugs and psychosurgery; the questionable validity of psychological testing and assessment; confidentiality; and voluntary versus involuntary treatment. With the importance of informed consent in mind, we will examine precisely how the child is viewed in the law.

The Child-Client and the Law. Even though changes may be soon in coming, children under eighteen still have very few rights under the law. One of the reasons why children find themselves deprived of certain basic legal protections is because the law allows parents great discretion in rearing their children.[1] In fact, the law becomes involved only when problems within the family unit spill over into the courts or public agencies. Once brought into the public arena, children are again denied basic protections guaranteed to adults by the United States Constitution, this time under two doctrines. Under he doctrine of *parens patriae,* the state refuses to provide civil rights for children because their supposed inability to wisely exercise those rights might result in their exploitation rather than their protection.[2] The second doctrine which applies to children is a simplistic, legal one which focuses on labels and holds that persons who are civilly adjudicated are not entitled to criminal due process protections. The courts therefore, in the personage of judges, are empowered to exercise their discretionary powers to protect children. Such a procedure places a tremendous responsibility on the judges, and can result in extremely subjective and inconsistent judgments. Thus, it would appear that even in court children are placed in a precarious position.

In partial recognition of these problems, the Supreme Court ruled in 1967 that children must be accorded due process protections in any juvenile hearing in which their freedom, and their parents' right to custody, are at stake.[3] Those protections are: (1) the right to notice of the charges and hearing; (2) the right to confront and cross-examine witnesses; (3) the right to counsel (appointed if necessary); and (4) the right to be informed of, and to exercise, the privilege against self-incrimination. In addition, a child's guilt must be determined beyond a reasonable doubt,[4] and he is entitled to the constitutional protection against double jeopardy.[5] However, children do *not* have the right to a jury trial,[6] and none of the aforementioned rights are afforded children who are hospitalized by their parents. The Supreme Court has, however, decided to hear arguments from children whose parents committed them to Pennsylvania state mental hospitals.[7] In the Pennsylvania case, it was argued that children should be guaranteed protections similar to those provided in juvenile delinquency proceedings.

Let us now turn to the question of whether children, under the law, can give informed consent to treatment. The contract of informed consent in medical cases is a relatively simple one: an agreement between doctor and patient that the patient, understanding the nature and consequences of the treatment, will undergo treatment by the doctor. The contract insulates the doctor from liability for performing a battery, since the touching has been consented to by the patient. It also protects the patient from consenting to a touching which might have consequences beyond those anticipated. As is obvious, the informed consent contract was designed for medical and surgical treatments, which by their nature require a touching. However, certain *psychiatric* treatments also require a touching, and cases do not distinguish the need for informed consent agreements between psychiatrist and patient from those between physician and patients. In the case of psychologists, where there is no touching, one might ask whether an informed consent agreement is even necessary.[8] However, such an interpretation of the purpose of the doctrine of informed consent would be unnecessarily shortsighted, since the doctrine was meant to protect *both* parties (patient and treator) in a treatment transaction.

Until recently children had no first amendment rights of free speech because they were not considered persons entitled to constitutional protections.[9] The idea that a child was not a person had its roots in the *parens patriae* aspects of pre-constitutional Anglo-Saxon law which saddled children with numerous disabilities, incapacitating children in law. This means, for example, that children could not contract. Even today, children cannot contract, except for "necessaries,"[10] and this seriously impedes a child's ability to give informed consent to treatment, since that agreement rests in contract. While there are those who argue for a more enlightened approach,[11] the general state of the law is such that a child cannot give informed consent. The consent of a parent, or someone standing *in loco parentis,* is thus necessary to avoid a battery, an unlawful or offensive touching.[12]

In some states, specific statutes allow children, above certain ages, to consent to medical services. However, the majority of these statutes are designed only to provide teenagers, engaged in adult activity, the benefit of sexual counseling. Thus, the statutes recognize that adolescents are capable of giving informed consent, within the limited sphere of venereal disease prevention and treatment or pregnancy counseling.[13] A limited number of states have also enacted laws allowing adolescents to consent to treatment of a mental or emotional disorder.[14] And the Supreme Court has recently ruled that a state may not constitutionally impose a blanket parental consent requirement as a condition for an unmarried minor's abortion during the first twelve weeks of her pregnancy, thus recognizing—albeit to a limited degree because of the nature of the particular case—that a minor can consent to that medical treatment.[15]

Aside from these statutory exceptions to the general rule, a judicial exception has been created in the case where the adolescent has demonstrated his ability to understand the nature and consequences of therapeutic treatment. So, for example, physicians have *not* been found liable of "unconsented touching" in cases where the adolescent is fifteen years of age or older,[16] suggesting that fifteen year-olds can indeed give consent to treatment in these circumstances. The most crucial element in this judicial exception is that the contemplated treatment must benefit the adolescent, rather than someone else (as would be the case which a child donates blood[17]). (Courts will also take into consideration the age and maturity of the adolescent, and the degree of emancipation from his parents.)

Another statutory exception becomes apparent in the statutes enacted in certain states allowing for the consent of married and emancipated minors to medical and surgical procedures.[18] Again, such statutes suggest that children under eighteen can legally, in some circumstances, give consent to treatment even without parental consent.

A further exception to the general rule that a minor's consent

is legally ineffective is encountered in the "emergency exceptions."
In an emergency situation the need for parental consent is vitiated.
However, the definition of emergency is narrowly construed in that
immediate treatment by a physician must be the *only* way to preserve the life or health of the young patient. Furthermore, the consent of a parent or guardian must be unobtainable.[19]

To summarize the legal status of children related to informed
consent, we might state, in spite of the exceptions mentioned above,
that "the law presumes a minor incapable of comprehending the
peril of his position, and, therefore, incompetent to consent to such
treatment" (Rosenberg & Katz, 1972, p. 54). As mentioned above,
it is, generally speaking, the parent or legal guardian who takes
responsibility for providing the child's consent to treatment. In
fact, as Rada (1976) points out, the situation involving the child-
client is not one in which the term "informed consent," even applies. Rather, he asserts, it is actually more appropriate to speak
of "vicarious consent" in describing "consent by a parent or legal
guardian for someone deemed legally incapable of giving consent
himself" (p. 9).

In conclusion, then, there are few legal precedents which
would presently warrant the conclusion that children, even adolescents under eighteen, can give legally effective informed consent
to treatment. Even in those exceptions to the law mentioned
above, the treatment referred to was medical rather than psychological treatment. Thus, the law currently provides little basis for
speaking of a child's "right" to give informed consent to treatment.
Perhaps the strongest argument for such a right emerges from a
consideration of the protections and benefits which might accrue
to the child-client if such a right can eventually be established.
An Argument for Informed Consent. The current legal status of
children related to informed consent need not be the final word.
Laws are subject to change, and legal precedents can be established, if strong arguments can be made on behalf of children that
allowing them the right to give informed consent to treatment
would benefit the child.

One important reason that a denial of informed consent to
children may be viewed as an especially onerous one is pointed out
by Rosenburg & Katz (1972), who suggest that the denial of
informed consent to minors may actually, on occasion, threaten
to undermine the effectiveness of therapy for these persons. As
these authors point out, "the law demands that consent, to be effective, must be 'informed.' Psychiatry, to be effective, to stimulate

trust, and to protect the patients cannot always provide details about the treatment to parents which would truly be sufficient to sustain a finding of 'informed consent'" (pp. 55–56). Thus, the legal restrictions of informed consent in minors may, when strictly adhered to, foster a very non-therapeutic atmosphere in which to conduct psychiatric treatment. In line with this possibility, LoCicero (1976, p. 15), has discussed the fact that children often invent explanations for being brought to see a mental health professional which are much worse than the actual reason, i.e., that they are "bad," "wild," "retarded," or as Chess (1969) has mentioned, "wicked" or "crazy." Given our knowledge about the importance of one's self-concept to one's overall adjustment (Bannister & Fransella, 1971), the danger of allowing such ideas to take root by silence seems quite obvious. Thus, according to the current assumptions underlying informed consent in children, a therapist could easily compound a child's problem and, just as unfortunately, forego an opportunity to show the child that "a well-respected and knowledgeable adult in the child's life sees the child in a more positive way than the child has anticipated ... [which can] in itself ... be therapeutic, and may initiate the process by which the child essentially achieves a better and a more acceptable view of himself or herself" (LoCicero, 1976, p. 15).

As several persons (Chess, 1969; Freud, 1946; LoCicero, 1976; Sylvester, 1952) have pointed out, the preparation for early stages of therapy often has profound effects upon the subsequent course of such treatment. With this consideration in mind, LoCicero (1976) has most aptly stressed the importance of providing the child with adequate and realistic information since

> such preparation can be of substantial help to the child, who can then mobilize resources to deal constructively with the treatment situation. The clinician must be careful to present the situation realistically to the child and avoid raising false hopes. The clinician who knows the child can help the child cope with any anxieties regarding treatment or changes necessary to implement the recommendations (p. 15).

Since "child psychotherapy rests on the assumption that children themselves, with help, can make changes in their own lives ... it seems reasonable, then, to share with the child any understanding that might help him or her to make decisions that could contribute to progress in healthy development" (LoCicero, 1976,

p. 14). In making a case for the therapeutic significance of providing information to the child, LoCicero has also pointed out the
advantages to be gained through the parents: "By indicating respect for the child as an individual with private experiences, the
clinician sets an example for parents; in some cases, parents are
encouraged to perceive the child in a new way" (pp. 15–16). With
regard to the importance of the parents' reactions to and appraisal
of the child in the growth or modifications of the child's self-concept, the potential advantages of the clinician's honesty toward
the child seem especially crucial. LoCicero (1976) points out one additional advantage: "By talking with the child about the results of
an evaluation, the clinician relieves the parents of the possible
burdens involved in deciding whether or what to tell the child, issues often cloaked in service" (p. 16). In summary, it seems quite
apparent that "if a child knows the method and the goals of treatment and if the child expects to receive answers to questions about
the treatment, the treatment process can be initiated and can
progress more smoothly. The well-informed and respected child is
in a sense invited to become a partner, an active participant in the
treatment process" (p. 16). Although resistance to treatment is
always possible, a healthier aspect is that children who construe
themselves as active participants in their own treatment are allied
with the therapist from the beginning, thus enhancing their own
development. Conversely, we can avoid the opposite situation, that
of the child pitted against the psychotherapist and, possibly, his or
her parents. In effect, then, a case may be made that an attempt
at informed consent for the child can serve as a very advantageous
tool in establishing a therapeutic atmosphere and, on the other
hand, the therapist's failure to provide such consent to the child
may actually serve to jeopardize his own efforts.

In addition to its implications for the efficacy of treatment,
the informed consent issue also is of importance for more ethical
reasons. APA's Ethical Standards for Psychologists (1975), for
example, address themselves to the clinician's responsibilities and
duties toward his/her "client." In cases involving the child-consumer, the question arises as to whom the term "client" actually
refers—the child himself or the child's parents or legal guardian?
Koocher (1976) points out the difficulties involved in such a situation: "On the one hand, the therapist is ethically bound to respect
the best interests of the child-client. On the other hand, the therapist is being paid to act as a kind of parental agent and parents are
[of course] responsible for their child's welfare in most cases"

(p. 26). Were it the case that the parents always know what is best for the child and always care about what is in his best interests, such a potential conflict of interest might be of little significance. However, as discussed above, parents and legal guardians often are either ignorant regarding such matters or simply do not have the child's best interests at heart. On occasion, it is possible that a well-intentioned but poorly informed parent may in fact, be pressured by larger segments of society (i.e., the school system, the courts) into securing for the child psychiatric treatment and/or institutionalization. As charged by Lowrey (1975), "services that are delivered to children are usually delivered based on the needs of the adults who are around them, based on the needs of the society at large troubled by a child who is dangerous on the street, by a parent who is troubled by a child out of control, by the school that wants the child who is a troublemaker excluded from class" (p. 480). With such considerations in mind, the denial of informed consent to the child seems both unethical and potentially dangerous for the child.

Worsfeld (1974) offers the following comments on this subject:

> Historically, rights in society have been ascribed only to adults. Children have been treated paternally, their conduct has been controlled by parents or others in authority. Such control has been justified, in the paternalistic view, by the need to protect children from themselves and others. It is argued that children cannot be responsible for their own welfare because by their nature they lack an adequate conception of their own present and future interests. They are said to want instant gratification and to be incapable of fully rational decisions.... Well intentioned though this view may be, its implicit claim that adults do have an adequate conception of children's interests, and that they are always willing to act upon this conception, is open to serious question. In fact, parents often do not know what is best for their children, and children often can make sensible decisions for themselves about their own lives (pp. 142–143).

Worsfeld's last point, that perhaps some children deserve more credit than is generally offered them with regard to their decision making capabilities has been also pointed out by Rosenberg & Katz (1972), who suggest that the denial of informed consent to minors rests upon a very questionable premise since "the assumption of the incompetency of minors to understand the nature of the proffered medical treatment is hardly accurate in a majority of cases" (p.

54). Cases in point would include, for example, self-supporting, financially independent "children" in their late teens who reside alone, or mature college students living away from home and supporting themselves with part-time jobs and student loans. Would it be reasonable, we must ask ourselves, to deny "children" of this particular level of maturity, responsibility, and sophistication the right to fully informed consent to treatment on the premise that they would somehow be incapable of adequately comprehending its nature, dangers, and implications? Reflection upon this and similar questions leads to the realization that there may be something quite unrealistic about the tendency of our legal system and our mental health agencies to treat all minors as though they are incapable of comprehending the essentials of psychiatric treatment. Certainly a mature college-aged "child" who lacks a few months to adulthood is not identical to a six-month-old or a six-year-old in his abilities to understand the procedures and implications of such treatment. And yet, legally, he is often treated as if he were.

The mere fact that one, technically, has not yet reached his legal majority does not necessarily insure his mental incompetency in such matters. Even a quick review of recent suggestions (Foster, 1974; Worsfeld, 1974) and attempts (Bartley v. Kremens; *in re* Gault; Wisconsin v. Yoder) to extend the rights of children to include more adult-like privileges reflect an overwhelming tendency to treat all minors as though they were a very homogeneous group.

With some exceptions (Beyer & Wilson, 1976; Kalogerakis, 1975; Koocher, 1976; Rodham, 1973) the majority of such examples seem, at best, to pay lip-service to the possibility that "children" possess greatly varying levels of reasoning, comprehension and sophistication. Yet, on the other hand, many children do indeed lack the intellectual equipment and skills needed to comprehend such matters. How should we go about deciding when a person can understand such factors sufficiently to allow him the right to make informed consent? At what point may we conclude safely that he is capable of making a truly intelligent and informed decision about his own treatment? To answer such questions and, thus, to avoid denying persons their rights while also assuring them our protection from the possible self-harm if forced to make a decision for which they lack sufficient comprehension, we should take a closer look at the information gathered by developmental psychologists about the intellectual development of children. We will argue that age should not be the exclusive determinant of intellectual maturity.

Cognitive Development as Related to the Child-Consumer

The intellectual skills which a child possesses at any given point in his development differ from those of the developmentally mature adult in certain specific and specifiable ways. Thus, children must not be viewed as miniature adults, but rather as being very different from adults in many of their abilities.

At the same time, however, a second conclusion may be drawn from the developmental literature. While the developmental evidence clearly points out that children, in general, differ greatly from adults, this same evidence also makes it impossible for us to think of all children as one homogeneous group. Rather, as many theorists have pointed out, children at different stages in their development differ greatly from each other in many ways, these differences manifesting themselves in terms of the child's emotional (Erikson, 1963; Goldstein, Freud & Solnit, 1973; Piaget, 1968) and intellectual (Piaget, 1970) capabilities. The reason for this, as Piaget (1970) and others (Kessen, 1962; Inhelder, & Piaget, 1969, 1964; White, 1965) have demonstrated, is that the cognitive development of the child involves a gradual process in which the child proceeds through a sequence of qualitatively differing stages which are invariant in order and hierarchical in arrangement with each successive stage evolving out of and building upon each preceding stage.

The child's progression from one stage to the next occurs as the result of the child's inherent activity which results in the child's constant interaction with his environment. Such interaction between the child's structures at each stage and the structures of the environment develop the child's cognitive structures toward greater and greater equilibrium in organism-environment interactions (Flavell, 1963). As greater equilibrium is attained at each successful stage in the child's cognitive development, the child can function in an increasingly more flexible, spontaneous, and sophisticated manner as he uses, applies, and structures his knowledge about the world (Inhelder & Piaget, 1964; Nelson & Kosslyn, 1975; Piaget & Inhelder, 1969). Thus, the child moves through qualitatively differing stages of logicomathematical development, each stage representing greater internalization and flexibility of his action-based thought structures.

The preoperational child's thought structures, while earlier having been based on the overt and similar action of the infant, undergo a gradual change; during this stage the child's actions become internalized, thus freeing him from the necessity of representing the world solely as overt activity. One manifestation of this internalization of action is the emergence of the symbolic function, which includes deferred imitation, mental imagery, modeling, drawing, and language, finally allowing the child to represent things symbolically rather than by overt action only and also to understand, at least rudimentarily, the symbolic representations of others (Piaget, Inhelder, 1969). Despite the great advancements of the preoperational stage, which generally spans the ages from about two to six or seven years—Piaget believes that ages are, at best, only approximations—the young child's thought structures are still highly inflexible and quite inefficient, owing to the fact that their reorganization on this new symbolic level is yet incomplete. As a result of the inflexibility and inefficiency of his cognitive skills, the child tends to center his attention on the perceptually salient qualities of things, people and situations. He can consider only one aspect of a situation at a time and, on an interpersonal level, everything is seen only from his point of view; the perspectives of others do not exist. Thus, he is a truly egocentric being, incapable of differentiating objective and subjective realities. People and situations are judged on the basis of their most outstanding characteristics, and, with regard to a child's own actions as well as the behavior of others, observable consequences rather than less obvious intentions are used as the basis for making interpersonal judgments.

The young child's tendency to center on and reason in terms of salient perceptual qualities has a profound influence upon his sociomoral judgments. He can reason only in absolute terms, i.e., this is good; that is bad (Piaget, 1932). Adults, being larger and more powerful than children, are viewed as omnipotent, omniscient persons whose pronunciations are seen as sacred, wholly beyond question (Aldrich & Mancuso, in press). Further his reasoning does not begin to allow him to consider the implications of the acts or ideas of himself or others, since everything is judged in terms of its observable consequences (Piaget, 1932).

Sometime between the ages of six and eight years (approximately), the preoperational stage gives way to the next stage—concrete operations—which is characterized by increased flexibility and sophistication in reasoning, a decrease in egocentrism, and the ability to deal quite efficiently with concrete situations. With the advent of these new thought structures, the child, on the interpersonal level, can, with his decreased egocentrism, consider the existence of viewpoints other than his own (Piaget & Inhelder, 1969). No longer tied to the perceptually salient and the superficial, he can now begin to separate subjective and objective reality and to consider the intentions, motivations, and mitigating circumstances underlying the behavior of others (Mancuso, Morrison & Aldrich, in press). In terms of moral judgments, he can now free himself from absolutes (he is "good"; she is "bad"), and from the belief that the moral good is a "given" of adult authority, and can now reason in terms of a morality based on mutual cooperation between equals (Piaget, 1932).

Despite the rather impressive and increasingly adult-like cognitive abilities demonstrated by the concrete operational child, relative to his preoperational predecessor—especially as related to personal perception within the social realm and moral judgment within the emotional realm—the concrete operational child is still tied to the "here-and-now," and cannot reason beyond the confines of concrete reality. Thus, he must treat each situation separately rather than being able to abstract the commonalities inherent in them (Ginsberg & Opper, 1969). Not until the advent of the final stage, that of "formal operations," anywhere from 12–15 years, can the child finally attain the ability to reason in an abstract, hypothetic-deductive manner, which enables him, at last, to transcend the confines of the concrete "here-and-now"; to consider the realm of ideals, principles, and implications; and to infer the causal relationships between several factors (Flavell, 1963).

Conclusions and Recommendations

We have attempted to establish that children, as consumers of mental health services, are a discrete, special-interest group which has generally been deprived of the privileges enjoyed by adult consumers. We have focused most on how child-consumers, even those who live away from home at colleges and universities, are generally deprived legally of the right to give informed consent to psychiatric treatment.

We have argued that the proliferating evidence from developmental research already allows us to draw a number of conclusions with a great deal of confidence. Age *per se* is not an adequate, first criterion for classification of a child's reasoning abilities. Rather, age is seen by Piaget and others as, at best, an approximation.

Cognitive stage is seen as *the* important factor in determining a person's ability to comprehend and reason. Second, despite the fact that children may be seen as sharing certain intellectual features or characteristics relative to adults, to think of children as a cognitively homogeneous group would be ludicrous since children, at different stages are very different people indeed! Third, some children, i.e., those who have attained the final stage, that of formal operational, are capable of reasoning in a highly abstract and adult-like manner and, therefore, can undoubtedly comprehend situations and make inferences on a par with their adult counterparts. (In fact some children are undoubtedly superior to a number of adults who never reach the final cognitive stage!) In summary, reflection upon these three conclusions, as well as consideration of the issues discussed above regarding treatment of the child-client, lead to the realization that our current methods of dealing with children both legally and, often, clinically—especially as reflected in the current practices involved in informed consent—fail to take into consideration a wealth of developmental evidence. The categorical denial of informed consent to all minors demonstrates the failure of persons in both the legal and the mental health professions to clearly consider and understand the significance of such developmental evidence. And, unfortunately, so do the overwhelming majority of recent attempts to extend such rights to minors (e.g., Bartley v. Kremens).

What seems to be needed, then, is a major revision in the current approaches to child rights. A revision which would include a concerted effort on the part of the interested parties in both the mental health and the legal professions so as to consider the developmental evidence in formulating both legislation and treatment procedures in dealing with the child-client. Using informed consent as a case in point, certain questions must be asked by both mental health and legal professionals. At which stage in cognitive development can the child truly comprehend the information involved in informed consent to treatment? Which cognitive skills would enable the child to understand the essentials of psychiatric treatment and its implications? Once these questions have been addressed, an attempt could be made to match the information given to children at various cognitive stages with the skills which they possess at these various levels. For example, a child at the most advanced stage might well be expected to comprehend any and all of the information about psychiatric treatment, including its most abstract present and future implications for his own well-being. A child at the concrete operational stage, while probably incapable of understanding any abstract implications, might still be able to understand the more concrete aspects of the treatment procedures, i.e., immediate goals, purposes, and techniques. A child below this stage might be expected to comprehend very little of the information that informed consent would entail. Thus, we suggest that the child's level of cognitive development be considered to determine the amount and kinds of information he should be presented about his treatment. In other words, a match between his intellectual capabilities and the information he is furnished should be sought. These considerations, should be used to guide further legal developments.

In the case of Yoder v. Wisconsin, Justice Douglas argued, in the minority, that "on the important and vital matter of education . . . children should be entitled to be heard" (in Rodham, 1974, p. 505). He based his opinion not only on available legal precedents, but on psychological and sociological findings that children of the relevant ages possess the moral and intellectual judgment necessary for making responsible decisions on matters of religion and education. To rebut the presumption that children lack sufficient maturity to make such decisions, Douglas relied on the works of Piaget, Kohlberg, Kay, Gesell, and Ilg (Rodham, 1974, p. 505). That his was a lone voice among the justices, the majority of whom chose to ignore the developmental considerations, is unfortunate, and yet, it might be viewed as a starting point; an example which might be followed by others.

We also would like to offer some specific, and practical recommendations for incorporating our knowledge of intellectual functioning into clinical interventions. First, it may be possible to develop a brief, easily administered (even by nonprofessionals) test of a child's level of intellectual functioning so that mental health professionals could determine, upon first encountering a potential child-client, whether that person is capable of informed consent or not; and if so, to what degree. Perhaps, with some adaptation, certain tests used by Piaget could be used to determine a child's ability to give informed consent. We strongly encourage researchers to explore the specific differences between informed consent as offered by children and adults. We would not be surprised if research demonstrated that many persons over eighteen, who now enjoy many adult privileges according to law, are really not capable of functioning as rational adults. And, correspondingly, we would not be surprised to discover many persons under eighteen who are actually capable of functioning as rational adults.

We further recommend making greater use of child advocates

in certain circumstances. As suggested by others (Koocher, 1976; McCoy & Koocher, 1976; Beyer, 1976; Foster, 1974), the child must have some idea who will take responsibility for seeing that his best interests are protected. Since practical considerations of time and money are of utmost importance in this matter, it would be quite impractical for legal or mental health professionals to be delegated such responsibility in all cases of clinical treatment. However, in those instances where psychosurgery, electroconvulsive therapy, and involuntary hospital commitment are being considered for the child, legal and mental health professionals not affiliated with the place of treatment might be asked to serve as advocates of the child. Since such radical clinical interventions call for more caution and safeguards, it is recommended that child advocates be required by state law to thoroughly review the necessity of those interventions *before* they are actually undertaken.

In cases where less radical clinical interventions (e.g., group therapy, play therapy, and so on) are contemplated for a child, but where some question exists as to the particular procedure to be used (e.g., a confrontative group approach for an eight-year-old), advocates might be appointed to review the case. Perhaps lay advocates might be helpful in some cases, provided that they are both informed and knowledgeable with regard to the issues central to children and that they are able to work from an objective position related to the child, his or her parents, and the legal and mental health personnel involved. Perhaps members of client advisory boards (Morrison, 1976) and citizen advisory boards might serve as such advocates.

A third suggestion merely reinforces what others (Koocher, 1976) have recommended: mental health professionals should attempt to explain to child-clients of all ages as much about a therapeutic intervention as they need to know and can actually understand. We cannot wait for changes in the law on a child's rights before we practice common sense: that a child can benefit more from an intervention if he can knowingly participate in that event.

Whether information revealed by a child to a therapist can and should be, at least in some circumstances, disclosed to parents is still a confusing issue. At present we can only recommend that this important issue be further studied and that every means possible be taken to protect the child-consumer.

A fifth recommendation emerges from the potential abuses in our system of computerized records. If a child can, as is presently the case, be taken for therapy at an early age, then usually there is a record that he had or has a "psychiatric problem." If, in later life, access can be gained legally or illegally to such information, could not a person be damaged for life? Could such a person, as an adult, sue a therapist, clinic and parents for taking him, as a child, for treatment when there was a strong risk of later stigma? Perhaps the only way around such issues is to recommend that the records of child and adolescent clients be routinely destroyed after the clients reach eighteen, unless the client would have it otherwise. A less extreme recommendation prevents the record of a child's client status from being computerized in any file outside the clinic or hospital where he is treated. The more persons who have access to such data, the greater the danger that such information can be obtained by those who have no right to this data.

A sixth recommendation is for attorneys. Considering the fact that lawsuits, especially a series of them, can often change mental health procedures, we would encourage attorneys to consider taking legal action on behalf of those adults, who, as children, were damaged mentally or physically due to a careless neglect of what we consider their rights. Such legal actions may result in the type of legal precedents which can establish, before the law, the right of the child-client to informed consent before the law.

A seventh and last recommendation centers on the need for information sharing between members of the legal and mental health professions, as well as between such professionals and the public at large. Community education workshops, interdisciplinary symposia at professional conventions (e.g., American Psychological Association, American Bar Association, American Psychiatric Association), and other educational efforts, all aimed at a discussion of the desirability and feasibility of extending the limits of children's rights, would give all of us a more accurate view of the new and possible horizons in the field of children's rights.

In summary, what is needed is an attempt by all parties involved to work for the rights of the child while keeping firmly in mind the special abilities and limitations of the child. Only in this way will the cause of the child-client best be served.

Notes

1. See Wisconsin v. Yoder, 406 U.S. 205 (1972).
2. See Andrew Jay Kleinfeld, The Balance of Power Among Infants, Their Parents and the State, 5 Family Law Quarterly 64 (1970).
3. In re Gault, 387 U.S. 1 (1967).
4. In re Winship, 397 U.S. 358 (1970).
5. Breed v. Jones, 421 U.S. 519 (1975).
6. McKeiver v. Penn., 403 U.S. 528 (1971).

7. Bartley v. Kremens, 402 F. Supp. 1039 (E.D. Pa. 1975).

8. Comment, Counseling the Counselors: Legal Implications of Counseling Minors Without Parental Consent, 31 Maryland Law Review 332, 347 (1971).

9. Tinker v. Des Moines Independent Community School District, 393 U.S. 503 (1969).

10. Necessaries include whatever is reasonably needed for the infant's subsistence, such as food and lodging; for his health, such as medicine, and services of a physician or nurse in case of sickness, for his comfort, and for his education. Laurence P. Simpson, Contracts, 2nd Ed. 104 (1965).

11. W. D. Nevin, Jr., The Contracts of Minors Viewed From the Perspective of Fair Exchange, 50 North Carolina Law Review 516 (1972).

12. Thomas A. Knapp, Problems of Consent in Medical Treatment, 62 Military Law Review 105, 121 (1973).

13. See H. Pilpel, Minors' Rights to Medical Care, 36 Albany Law Review 462, 467 (1972).

14. Md. Annot. Code, Art. 43, 135 (A) (Supp. 1971).

15. Planned Parenthood of Central Missouri et. al. v. Danforth, 44 U.S. Law Week 5197 (July 1, 1976).

16. Note, Parental Consent Requirements and Privacy Rights of Minors: The Contraceptive Controversy, 88 Harvard Law Review 1001, 1005 (1975); see also, T. Knapp, Problems of Consent in Medical Treatment, 62 Military Law Review 105, 123 (1973).

17. Zaman v. Schultz, 19 Pa. D. and c. 309 (Cambria County Ct. 1933) (Blood donation for benefit of another held non-therapeutic and minor's consent legally insufficient); Bonner v. Moran, 126 F. 2d (D.C. Cir. 1941) (donation of skin graft held non-therapeutic and minor's consent legally insufficient); Gulf and Ship Island R.R. v. Sullivan, 119 So. 501 (Miss. 1928) (17 year old boy could consent to smallpox vaccination); Lacey v. Laird, 166 Ohio St. 12, 139 N.E. 2d 25 (1956) (18 year old girl could consent to simple plastic surgery to her nose); Younts v. St. Francis Hospital and School of Nursing, Inc., 250 Kan. 292, 469 P. 2d 330 (1970) (17 year old girl could consent to emergency surgical repair of injured finger when mother unconscious and divorced father unavailable).

18. Thomas A. Knapp, Id., 124.

19. Thomas A. Knapp, Id., 126.

References

American Psychological Association, *Ethical standards of psychologists.* (Draft No. 7) Washington, D.C., 1975.

Bannister, D., & Fransella, F. *Inquiring man: The theory of personal constructs.* Middlesex, England: Penguin Books, 1971.

Beit-Hellahmi, B. Salvation and its vicissitudes: Clinical psychology and political values. *American Psychologist*, 1974, *29*, 124–129.

Beyer, H. A., & Wilson, J. P. The reluctant volunteer: A child's right to resist commitment. In G. P. Koocher (Ed.), *Children's rights and the mental health professions*. New York: Wiley, 1976.

Brodsky, S. L. Shared results and open files with the client, *Professional Psychology*, 1972, *4*, 362–364.

Brown, B. S. The life of psychiatry. *The American Journal of Psychotherapy*, 1976, *133*, 489–495.

Brown, J. L., & Bing, S. R. Drugging children: Child abuse by professionals. In G. P. Koocher (Ed.), *Children's rights and the mental health professions*, New York: Wiley, 1976.

Burg, S. R., & Brown, J. L. The juvenile court: Ideology of Pathology. In G. P. Koocher (Ed.), *Children's rights and the mental health professions*. New York: Wiley, 1976.

Campbell, B. Children's rights drive centered in courtroom. *New York Times*, October 31, 1976, p. 26.

Chess, S. *An introduction to child psychiatry* (2nd ed.) New York: Grune and Stratton, 1969.

Daniels, A. K. The captive professional: Bureaucratic limitations in the practice of military psychiatry. *Journal of Health and Social Behavior*, 1969, *10*, 255–265.

Ennis, B. J. Legal rights of the voluntary patient. *The National Association of private psychiatric hospitals*, 1976, *8*, 4–8.

Erikson, E. *Childhood and society*. New York: W. W. Norton & Co., 1963.

Eysenck, H. S. The effects of psychotherapy: An evaluation. *Journal of Consulting Psychology*, 1952, *16*, 319–324.

Ferleger, D. Kremens v. Bartley: The right to be free. *Hospital and Community Psychiatry*, 1976, *27*, 708–712.

Flavell, J. *The developmental psychology of Jean Piaget*. Princeton, N.J.: Van Nostrand, 1963.

Foster, H. H., Jr. *A "Bill of Rights" for children*. Springfield, Ill.: Charles C. Thomas, 1974.

Freud, A. The psychoanalytical treatment of children. *Psychoanalytic Study on Children*, 1945, *1*, 233–246.

Ginsberg, A. An examination of the civil rights of mentally ill children. *Child Welfare*, 1973, *52*, 14–15.

Ginsberg, H., & Opper, S. *Piaget's theory of intellectual development: An introduction*. Englewood Cliffs, N.J.: Prentice-Hall, Inc., 1969.

Goldstein, J., Freud, A., & Solnit, A. J. *Beyond the best interests of the child*. New York: Macmillan, 1973.

Grunspoon, L. & Singer, S. B. Amphetamines in the treatment of hyperkinetic children. *Harvard Educational Review*, 1973, *43*, 514–523.

Inhelder, B., & Piaget, J. *The early growth of logic in the child*. London: Rutledge and Kegan Paul, 1964.

Kalogerakis, M. G. In A. Levy (Moderator), Symposium: Children's rights-psychiatry and the law. *Journal of Psychiatry and Law*, 1975, *3*, 475–499.

Kessen, W. "Stage" and "structure" in the study of children. *Monographs of the society for research in child development*, 1962, *27*, 65–82.

Kohlberg, L. The development of children's orientations toward a moral order: I. Sequences in the development of moral thought, *Vita Humana*, 1963, *6*, 11–23.

Koocher, G. P. (Ed.), *Children's rights and the mental health profession*. New York: Wiley, 1976.

Levitt, E. E. The results of psychotherapy with children: An evaluation. *Journal of Consulting Psychology*, 1957, *21*, 189–196.

LoCicero, A. The right to know: Telling children the results of clinical evaluations. In G. P. Koocher (Ed.), *Children's rights and the mental health profession*, New York: Wiley, 1976.

Lowery, M. In A. Levy (Moderator), Symposium: Children's rights— psychiatry and the law. *Journal of Psychiatry and Law*, 1975, *3*, 475–499.

Mancuso, J. C., Morrison, J. K., & Aldrich, C. C. Developmental changes in social-moral perception: Some factors affecting children's evaluations and predictions of the behavior of a "transgressor". *Journal of Genetic Psychology*, in press.

McCoy, R., & Koocher, G. P. Needed: A public policy for psychotropic drug use with children. In G. P. Koocher (Ed.), *Children's rights and the mental health professions*. New York: Wiley, 1976.

McGuire, J. M. Confidentiality and the child in psychotherapy. *Professional Psychology*, 1974, *5*, 374–379.

Mercer, J. R. A policy statement on assessment procedures and the rights of children. *Harvard Educational Review*, 1974, *44*, 125–141.

Mischel, W. *Personality and assessment*. New York: Wiley, 1968.

Moore, R. Y., & Glickstein, M. Biological factors in development. In H. W. Reese and L. P. Lipsitt (Eds.), *Experimental child psychology*, New York: Academic Press, 1970.

Morrison, J. K. Developmental study of the person perception of young children. *Proceedings, 81st Annual Convention, American Psychological Association*, 1973, *8*, 101–102.

Morrison, J. K. An argument for mental patient advisory boards. *Professional Psychology*, 1976, *7*, 1–6.

Morrison, J. K. The client as consumer and evaluator of community mental health services. *American Journal of Community Psychology*, in press.

Morrison, J. K., Federico, M., & Rosenthal, H. J. Contracting confidentiality in group psychotherapy. *Journal of Forensic Psychology*, 1975, *7*, 1–6.

Nelson, K., & Kosslyn, S. Semantic retrieval in children and adults. *Developmental Psychology*, 1975, *11*, 807–813.

National Institute of Mental Health. Hospital inpatient treatment units for emotionally disturbed children: United States, 1971–1972, Department of Health, Education and Welfare, Pub. No. (ADM) (1974A), 74–82.

NIMH Residential psychiatric facilities for children and adolescents: United States, 1971–1972. Department of Health, Education and Welfare Pub. No. (ADM) (1974B), 74–78.

Office of Children's Services. The PINS child: A plethora of problems. New York: Office of Children's Services, Judicial Conference of the State of New York, September, 1973B. *In re Ellery c.* 32 New York, second district, 588 (1973).

Older, J. Psychosurgery: Ethical issues and a proposal for control. *American Journal of Orthopsychiatry*, 1974, *44*, 661–674.

Piaget, J. *The moral judgment of the child.* London: Kegan Paul, 1932.

Piaget, J. *Six psychological studies.* New York: Random House, 1968.

Piaget, J. *The judgment and reasoning of the child.* Toronto: Littlefield, 1969.

Piaget, J. Piaget's theory. In P. Mussen (Ed.), *Carmichael's manual of child psychology* (3rd ed.). New York: Wiley, 1970.

Piaget, J., & Inhelder, B. *The psychology of the child.* New York: Basic Books, 1969.

Pond, D. Behavior disorders in brain-damaged children. In D. Williams (Ed.), *Modern trends in neurology.* (Series 4): Washington, D.C.: Butterworth, 1967.

Rada, R. T. Informed consent in the care of psychiatric patients. *The National Association of Private Psychiatric Hospitals*, 1976, *8*, 9–12.

Rodham, H. Children under the law. *Harvard Educational Review*, 1973, *43*, 487–514.

Rosen, B. M., Bahn, A. K., & Kramer, M. Demographic and diagnostic characteristics of psychiatric clinic outpatients in the U.S.A. *American Journal of Orthopsychiatry*, 1964, *24*, 455–467.

Rosenberg, A. H., & Katz, A. S. Legal issues in psychiatric treatment of minors. *Mental Health Digest*, 1972, *4*, 54–56.

Rosenhan, D. L. On being sane in insane places. *Science*, 1973, *179*, 250–257.

Rosenthal, R., & Jacobsen, L. F. *Pygmalion in the classroom: Teacher expectation and pupils' intellectual development.* New York: Holt, Rinehart & Winston, 1968.

Schrag, P., & Divoky, D. *The myth of the hyperactive child and other means of child control.* New York: Pantheon Books, 1976.

Shore, M. F., & Golann, S. E. Problems of ethics in community mental health: A survey of community psychologists. *Community Mental Health Journal*, 1969, *5*, 452–560.

Simmonds, D. D. Client attitudes toward release of confidential information without consent. *Journal of Clinical Psychology*, 1968, *24*, 364–365.

Simmonds, D. W. Children's rights and family dysfunction: "Daddy, why do I have to be the crazy one?" In G. P. Koocher (Ed.), *Children's rights and the mental health professions*. New York: Wiley, 1976.

Sinclair, H. Developmental psycholinguistic. In D. Elkind and J. H. Flavell (Eds.), *Studies in cognitive development*, New York: Oxford University Press, 1969.

Sussman, A. N. *The rights of young people*. New York: Avon Books, 1977.

Sylvester, E. Discussion of techniques used to prepare young children for analysis. *Psychoanalytic Studies of Children*, 1957, *7*, 306–321.

Szasz, T. S. *The myth of mental illness*. New York: Hoeber-Harper, 1961.

Szasz, T. S. *Psychiatric justice*. New York: MacMillan, 1965.

Szasz, T. S. *The manufacture of madness*. New York: Delta, 1970 (a).

Szasz, T. S. *Ideology, and insanity*. New York: Doubleday, 1970(b).

Tanner, J. M. Physical growth. In J. Carmichael's *Manual of Child Psychology*, New York: Wiley, 1971.

Walker, S. III Drugging the American child. We're too cavalier about hyperactivity. *Psychology Today*, December 1974, 43–48.

White, S. H. Evidence for a hierarchical arrangement of learning processes. In L. P. Lipsitt and C. C. Spiker (Eds.), *Advances in child development and behavior*, Vol. 23, Academic Press, 1965.

Worsfeld, V. L. A philosophical justification for children's rights. *Harvard Educational Review*, 1974, *44*, 142–157.

Appendices
Research Instruments

Appendix A:
The Client Attitude Questionnaire: Brief Manual
James K. Morrison

There are *two versions* of the *Client Attitude Questionnaire* (CAQ). The first version, *CAQ-A*,[1] was developed by James K. Morrison in 1973. The CAQ-A has a test–retest reliability coefficient of .81 over three months. Total scores on the CAQ-A correlate .59 ($p < .01, n = 26$) with total scores on a revised, 30 item version of the original *Patient Attitude Test* (Braginsky, Braginsky & Ring, 1962[2]). The CAQ-A has been successfully used in a number of predictive studies (Morrison & Becker, 1975; Morrison, 1976; Morrison & Nevid, 1976a; Morrison & Nevid, 1976b) which have demonstrated that attitudes toward mental illness can be changed by means of educative seminars. (Such attitude change appeared to be stable as indicated by 3 and 9 months posttests with the CAQ-A.) It was also demonstrated that the CAQ is a useful instrument in distinguishing interprofessional differences in attitudes toward mental illness (Morrison & Nevid, 1976; Morrison, Yablonovitz, Harris & Nevid, 1976).

---

1. In the literature the CAQ-A is referred to simply as the CAQ, since the second version (CAQ-B) of the instrument had not been developed when studies had been completed.
2. Braginsky, B., Braginsky, D., & Ring, K. *Methods of madness*. New York: Holt, Rinehart, & Winston, 1969.

The *CAQ-B,* also developed by James K. Morrison, is a revised version of the CAQ-A, containing 7 identical items, 3 similar but reworded items, and 10 new items considered more discriminative in terms of interprofessional attitude differences. The total scores of the CAQ-B correlate .77 ($n =27$, $p <.001$) with total scores on the CAQ-A, suggesting that although both measures tap somewhat the same attitudes, they also, to some extent, tap different attitudes. The test-retest reliability coefficient of the CAQ-B is .90 over six weeks. Total scores on the CAQ-B correlate .60 ($n = 58$, $p <.001$) with total scores on the *Client Independence Questionnaire,*[3] indicating that "psychosocial" attitudes toward mental illness are related to client attitudes of independence, and that attitudes toward mental illness characteristic of the medical model are related to client attitudes of dependence (Morrison, Bushell, Hanson, Fentiman & Holdridge-Crane, 1977). The CAQ-B appears to distinguish professionals' attitudes toward mental illness as a function of agency affiliation (Morrison, Schwartz & Holdridge-Crane 1977), to be useful in predicting attitude change as a result of educative seminars (Morrison, Cocozza & Vanderwyst, 1977; Morrison & Teta, 1978; Morrison & Teta, 1977), and to distinguish the attitudes of professionals from those of students in the same disciplines (Morrison, Madrazo-Peterson, Simons & Gold, 1977).

Both versions of the CAQ consist of 20 items designed to tap a respondent's attitudes toward "mental illness." Among the items are statements worded so as to determine whether or not respondents' attitudes reflect the views ("psychosocial") of Szasz and others who have adopted an anti-medical model position. Items are both positively and negatively keyed to avoid response bias. The scale was constructed in a three-point format, with provision for the respondent to answer either true, false, or not sure. This simplified response mode was chosen so that the questionnaire could be used with institutionalized mental patients as well as with persons of limited formal education.

The maximum score on both versions is 60; the minimum 20. Items are scored 3, 2, and 1, respectively, for items positively keyed in terms of the psychosocial model (e.g., answering "true" to the statement, "There is no such thing as 'mental illness'; just people

---

3. Morrison, J. K., & Yablonovitz, H. Increased clinic awareness and attitudes of independence through client advisory board membership. *American Journal of Community Psychology,* 1978, *6,* 363–369.

with problems" obtains a score of 3). (The scoring key is available from the author.)

References

CAQ-A

Morrison, J. K., & Becker, R. E. Seminar-induced change in a community psychiatric team's reported attitudes toward mental illness. *Journal of Community Psychology*, 1975, *3*, 281–284.

Morrison, J. K. Demythologizing mental patients' attitudes toward mental illness: An empirical study. *Journal of Community Psychology*, 1976, *4*, 181–185.

Morrison, J. K., & Nevid, J. S. Demythologizing the attitudes of family caretakers about mental illness. *Journal of Family Counseling*, 1976, *4*, 43–49.(a)

Morrison, J. K., & Nevid, J. S. Demythologizing the service expectations of psychiatric patients in the community. *Psychology*, 1976, *13*, 26–29.(b)

Morrison, J. K., & Nevid, J. S. The attitudes of mental patients and mental health professionals about mental illness. *Psychological Reports*, 1976, *38*, 565–566.(c)

Morrison, J. K., Yablonovitz, H., Harris, M., & Nevid, J. S. The attitudes of nursing students and others about mental illness. *Journal of Psychiatric Nursing and Mental Health Services*, 1976, *14*, 17–19.

CAQ-B

Morrison, J. K., Bushell, J. D., Hanson, G. D., Fentiman, J., & Holdridge-Crane, S. Relationship between psychiatric patients' attitudes toward mental illness and attitudes of dependence. *Psychological Reports*, 1977, *41*, 1194.

Morrison, J. K., Cocozza, J., and Vanderwyst, O. Changing students' constructs of mental patients by means of educative seminars. *Journal of Clinical Psychology*, 1978, *34*, 482–483.

Morrison, J. K., Madrazo-Peterson, Simons, P., & Gold, B. A. Attitudes toward mental illness: A conflict between professionals and students. *Psychological Repports*, 1977, *41*, 1013–1014.

Morrison, J. K., Schwartz, M. P., & Holdridge-Crane, S. Differential attitudes of community agencies toward mental illness: A new dilemma for the psychiatric nurse. *Journal of Psychiatric Nursing and Mental Health Services*, 1977, *15*, 25–29.

Morrison, J. K., & Teta, D. C. Effect of demythologizing seminars on attributions to mental health professionals. *Psychological Reports*, 1978, *43*, 493–494.

Morrison, J. K., & Teta, D. C. Increase of positive self-attributions by means of demythologizing seminars. *Journal of Clinical Psychology*, in press.

Client Attitude Questionnaire (Version A)

Answer true (T), false (F), or not sure to the following statements by circling the answer which best describes how you feel about each statement.

1. I believe that mental patients have an illness like any other illness.

    T   F   Not Sure

2. I believe that mental problems are usually caused by something physical which has gone wrong inside the person's brain.

    T   F   Not Sure

3. No one can really do anything to solve a mental patient's problems.

    T   F   Not Sure

4. People have been duped or fooled into believing that there is such a thing as "mental illness."

    T   F   Not Sure

5. Psychiatrists and psychologists can tell what kind of illness a person has by giving him certain psychological tests (e.g., Rorschach, MMPI, etc.).

    T   F   Not Sure

6. Pills (e.g., Thorazine, Stellazine, Prolixin, etc.) by themselves do *not* solve a mental patient's problems, as a rule.

    T   F   Not Sure

7. Most mental patients at one time or another really should go to a psychiatric hospital for help.

    T   F   Not Sure

8. Most psychiatrists and psychologists agree on what "mental illness" is.

    T   F   Not Sure

9. Some psychologists believe that mental patients are even superior to "normal" people.

    T   F   Not Sure

10. Most people in mental hospitals are among society's poor and unwanted.

    T   F   Not Sure

11. Psychiatrists and psychologists almost always can tell a "mentally ill" person from a "normal" person.

    T   F   Not Sure

12. Mostly women, rather than men, end up being diagnosed as "schizophrenic" and "psychotic."

    T   F   Not Sure

13. Mental patients have the same rights in our society as do so called "normal" people.

    T   F   Not Sure

14. There is really no such thing as "mental illness," just people with problems.

    T   F   Not Sure

15. Mental hospitals should be abolished.

    T   F   Not Sure

16. People with psychiatric problems should have a nice, comfortable place to go for a rest or vacation; not mental hospitals with locked wards.

    T   F   Not Sure

17. Mental patients do not know how to get out of the hospital except by really getting better.

    T   F   Not Sure

18. Mental patients are not able to fool a psychiatrist.

    T   F   Not Sure

19. Mental patients should work harder to solve their own problems, rather than waiting for a psychiatrist to "cure" them.

    T   F   Not Sure

20. Families can usually be blamed for children who grow up to become mental patients.

    T   F   Not Sure

Client Attitude Questionnaire (Version B)

Please answer true (T), false (F), or not sure to the following statements by *circling* the answer which best describes how you feel about each statement.

1. There are some people who clearly suffer from "schizophrenia."

    T   F   Not Sure

2. People have been duped or fooled into believing that there is such a thing as "mental illness."

    T   F   Not Sure

3. Psychiatrists and psychologists can tell what kind of illness a person has by giving him/her certain psychological tests (i.e., Rorschach, MMPI).

    T   F   Not Sure

4. You can predict a mental patient's behavior about as well (or as poorly) as you can predict anyone's behavior.

    T   F   Not Sure

5. Mental problems are quite often caused by some disorder of the body.

    T   F   Not Sure

6. In contrast to men, women get "ripped off" (treated unfairly), when they come for psychiatric services.

    T   F   Not Sure

7. Mental patients are less dangerous than the average citizen.

    T   F   Not Sure

8. Psychiatric diagnosis (for example, determining whether a person is a "paranoid schizophrenic" or not) is an important first step in the proper treatment of psychiatric problems.

    T   F   Not Sure

9. A mental hospital is often a place where society dumps its poor.

    T   F   Not Sure

10. Psychiatrists and psychologists almost always can tell a "mentally ill" person from a "normal" person.

    T   F   Not Sure

11. There is really no such thing as "mental illness"; just people with problems.

    T   F   Not Sure

12. Mental hospitals should be abolished.

    T   F   Not Sure

13. People with psychiatric problems should have a comfortable place to which to go for a rest, rather than mental hospitals with locked wards.

    T   F   Not Sure

14. Mental patients should work harder to solve their own problems, rather than waiting for a psychiatrist to "cure" them.

    T   F   Not Sure

15. Electroshock Therapy is the best treatment for some very depressed patients.

    T   F   Not Sure

16. Mental patients can and should pretend to be "normal" in order to get out of large state mental hospitals.

    T   F   Not Sure

17. Medication (e.g., Thorazine) is often the only way to keep mental patients from having to go back to the mental hospital.

    T   F   Not Sure

18. A mental hospital is usually very helpful to patients in resolving their problems.

    T   F   Not Sure

19. Knowing the way the family of a mental patient has treated him/her in the past can usually explain why the patient has problems today.

    T   F   Not Sure

20. People in the community should be taught that being "mentally ill" is like having any other kind of sickness.

    T   F   Not Sure

Appendix B: Semantic Differential

I believe that _____ can be described as follows:

intimate — — — — — — — remote
light — — — — — — — heavy
foolish — — — — — — — wise
intelligent — — — — — — — ignorant
strange — — — — — — — familiar
active — — — — — — — passive
sincere — — — — — — — insincere
predictable — — — — — — — unpredictable
weak — — — — — — — strong
slow — — — — — — — fast
understandable — — — — — — — mysterious
rugged — — — — — — — delicate
warm — — — — — — — cold
clean — — — — — — — dirty
safe — — — — — — — dangerous
relaxed — — — — — — — tense
valuable — — — — — — — worthless
sick — — — — — — — healthy
good — — — — — — — bad
sociable — — — — — — — unsociable
nice — — — — — — — awful
brave — — — — — — — cowardly
constrained — — — — — — — free
fair — — — — — — — unfair
happy — — — — — — — sad
deep — — — — — — — shallow
excitable — — — — — — — calm
aggressive — — — — — — — defensive
hard — — — — — — — soft
involved — — — — — — — uninvolved

Appendix C: CAB Staff Evaluation Index

Please use this rating scale to indicate the level of your agreement with the following statements concerning the Client Advisory Board (CAB). After each statement, *circle* the number corresponding to the following scale:

7	6	5	4	3	2	1
Strongly agree	Moderately agree	Slightly agree	Not sure	Slightly disagree	Moderately disagree	Strongly disagree

A. Despite beneficial aspects of the CAB, I feel that staff members have experienced unnecessary discomfort at having to justify their programs to the CAB. 7 6 5 4 3 2 1

B. The CAB has definitely provided clients with a means of expressing their feelings (pro and con) about our services and programs 7 6 5 4 3 2 1

C. CAB has allowed clients to assume more control over the course of their treatment than is often desireable. 7 6 5 4 3 2 1

D. At the present time, CAB members don't reflect the opinions of our total clientele. 7 6 5 4 3 2 1

E. CAB has resulted in a large number of valuable suggestions regarding the improvement of our services. 7 6 5 4 3 2 1

F. In general, CAB clients are able to provide assessments and suggestions—and to note areas of concern —in a manner comparable to that of our staff members. 7 6 5 4 3 2 1

G. I have found all of the CAB's suggestions to be quite reasonable and acceptable.   7 6 5 4 3 2 1

H. I'm afraid that a manipulative client on the CAB could get a staff member fired without real justification.   7 6 5 4 3 2 1

I. After exposure to CAB, I feel I have more respect for clients in terms of their awareness of problems and issues.   7 6 5 4 3 2 1

J. My experiences with CAB have, unfortunately, tended to make me too guarded in my interactions with clients.   7 6 5 4 3 2 1

K. The CAB has no real power.   7 6 5 4 3 2 1

L. Given the fact that clients do not have the training/experience of staff, I do *not* approve of staff being subject to client grievances.   7 6 5 4 3 2 1

M. Due to the CAB, I have more respect for a client's ability to assume responsibility.   7 6 5 4 3 2 1

N. CAB has definitely been successful in making many changes in the clinic.   7 6 5 4 3 2 1

O. Clients involved in CAB (i.e., those whom I see individually) seem to have improved their self-concept as a result of CAB membership.   7 6 5 4 3 2 1

P. In a vast majority of cases, a client is better able to assess the value of programs than are staff members.   7 6 5 4 3 2 1

Q. The CAB is actually a mere token gesture since board members do not have an important role in the clinic.   7 6 5 4 3 2 1

R. Staff members (myself in particular) have received valuable "feedback" about their programs through CAB meetings.   7 6 5 4 3 2 1

S. I only pretend that I'll follow CAB program recommendations.   7 6 5 4 3 2 1

T. The CAB is clearly the most valuable program at the clinic.   7 6 5 4 3 2 1

1. Please estimate the number of CAB sessions that you have attended. _____

2. How many of your personal programs have been presented to CAB for program evaluation? _____

3. How often have you read the minutes of CAB meetings? (Circle one.)

1	2	3	4	5
Never	Rarely	Sometimes	Frequently	Always

Appendix D: Client Independence Questionnaire

Answer true (T) or false (F) to the following statements by circling the answer which best describes how you feel about each statement:

1. Whatever happens to me in the future depends mostly on the psychiatric help I receive.

    T   F

2. I feel angry when I think of how I must wait for my advisor to do something before I can get better.

    T   F

3. When I need help (money, legal advice, place to live, etc.) I like to do things on my own.

    T   F

4. I should have the right to tell staff which programs (social club, group therapy, etc.) are good, and which are bad.

    T   F

5. The clinic staff should ask me more often about what I think should be done about my problems.

    T   F

6. I should seldom question the type of treatment which my advisor suggests for me.

    T   F

7. I have no real right to disagree with psychiatric staff.

    T   F

8. I will just have to wait for a real cure for whatever is bothering me.

    T   F

9. Sometimes I wish my advisor would hurry up and solve my problems.

    T   F

10. When I come to the psychiatric clinic, I know that all the staff will always take good care of me.

   T   F

11. Clients can change many things (programs, treatment, etc.) about the psychiatric clinic, if they try.

   T   F

12. I would come to the clinic, even when I don't want to, if my advisor asked me to.

   T   F

13. I'm afraid I'll always need the help of a psychiatric clinic.

   T   F

14. I definitely want more say about the treatment (medication, therapy, etc.) I get at the clinic.

   T   F

15. I would come to the clinic's programs, even when I do not want to, if someone tells me to.

   T   F

16. When I feel good, I have to give most of the credit to my advisor.

   T   F

Appendix E: Individualized Problem Resolution Checklist

The following is a list of those *specific* (e.g., "anxious *about* being with a group of people," *not* simply "anxious") problems which I hope to at least partially resolve in group therapy. Using the rating system listed below I estimate that on the above-mentioned date each of these problems is in a certain state of resolution or unresolution (Resolution Rating).

Rating Number	Resolution State
1	= 100 percent (completely resolved)
2	= 75–99 percent (partially resolved)
3	= 50–74 percent (partially resolved)
4	= 25–49 percent (partially resolved)
5	= 1–24 percent (partially resolved)
6	= 0 percent (completely *un*resolved)

No.	Specific Problem	Current Resolution Rating
1.		
2.		
3.		
4.		
5.		
6.		
7.		

Appendix F: Interpersonal Improvement Scale

Using the 1—6 Resolution Rating Scale listed below estimate your *present* point of resolution of the following problems.

   1 = 100 percent (complete resolution)
   2 = 75–99 percent (partial resolution)
   3 = 50–74 percent (partial resolution)
   4 = 25–49 percent (partial resolution)
   5 = 1–24 percent (partial resolution)
   6 = 0 percent (complete lack of resolution)

Item	Problem	Resolution Rating
1.	Anxiety when talking in a group of people.	_____
2.	Fear of confronting someone with whom I disagree strongly.	_____
3.	Apparent inability to clearly define my feelings at a given moment.	_____
4.	Discomfort in the presence of psychologists and psychiatrists.	_____
5.	A sense of loneliness even with people around me.	_____
6.	A feeling that others do not know the real me.	_____
7.	A feeling that others do not like the person they feel I am.	_____
8.	Confusion as to how others feel about me.	_____
9.	A reluctance to express anger, even when it is justified.	_____
10.	A reluctance to express tenderness, even when I want to.	_____
11.	Discomfort during silences in group discussions.	_____
12.	Fear of confronting authority figures.	_____
13.	An apparent inability to feel empathy for others.	_____
14.	A lack of understanding as to why others treat me the way they do.	_____
15.	A sense of discomfort around people of the opposite sex.	_____
16.	A fear of being exposed by others for what I am.	_____
17.	A reluctance to touch others I don't know extremely well, even when appropriate.	_____

Appendix G: Psychotherapy Problem Checklist

Circle yes or no in answering *all* of the following questions. Please answer
each question honestly.

1. Do you frequently have headaches?

   Yes   No

2. Does your stomach often feel like it is tied up in knots?

   Yes   No

3. Does your chest often feel tight and constricted?

   Yes   No

4. Are you easily depressed?

   Yes   No

5. Do you feel anxious a great deal of the time?

   Yes   No

6. Do you often have problems getting to sleep?

   Yes   No

7. Do you frequently toss and turn at night?

   Yes   No

8. Do you usually wake up feeling rested?

   Yes   No

9. Do you often wake up early and are not able to get back to sleep?

   Yes   No

10. Are you a heavy smoker (more than one pack a day)?

    Yes   No

11. Do you often drink alcohol to excess?

    Yes   No

12. Do you always try to keep busy with something?
                    Yes   No

13. Do you ever seriously consider suicide?
                    Yes   No

14. Do you bite your fingernails?
                    Yes   No

15. Do you easily lose your temper?
                    Yes   No

16. Do you take tranquilizers and pills to "calm your nerves"?
                    Yes   No

17. Do you often use any drugs (marijuana, heroin, LSD, etc.)?
                    Yes   No

18. Do you consider your life happy?
                    Yes   No

19. Do you think about the past much?
                    Yes   No

20. Do you worry about the future a great deal?
                    Yes   No

21. In your estimation, do you have any serious sexual problems?
                    Yes   No

Appendix H: Client Service Questionnaire

The questions below are meant to find out simply and honestly how you feel about yourself and your treatment. Nothing you say here will in any way be used against you. The information is for a research project which will help us to give you better service. You will take this questionnaire again in two months.

Please answer true or false to the following questions by circling either T (true) or F (false), according to how you *feel right now*. *Answer all questions*, even if it seems difficult.

1. Often I call the CDPC staff when it turns out I really didn't need to.   1.   T   F
2. I feel comfortable calling the CDPC staff in Cohoes when I have problems.   2.   T   F
3. I rarely feel afraid.   3.   T   F
4. I call the CDPC staff whenever I have real problems.   4.   T   F
5. I am quite sure that someone at the CDPC in Cohoes will try to send me to the mental hospital in the next 5 months.   5.   T   F
6. I am really anxious lately; my nerves really bother me.   6.   T   F
7. I really look forward to each day lately.   7.   T   F
8. I'm sure that no one at the CDPC will try to send me to the mental hospital in the next 5 months.   8.   T   F
9. When I have problems, I do not feel comfortable calling the CDPC staff in Cohoes.   9.   T   F
10. I seldom get really depressed anymore.   10.   T   F
11. Since coming to the CDPC, I have more problems than before.   11.   T   F

12. I am hearing a lot of "voices" lately.   12.   T   F
13. Sometimes I feel like taking my life.   13.   T   F
14. I could never actually try to kill myself.   14.   T   F
15. There is always someone who can help me with my problems.   15.   T   F
16. At least one person at the CDPC in Cohoes really cares about me.   16.   T   F
17. Generally, no one in my family complains to the CDPC about my behavior.   17.   T   F
18. No one at the CDPC really cares about me.   18.   T   F
19. Someone in my family often complains to the CDPC about my behavior.   19.   T   F
20. Lately I see things which I am not sure are there.   20.   T   F
21. I am pessimistic about what will happen to me in the future.   21.   T   F
22. I want to be independent to live my life the way I choose.   22.   T   F
23. I think I would rather be dead than alive.   23.   T   F
24. I have received poor treatment for my problems since coming to CDPC in Cohoes.   24.   T   F
25. I don't get along with the people I live with.   25.   T   F
26. I sleep quite well at night now.   26.   T   F
27. I have received excellent treatment for my problems since coming to CDPC in Cohoes.   27.   T   F
28. Since coming to the CDPC, I have fewer problems than before.   28.   T   F

Answer if applicable to you:

29. If I could, I would like to remain completely silent in group therapy.   29.   T   F
30. I really like my job.   30.   T   F
31. Often I don't take my medication as directed.   31.   T   F
32. I don't really like my job.   32.   T   F
33. I try not to miss my therapy sessions.   33.   T   F
34. I enjoy telling about my problems in group therapy.   34.   T   F
35. I usually take my medication as directed.   35.   T   F
36. I often find excuses for not going to my therapy session.   36.   T   F

Suggestions: How can we better help you to cope with your problems?

Index